CONCEPTS IN GENETIC MEDICINE

CONCEPTS IN GENETIC MEDICINE

Edited by

Boro Dropulic
Lentigen Corporation

Barrie Carter
Targeted Genetics Corporation

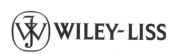 **WILEY-LISS**

A JOHN WILEY & SONS, INC., PUBLICATION

Published by John Wiley & Sons, Inc., Hoboken, New Jersey.
Published simultaneously in Canada.

For general information on our other products and services or for technical support, please contact our Customer Care Department within the United States at (800) 762-2974, outside the United States at (317) 572-3993 or fax (317) 572-4002.

Wiley also publishes its books in a variety of electronic formats. Some content that appears in print may not be available in electronic formats. For more information about Wiley products, visit our web site at www.wiley.com.

Library of Congress Cataloging-in-Publication Data:

Concepts in genetic medicine / [edited by] Boro Dropulic, Barrie Carter.
    p. ; cm.
   Includes bibliographical references.
   ISBN 978-0-471-70320-4 (cloth)
  1.   Medical genetics. 2. Gene therapy. I. Dropulic, Boro. II. Carter, Barrie
   [DNLM: 1. Gene Therapy—methods—Review. 2. Gene Transfer Techniques—Review. 3. Genetic Vectors—Review. 4. Viruses—genetics—Review. QZ 52 c744 2007]
   RB155.C597 2007
   616'.042—dc22

                                            2007008049

Printed in the United States of America

10 9 8 7 6 5 4 3 2 1

CONTENTS

APPLICATIONS

THE MANUFACTURE OF GENE THERAPY PRODUCTS

CONTRIBUTORS

ANNA-MARIA ANESTI, BioVex Ltd, The Windeyer Institute, London, UK

LAURA K. AGUILAR, Advantagene, Inc., Waban, Massachusetts

ESTUARDO AGUILAR-CORDOVA, Advantagene, Inc., Waban, Massachusetts

GWENDOLYN K. BINDER, Abramson Family Cancer Research Institute, School of Medicine, University of Pennsylvania, Philadelphia, Pennsylvania

FLAVIA BORELLINI, Genentech, South San Francisco, California

CHRISTIAN J. BUCHHOLZ, Division of Medical Biotechnology, Paul-Ehrlich-Institut, Langen, Germany

HAIM BURSTEIN, Targeted Genetics Corporation, Seattle, Washington

BARRY J. BYRNE, Department of Molecular Genetics and Microbiology, Gene Therapy Center, University of Florida, Gainesville, Florida

BARRIE J. CARTER, Targeted Genetics Corporation, Seattle, Washington

MARIA G. CASTRO, Gene Therapeutics Research Institute, Cedars-Sinai Medical Center, and Department of Molecular and Medical Pharmacology, University of California–Los Angeles, Los Angeles, California

JEFFREY S. CHAMBERLAIN, Department of Neurology, Division of Neurogenetics, The University of Washington School of Medicine, Seattle, Washington

KLAUS CICHUTEK, Division of Medical Biotechnology, Paul-Ehrlich-Institut, Langen, Germany

ROBERT S. COFFIN, BioVex Advanced Vaccines, Abingdon, Oxford, UK

KENNETH CORNETTA, Department of Medical and Molecular Genetics, Indiana University School of Medicine, Indianapolis, Indiana

KERRY O. CRESAWN, Department of Molecular Genetics and Microbiology, Gene Therapy Center, University of Florida, Gainesville, Florida

PHILIP J. CROSS, Harvard Gene Theraphy Initiative, Boston, Massachusetts, and Philip J. Cross & Associates, Inc., Wilmington, Delaware

DAVID T. CURIEL, Division of Human Gene Therapy, Gene Therapy Center, University of Alabama at Birmingham, Birmingham, Alabama

BORO DROPULIC, Lentigen Corporation, Baltimore, Maryland

THEODORE FRIEDMANN, Center for Molecular Genetics, School of Medicine, University of California at San Diego, La Jolla, California

MARTIN GOLD, Technology Access Partners, LLC, Suffern, New York

PAUL GREGOREVIC, Department of Neurology, Division of Neurogenetics, University of Washington School of Medicine, Seattle, Washington

DOUGLAS J. JOLLY, Advantagene, Inc., Encinitas, California

CARL H. JUNE, Abramson Family Cancer Research Institute, and Department of Pathology and Laboratory Medicine, School of Medicine, University of Pennsylvania, Philadelphia, Pennsylvania

SUSAN M. KINGSMAN, Oxford BioMedica, Oxford, UK

BRUCE L. LEVINE, Clinical Cell and Vaccine Production Facility and Department of Pathology and Laboratory Medicine, University of Pennsylvania, Philadelphia, Pennsylvania

DOUGLAS D. LIND, GBP Capital, Greenwich, Connecticut

DEXI LIU, Department of Pharmaceutical Sciences, University of Pittsburgh School of Pharmacy, Pittsburgh, Pennsylvania

PEDRO R. LOWENSTEIN, Gene Therapeutics Research Institute, Cedars-Sinai Medical Center, and Deparment of Molecular and Medical Pharmacology, University of California–Los Angeles, Los Angeles, California

RUSSETTE M. LYONS, Novartis Vaccines and Diagnostics, Cambridge, Massachusetts

QIANA L. MATTHEWS, Division of Human Gene Therapy, Gene Therapy Center, University of Alabama at Birmingham, Birmingham, Alabama

JAMES E. MISKIN, Oxford BioMedica, Oxford, UK

KYRIACOS A. MITROPHANOUS, Oxford BioMedica, Oxford, UK

KEVIN V. MORRIS, Department of Molecular and Experimental Medicine, The Scripps Research Institute, La Jolla, California

RIMAS J. ORENTAS, Department of Pediatrics, Medicine, Microbiology and Molecular Genetics, Medical College of Wisconsin, and the Children's Research Institute of the Children's Hospital of Wisconsin, Milwaukee, Wisconsin

CHRISTINA A. PACAK, Department of Molecular Genetics and Microbiology, Gene Therapy Center, University of Florida, Gainesville, Florida

RALPH W. PAUL, Targeted Genetics Corporation, Seattle, Washington

RICHARD PELUSO, Targeted Genetics Corporation, Seattle, Washington

JAMES L. RILEY, Abramson Family Cancer Research Institute, and Department of Pathology and Laboratory Medicine, School of Medicine, University of Pennsylvania, Philadelphia, Pennsylvania

JOHN J. ROSSI, Division of Molecular Biology, Beckman Research Institute of the City of Hope, Duarte, California

MATTHIAS SCHWEIZER, Division of Medical Biotechnology, Paul-Ehrlich-Institut, Langen, Germany

DAVID S. STRAYER, Department of Pathology and Cell Biology, Jefferson Medical College, Philadelphia, Pennsylvania

TAKESHI SUDA, Department of Pharmaceutical Sciences, University of Pittsburgh School of Pharmacy, Pittsburgh, Pennsylvania

DOUGLAS J. SWIRSKY, GenVec, Inc., Gaithersburg, Maryland

CAROLYN A. WILSON, Division of Cellular and Gene Therapies, Center for Biologics Evaluation and Research, U.S. FDA, Bethesda, Maryland

PREFACE

Our goal in compiling *Concepts in Genetic Medicine* was to produce a book that looked broadly at the issues surrounding the development of gene-based therapies. Consequently, topics include new developments in vector design and methods for their application to various disease states, the manufacture and testing of gene transfer products; understanding the regulatory environment for development of gene therapy products; some considerations as to how the development of gene therapy products financed toward commercialization, and finally how companies commercializing gene therapeutic products will ultimately realize returns on their investment.

The organization of the chapters approximates the chronological order of product development. After an insightful introduction by Theodore Friedmann, we start with vector design by focusing on select examples and their potential utility for the treatment of specific diseases. The selection is by no means exhaustive, but provides the reader with some background as to the major vector classes in development and the specific diseases for which they are being targeted for therapy. The subsequent set of chapters summarize methods for the manufacture and release testing of some of these vectors, emphasizing methods and processes that are relevant for their application in human clinical trials. The following chapters expand on the regulatory theme, providing key concepts for preclinical studies and clinical trial design. The final chapters provide important insights as how to finance the development of gene therapy products using private equity investment as a vehicle, and how the return on investment in these companies will be actualized by new reimbursement strategies for cellular and gene therapy products.

It is important to note that *Concepts in Genetic Medicine* is not designed to be a thorough review of every potential gene therapeutic strategy currently in development in numerous laboratories around the world. Rather, its aim is to provide salient examples of such strategies so that the book can broadly cover many of the *concepts* that need to be taken into consideration when developing gene therapy products: from basic research in the laboratory to full commercialization by companies. We believe that successful development of these new revolutionary products will happen only when these considerations are taken into account early in the product development cycle. Only then will the goals of this field be realized: revolutionary treatments for serious diseases and unmet medical needs where other approaches have failed to provide a satisfactory outcome or cure.

BARRIE CARTER
BORO DROPULIC

xiii

1 The Evolution of Human Gene Therapy: A Journey from Excessive Hype to Excessive Diffidence to Reality

THEODORE FRIEDMANN

Center for Molecular Genetics, School of Medicine,
University of California at San Diego, La Jolla, California

Unlike Athena, who emerged from the brow of Zeus fully armed and ready for her godly duties, advances in biomedicine are not born fully formed and mature. Virtually all of the therapies and preventive methods that we take for granted—cancer chemotherapy, immunization techniques, tissue transplantation, management of cardiovascular disease, and treatment of diabetes and many other metabolic and degenerative diseases—have required decades of development and incremental advance from initial concept and early proof of concept to truly effective and widely applicable clinical application. They are all still imperfect but are evolving rapidly, and their practitioners are learning from false starts, detours, reversals, and missteps. In most cases, scientists, the public, policymakers, and the media understand and accept what is often a discouragingly slow pace of advance in a difficult new science. In contrast and for many reasons, the field of gene therapy found itself in its early stages on a somewhat unusual path, with many segments of the community—basic and clinical scientists and their institutions, the public and its agents, disease foundations and patients' interest groups, the media, and the biotechnology and pharmaceutical industries—too often expecting immediate success and not appreciating the inevitable need for slow, incremental evolutionary growth.

There have been enough reviews of the history of gene therapy from concept to clinical application to establish the fact that it is still a very young discipline [1,2]. Its most obvious conceptual origins date back no further than the late 1960s and early 1970s [3], and its clinical applications began only in 1989–1990 [4,5]: a clinical history of a mere 15 to 16 years. In that relatively short period of time, the birth and development of the field of human gene therapy have been characterized not only by impressive scientific and medical innovation but also by controversy and missteps that have at times inappropriately overshadowed the impressive scientific and medical achievements that have already begun to convert basic gene transfer technology into truly effective therapy. Fortunately, most of us now understand that human gene therapy is no Athena, but rather, is at the very earliest stages of its evolutionary process. Even so, there have been frequent reminders from parts of the scientific and biomedical communities and from the media that the gene therapy community has largely failed to deliver on its stated and implied promises of rapid and even imminent clinical benefits of gene transfer technology delivered by the gene therapy community itself and by research institutions, disease foundations and funding agencies, and private industry.

Without doubt, the early and often overstated clinical promise of gene therapy has been largely unfulfilled—we can all agree on that. But that fact speaks less to the merits of the scientific and medical results than to the exaggeration and unattainable goals of many early expectations as well as to the extreme difficulty of the task. Disappointment does not occur in a vacuum—it is always a result of unmet expectations. It has obviously been the unrealistic expectations that have been most responsible for the widespread disappointment in the achievements of gene therapy until now. The unrealistic early clinical claims have produced unattainable goals that in turn led to disappointment with the apparent slow pace of clinical success and to the common reflexive preoccupation on the part of many critical observers with the trees and not the forest. What is this forest, and has the field of gene therapy actually achieved something important even so early in its life?

The forest is the fact that a conceptually new form of medicine has been born, that it is still very immature, but that like human infants, it is beginning to show hints of future maturity. A number of recent studies have indicated without any doubt that clinical applications of basic clinical gene transfer studies can indeed improve the course of disease and ameliorate suffering. Such improvements have not been trouble-free and have come at some great cost, but in several instances they have constituted undeniable savings of lives and improvements in quality of life. Without disregarding the reversals and difficulties of the past, that development must be called therapy. Some of the most convincing objective therapeutic results have come in the gene transfer studies of the monogenic immunodeficiency inborn errors of metabolism, a group of several distinct lethal diseases for which therapy has remained largely inadequate. For some of these disorders, such as the inborn errors of metabolism that cause severe combined immunodeficiency disease (SCID), bone marrow transplantation has, when feasible, allowed excellent and even definitive treatment. But for the many patients with one or another form of SCID for whom this option is not available, far less effective symptomatic therapies have been used but generally not with uniform success. The new form of treatment represented by gene transfer studies for several of these disorders, especially X-linked SCID (X-SCID) [6], adenosine deaminase deficiency SCID (ADA-SCID) [7], and most recently, chronic granulomatous disease (CGD) [8], has allowed patients to achieve virtually full immunological reconstitution and thereby to survive and even thrive for up to and exceeding six years after treatment: to attend school and to roll around in the dirt with their playmates, that is, to lead the perfectly normal childhood lives previously not possible for them.

We are all painfully aware that the treatment has been clouded by the development of a leukemialike disease in three of the children and the death of one child as a direct result of the therapy. So we have relearned the lesson that we have learned from many other early and still developing therapies: that even undeniably effective but imperfectly understood therapeutic procedures can, and do, lead to serious adverse and even lethal consequences. In the case of the X-SCID disease model, we have learned of the technical problems caused by integration of vectors into unforgiving regions of the genome in recipient children, and there is evidence that the X-SCID model itself may be severely complicated conceptually by the possibility that the γ-C gene, the gene responsible for X-SCID and that must be reconstituted in patients, can itself be an oncogene. Fortunately, the results with ADA-SCID have not yet been reported to produce similar adverse consequences, possibly because the ADA gene does not have similar oncogenic properties. There are other tantalizingly promising early results in other human disease settings, including forms of cancer, cardiovascular disease, blindness, and others [9–14].

At the clinical level, this evolution from the first gene transfer studies in human subjects to the present time of unequivocal clinical therapeutic efficacy has taken approximately 16 to 17 years, a remarkably rapid course compared with many technically complex areas of therapy. Therapeutic success stories usually develop slowly and with incremental advances over several decades, usually through stages of severe conceptual and technical setbacks and failures. For instance, the beginnings of antimetabolite treatment for childhood leukemia with the introduction of the folic acid antagonist aminopterin by Sidney Farber and colleagues in 1948 [15] came at a time when successful salvage from childhood T-cell leukemia occurred at a rate below several percent. With additional drug discovery and refinements in delivery, therapeutic success increased inexorably to its current level of 90% or greater, but that change required 30 to 40 years. Similarly, there are numerous other examples of decades-long development and maturation times required for other, now standard forms of therapy to progress from conception to initial glimmerings of treatment success to truly effective and widespread application. Consider, for instance, the histories of cancer chemotherapy, organ and tissue transplantation, and the clinical application of monoclonal antibodies. Every one of these and many other therapies came only after several decades of incremental advances, incorporating lessons learned from many false starts, errors, and setbacks.

Not only does it take time for new concepts to mature into effective therapy, but it also evident that it can be precisely at the time when gene transfer begins to be efficient and therapeutically effective that serious clinical setbacks may first appear. Consider the well-known induction of secondary tumors during successful and lifesaving chemotherapy and radiotherapy of cancer. It is with increasing efficacy of aggressive treatment that the induction of secondary tumors came to be revealed. These and other types of adverse events may therefore not necessarily represent conceptual errors or flaws in the experimental design so much as the harm inherent in effective, yet imperfect therapy itself. In that regard, the induction of leukemia in some patients in the X-SCID study might be seen to represent harm intrinsic to effective therapy in the same way that secondary tumors are an intrinsic and inevitable consequence of effective but still flawed therapy for cancer. It seems very likely that leukemias or other unwanted consequences for retrovirus-mediated gene transfer studies have not been seen in previous studies at least partially because gene transfer and transgene expression have previously simply been too inefficient. Once gene transfer became efficient enough to permit frequent provirus integration near oncogenes and to lead to stable and efficient expression of the therapeutic transgene, tumorigenesis occurred in transduced cells. In the case of retrovirus vectors, it is difficult at the present time to envision a solution to this problem short of site-specific integration of the transgene, but methods are emerging that begin to make the possibility of definitive sequence correction of mutations through site-specific genetic modification seem feasible [16]. Similarly important new methods are emerging that promise specific control of gene expression through modulation of RNA expression [17].

At the clinical level, gene therapy has had an unusually short history of merely 15 to 16 years, admittedly to enormous publicity and great early academic and commercial expectations of imminent success. However, consider what has occurred in that short time. Not only has this completely theoretical approach to disease treatment established itself as a powerful new concept in medicine, but it has also become a very large worldwide effort in academia and industry. Furthermore it has delivered a handful of results that provide inescapable proof of the concept that human disease can indeed be treated at the level of the underlying genetic defects and not only at the symptomatic or metabolic level. Its course has certainly been irregular and even contentious because of missteps and setbacks, overstated early progress, and therapeutic claims. But the field as a whole has learned well from these experiences and has clearly recognized the need for greater care and rigor than was evident at times during the earliest clinical period of the field of gene therapy. Most investigators understand well the hazards of shortcuts and appreciate that studies in this field of biomedicine should be carried out with all the rigorous care required of other areas of clinical research.

Notwithstanding setbacks and treatment-associated harm, progress has been real, and the time has arrived for a more realistic and sober appreciation of the field of gene therapy. Some critics might well be advised to temper their reflexive preoccupation with past difficulties with a more realistic recognition of the important advances in the field and of the undeniable clinical benefits in some studies. Just as important, it is an appropriate time for proponents and advocates of gene therapy to put aside what has become almost timidity in the face of the admitted difficulties and setbacks and begin to point more effectively to the real successes and achievements of the field—to point justifiably to the important achievements in the field and to do so with an appreciation not only of the conceptual and technical missteps of the past but also of the great conceptual and technical advances that have been made.

As this volume attests, gene therapy is no will-of-the wisp and no mirage, either as a stand-alone approach to treatment of some disorders or as adjunct treatment for many other common and widespread disorders, such as most forms of cancer. Those who have conceived and shaped this field and who are working to bring it to the relief of illness have good reason to be pleased with the recent progress and with the future promise.

REFERENCES

1. Friedmann T. *The Development of Human Gene Therapy*. Woodburg, NY: Cold Spring Harbor Laboratory Press; 1999.
2. Verma IM, Weitzman MD. Gene therapy: twenty-first century medicine. *Annu Rev Biochem*. 2005;74:711–738.
3. Friedmann T, Roblin R. Gene therapy for human genetic disease? *Science*. 1972; 175:949–955.
4. Rosenberg SA, Aebersold P, Cornetta K, et al. Gene transfer into humans: immunotherapy of patients with advanced melanoma, using tumor-infiltrating lymphocytes modified by retroviral gene transduction. *N Engl J Med*. 1990;323:570–578.
5. Anderson WF, Blaese RM, Culver K. The ADA human gene therapy clinical protocol: points to consider response with clinical protocol, July 6, 1990. *Hum Gene Ther*.Fall 1990;1:331–362.
6. Fischer A, Hacein-Bey-Abina S, Lagresle C, Garrigue A, Cavazana-Calvo M. Gene therapy of severe combined immunodeficiency disease: proof of principle of efficiency and safety issues—gene therapy, primary immunodeficiencies, retrovirus, lentivirus, genome. *Bull Acad Natl Med*. 2005;189(5):779–785.
7. Aiuti A, Ficara F, Cattaneo F, Bordignon C, Roncarolo MG. Gene therapy for adenosine deaminase deficiency. *Curr Opin Allergy Clin Immunol*. December 2003;3(6):461–466.
8. Ott MG, Schmidt M, Schwarzwaelder K, et al. Correction of X-linked chronic granulomatous disease by gene therapy, augmented by insertional activation of *MDS1-EVI1, PRDM16* or *SETBP1*. *Nat Med*. Apr 2006;12:401–409. Epub: April 2, 2006.
9. Acland GM, Aguirre GD, Bennett J, et al. Long-term restoration of rod and cone vision by single dose *rAAV*-mediated gene transfer to the retina in a canine model of childhood blindness. *Mol Ther*. 2005;12:1072–1082. Epub: October 14, 2005.
10. Nemunaitis J. Vaccines in cancer: GVAX, a *GM-CSF* gene vaccine. *Expert Rev Vaccines*. 2005;4(3):259–274.
11. Roth JA. Adenovirus p53 gene therapy. *Expert Opin Biol Ther*. 2006;6:55–61.
12. Peng Z. Current status of gendicine in China: recombinant human Ad-p53 agent for treatment of cancers. *Hum Gene Ther*. 2005;16:1016–1027.
13. Samakoglu S, Lisowski L, Budak-Alpdogan T, et al. A genetic strategy to treat sickle cell anemia by coregulating globin transgene expression and RNA interference. *Nat Biotechnol*. 2006;24:89–94. Epub: December 25, 2005.

14. Vahakangas E, Yla-Herttuala S. Gene therapy of atherosclerosis. *Handb Exp Pharmacol.* 2005;170:785–807.

15. Farber S, Diamond LK, Mercer R, Sylvester R, Wolff J. Temporary remissions in acute leukemia in children produced by folic acid antagonist, 4-aminopteroyl-glutamic acid (aminopterin). *New Engl J Med.* 1948;238(23).

16. Urnov FD, Miller JC, Lee YL, et al. Highly efficient endogenous human gene correction using designed zinc-finger nucleases. *Nature.* 2005;435:646–651. Epub: April 3, 2005.

17. Dykxhoorn DM, Palliser D, Lieberman J. The silent treatment: siRNAs as small molecule drugs. *Gene Ther.* 2006;13:541–552.

2 Murine Leukemia Virus–Based Retroviral Vectors

KENNETH CORNETTA

Department of Medical and Molecular Genetics,
Indiana University School of Medicine, Indianapolis, Indiana

Gamma retrovirus–based retroviral vectors can efficiently integrate into the target cell genome, thus conferring the transgene to the transduced cell and all subsequent progeny. The integrating property of these vectors makes them an ideal system for altering stem cells, progenitor cells, or other cells that are expected to expand in great number. Other advantages include a gene transfer efficiency significantly greater than that of non viral gene transfer techniques and manufacturing methods that produce vector in quantities suitable for clinical use.

Retroviral vectors do have a number of disadvantages. Retroviral vectors require cell division for integration, so quiescent cells must be induced to cycle to obtain significant transduction. Also, integration has been associated with insertional mutagenesis, a rare and complex process whereby vector integration leads to malignant transformation of the target cell. Finally, vector particles can be inactivated by human serum and require modification for in vivo administration. Despite these limitations, retroviral vectors are a well-defined system with many useful reagents that have been developed over the past two decades. These vectors remain an attractive system when stable integration of target cells is desired.

MURINE-BASED RETROVIRAL VECTORS

Gamma retrovirus–based retroviral vectors (subsequently referred to as *retroviral vectors*) were the first viral vectors developed [1–3] and the first to enter clinical trials [4]. The initial retroviral vectors were based on the murine leukemia viruses, which are membrane-bound RNA viruses. The viral genes of these viruses are relatively simple and include the *gag* region, which includes structural proteins involved with capsid formation. The *pol* region encodes proteins with enzymatic functions, including reverse transcriptase and integrase. The viruses also contain

Concepts in Genetic Medicine, Edited by Boro Dropulic and Barrie Carter
Copyright © 2008 John Wiley & Sons, Inc.

an *env* gene that encodes a membrane-associated glycoprotein that targets the particles to specific cell receptors. Retroviruses are attractive gene delivery vehicles related to certain unique features of their life cycle. Understanding these feature is important when designing vector constructs and generating vector particles [5]. As shown in Figure 2.1, vector constructs generally retain the retroviral long terminal repeats (LTRs), as these sequences are required for vector integration. The LTRs also contain promoter and enhancer functions which drive vector expression. A packaging (ψ) sequence is also needed to facilitate efficient uptake of vector RNA into the virion. In contrast, most vectors are designed with complete deletions in the *pol* and *env* regions. Only a small portion of the *gag* region is retained, since complete deletion of *gag* is associated with a marked decrease in vector titer [6].

Deletion of the viral genes generates a vector genome that is replication defective. Therefore, a system is required that produces the viral gene products in the

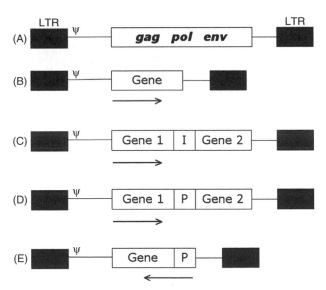

Figure 2.1   Options in designing retroviral vector constructs. (A) Schematic representation of the Moloney murine leukemia virus, from which most retroviral vector constructs are derived. The three viral gene regions *gag, pol*, and *env* are flanked by long terminal repeats (LTRs), which contain promoter and enhancer functions. The psi (ψ) sequence is required for efficient packaging of viral RNA into virions. (B) A vector construct retains the LTR and ψ sequence with deletion of the majority of the viral gene region. The promoter in the 5′ LTR is used to express the gene of interest. (C,D) More than one gene product or sequence can be expressed by use of an IRES sequences (I) or introduction of a second promoter (P). (E) When the sequence to be expressed contains introns or other sequences that may interfere with production of a full-length vector transcript, a promoter–transgene cassette can be created, then placed in opposite orientation. This allows the full-length transcript to be incorporated into virions, and the gene of interest will be expressed after integration into target cells.

absence of replication-competent virus. This is accomplished by expressing the viral genes using plasmids that lack the psi sequence for efficient virion incorporation and lack LTRs for efficient integration. Segregating the vector, the *gag* and *pol* genes, and the viral envelope onto three distinct plasmids also decreases the incidence of recombination that could generate a replication-competent virus. These plasmids have been used to produce vectors by transient transfection and have also been used in the generation of retroviral packaging cell lines (see Figure 2.2).

GENERATING VECTOR CONSTRUCTS

Four important issues should be considered when constructing retroviral vectors: selection of viral backbone sequences, transgene orientation, the risk of insertional mutagenesis, and virion pseudotyping. The majority of initial studies in retroviral gene transfer utilized vectors derived from the Moloney murine leukemia virus (MoMLV). The promoter and enhancer regions within the MoMLV LTR can be used to drive transgene expression, and this works well in most cell lines and differentiated primary cells. A limitation of the MoMLV LTR is relatively poor expression in preimplantation embryos, embryonic stem cells, and primitive hematopoietic progenitors [7,8]. It is now known that the MoMLV LTR and primer binding site contain at least four silencer elements active in many primitive cell populations. The mechanisms by which vectors are silenced is complex and not completely understood, but a significant number of vector backbones have been generated in which the MoMLV sequences prone to silencing have been mutated or replaced with sequences from alternative retroviruses (for a review, see ref. [9]). These novel LTRs have been shown to improve expression in specific cell types (eg., hematopoietic cells of myeloid lineage); there is a decrease in in vivo silencing due to methylation or other cellular mechanisms, although silencing is not eliminated completely (for a review, see ref. [10]).

As mentioned above, the most simplistic vector design utilizes the LTR promoter to express the transgene. Generally, transgenes derived from cDNA sequences lack introns and therefore are generally not spliced during RNA processing. In situations where intron sequences are important for transgene expression, or in situations where tissue-specific promoters are preferred to the nonspecific expression associated with the viral LTR, the transgene cassette can be placed in reverse orientation (Figure 2.1). Placing sequences in reverse orientation may require the addition of a poly-A signal onto the transgene, whereas the 3′ LTR may serve this function for some transgenes placed in the normal orientation.

Recently, the risk of insertional mutagenesis has led to further considerations of vector design [11–14]. Insertional mutagenesis can occur when retroviral regulatory sequences (most commonly, the enhancer) integrate near susceptible oncogenes, leading to overexpression, or when integration occurs that disrupts the normal expression of tumor suppressor genes. Insertional mutagenesis is complex and discussed at length in Chapter 23. For this discussion it is important to note

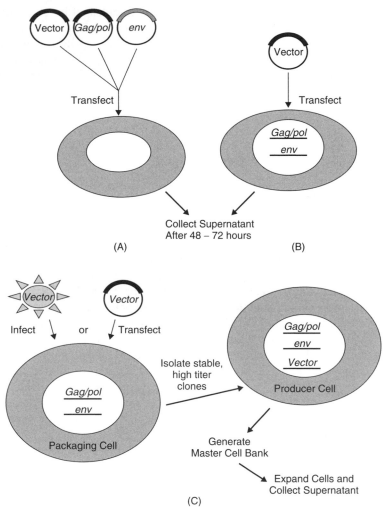

Figure 2.2 Vector production options. There are a number of options when generating retroviral vectors. (A) Production is accomplished using the transient transfection method. Plasmids expressing the vector, the viral *gag* and *pol* gene, and a viral envelope are introduced into a cell that transfects with high efficiency (e.g., HEK293T cells). Vector supernatant is harvested after 48 to 72 hours. (B) Packaging cells lines stably expressed the viral genes are used. In this case, only the vector plasmid is introduced during the production procedure. (C) The vector plasmid is introduced into the packaging cell and a stable high-titer clone is isolated, allowing a cell bank of vector-producing cells to be established. Generally, a selectable marker is incorporated into a vector to aid in selecting vector producer cells. The construct can be introduced by transient transfection of plasmid or by infecting the packaging cell line with a vector-containing virion (*trans-infection*). Expression of the construct after viral integration does appear to provide a higher titer than that obtained by transfection. *Note:* The virion used for trans-infection should be pseudotyped with a different envelope than that expressed by the packaging cell line, to minimize receptor interference (blocking of the receptor by the env protein).

that integration per se may not be oncogenic, but the insertion of regulatory elements, in particular the MoMLV enhancer, may be a major contributor to gene deregulation of certain susceptible oncogenes. As a means of addressing insertional mutagenesis, a number of novel approaches are being explored. These include insulator sequences, matrix attachment regions, and locus control regions that seek to limit the influence on surrounding DNA of the inserted vector. Another approach is the use of self-inactivating (SIN) vectors, which eliminate the regulator regions within the LTR [15,16]. Such sequences have the potential to prevent undesired activation of surrounding genetic sequences and may also protect the transgene cassette from silencing due to positional effects related to the site of integration. Whether these vector modifications will improve the safety of retroviral gene transfer is an avenue of active investigation.

The fourth factor to consider when designing retroviral vectors is the envelope glycoprotein that will serve as the viral envelope (Table 2.1). The *env* gene from MoMLV is considered an ecotropic glycoprotein, as it binds to receptors that are only present on murine and other rodent cells. If all work is to be done in murine models, the ecotropically packaged vectors have a potential biosafety advantage in terms of exposure to laboratory workers and animal caretakers. If human cells are to be targeted, the MoMLV *env* must be replaced with an envelope that recognizes a broader spectrum of receptors. Reengineering virions to contain alternative envelopes is termed *pseudotyping*. Options include amphotropic envelopes derived from viruses such as the murine 4070A

TABLE 2.1   Retroviral Packaging Cell Lines

Parent Viral Envelope[a]	Target Cell Species	Cell Line[b]	Parent Cell Line	Ref.
Moloney ecotropic MLV	Rodent	GPE + 86	Murine NIH 3T3	31
	Rodent	EcoPhoenix	Human HEK293T	c
4070A MLV	Rodent, primate	PA317	Murine NIH3T3	32
	Rodent, primate	GP + *env* AM12	Murine NIH3T3	33
	Rodent, primate	AmphoPhoenix	Human HEK293T	c
	Rodent, primate	FLYA13	Human HT-1080	18
Gibbon ape leukemia virus	Primate	PG13	Murine NIH 3T3	34
Cat endogenous virus RD114	Primate	FLYRD18	Human HT-1080	18
	Primate	Phoenix RD114	Human HEK293T	35
None		PhoenixGP	Human HEK293T	c

[a]MS, murine leukemia virus.
[b]The PhoenixGP cells express Moloney *gag* and *pol* and can be engineered to express additional pseudotypes by introducing the viral envelope desired.
[c]Information regarding the Phoenix cell lines can be found at www.stanford.edu/group/nolan; cells are also available at the American Tissue Culture Collection, Manassas, VA (www.atcc.org).

and 10A1 that can bind to receptors on murine, human, and many other cell types. Alternatively, xenotropic viruses, which do not infect murine cells but can infect human cells, have been used successfully for pseudotyping. Examples of xenotropic envelopes include those derived from the gibbon ape leukemia virus (GALV) and the feline endogenous virus RD114. Vectors pseudotyped with the amphotropic and xenotropic envelopes have been used in clinical trials. More recently, pseudotyping using nonretroviral envelopes have been successful for the vesicular stomatitis virus G protein and the alphaviruses Ross River virus and Simliki Forest virus.

VECTOR PRODUCTION

Once the vector construct has been created, there are a number of options for generating vector particles. The simplest and quickest method is utilizing the transient transfection method in which three plasmids, encoding the vector sequence, the viral *gag* and *pol* regions, and the envelope gene are introduced into cell lines such as HEK293 and HT1080 cells (Figure 2.2A). These cell lines have a high transfection efficiency and are capable of producing vectors at high titer. This process can be simplified slightly by utilizing packaging cell lines, such as the Phoenix cell lines, which are HEK293 cell lines that stably express *gag/pol* and an envelope plasmid, so only the vector construct need be introduced (Figure 2.2B). Transient transfection methods allow rapid screening of vector constructs and facilitate a quick comparison of different envelopes when seeking to optimize gene transfer.

Disadvantages of transient transfection methods are (1) the need for high-quality plasmid preparations, (2) variability in vector titer from batch to batch, (3) the potential of residual plasmids to yield false positive results when using DNA detection methods for vector integration, and (4) the limited volumes that can be obtained in each production batch. An attractive alternative has been the generation of stable vector producer cell lines. In this approach, retroviral packaging cell lines stably expressing *gag/pol* and an envelope gene are transfected with the vector plasmid. A stable high-titer producer cell clone is isolated and expanded into a cell bank. Often, a higher-titer cell clone can produce vector at titers similar to that obtained by transient transfection methods. Also, the lack of plasmid transfection significantly decreases the amount of non-particle-associated vector sequences in the vector preparation (i.e., decreasing the inadvertent transfer of viral gene sequences to target cells). As indicated in Table 2.1, a wide variety of packaging cell lines are available. Cell lines derived from murine NIH3T3 cells were the initial packaging cell lines created and have been used extensively in clinical trials. Murine cell lines do pose the risk of inadvertent transfer of VL30 and other endogenous retroviral sequences [17]. The development of packaging cell lines using cells of human origin does address this theoretical safety concern and also generates particles that are less likely to be inactivated by human serum [18].

VECTOR CHARACTERIZATION

The level of characterization of retroviral vectors varies with the intended use. For most research purposes, the vector supernatant is evaluated for physical titer using assays such as quantitative polymerase chain reaction (PCR) (i.e., the number of RNA genomes) [19] or the product enhance reverse transcriptase (PERT) assay, which measures the amount of reverse transcriptase) [20,21]. As physical titer methods do not assess vector infectivity, most laboratories confirm physical titers with a function titer assay. In this assessment, a vector is subjected to serial dilutions and the level of gene transfer at the various dilutions is used to calculate the number of infectious vector particles. Functional titer assays ensure that accurate virion assembly has occurred and demonstrate that vector particles are infectious. As the level of gene transfer is often cell line and assay dependent, infectious titer reported by various laboratories can vary widely even though the biological activity of the vector may be similar.

In addition to titer (potency), cell lines used in vector production should be screened for sterility and *Mycoplasma* contamination. Also, packaging cell lines, especially those packaged for long periods of time, can develop recombinations that lead to development of replication-competent retroviruses. When generating material for clinical use, an extensive series of testing is required to detect infectious contaminants as well as to characterize the vector product (discussed in detail in Chapter 23). In general, limiting the number of passages for vector producer cells minimizes the incidence of recombination-competent retrovirus development and helps to decrease clonal drift and maintain titer.

VECTOR TRANSDUCTION

Transduction of target cells with retroviral vector is generally performed ex vivo, due to the neutralizing effects of serum components on vector particles. When performing transduction ex vivo, the process can be relatively straightforward for most cell lines. Briefly, (1) cells are maintained in log phase growth, (2) the medium replaced or mixed with retroviral vector, (3) a polycation is added (such as Polybrene or protamine sulfate [22]) to promote vector cell interaction, (4) the cells are incubated from 4 to 24 hours at their normal growth conditions, and (5) the vector medium is removed and replaced with fresh culture medium. Integration and expression is usually detectable within 24 to 48 hours and generally plateaus after 72 hours. This simple method works extremely well for many adherent cell lines, but transduction of primary cells is generally less efficient.

In general, immortalized cells transduce efficiently, probably due to their proliferating activity. In contrast, primary cells have a lower gene transfer efficiency, and noncycling cells are relatively resistant to transduction with retroviral vectors. Retroviral vectors lack nuclear localization sequences and therefore move into the nucleus predominantly during dissolution of the nuclear membrane during cell division. The relationship of vector integration and cell cycle has been evaluated extensively in hematopoietic progenitor cells, and a variety of interventions can be used alone or in combination to maximize gene transfer. First, cytokines and other growth factors can be used to stimulate cell cycling and markedly increase gene transfer efficiency [23–26]. Second, matrix proteins such as fibronectin and the recombinant fibronectin molecule CH-296 (Retronectin) have proven important in maximizing gene transfer by colocalizing target cells (via VLA-4- and VLA-5- binding sites) and vector particles (via heparin-binding sites) [27,28]. Also, transduction rates can be increased by repeating the transduction daily for two or three consecutive days. This presumably increases the number of target cells exposed to vector during a susceptible time in the cell cycle. Finally, low-speed centrifugation of vector and cells, termed *spinoculation*, can improve gene transfer efficiency [29].

When attempting to maximize gene transfer efficiency, three additional factors should be considered: multiplicity of infection (MOI), vector titer, and cell density at the time of transduction. The optimal MOI varies with each cell line, but an MOI of 10 to 20 infectious vector particles per cell is more than adequate for most immortalized cell lines, especially for adherent cell lines. Above the optimal MOI the transduction efficiency tends to plateau (i.e., the percentage of cells transduced plateaus), although the number of integrations per cell can continue to increase (theoretically increasing the risk of insertional mutagenesis) [30]. In addition, MOI alone cannot be considered when attempting to maximize gene transfer, as the vector titer (concentration) is also important. In general, the higher the number of vector particles per milliliter, the more efficient the level of gene transfer. It should be noted that maximal gene transfer, especially gene transfer into primary cells, requires evaluation of various envelopes along with assessment of a variety of culture conditions and transduction procedures when seeking the highest level of gene transfer.

FUTURE DIRECTIONS

Retroviral vectors based on mouse gammaretroviruses remain attractive gene transfer vectors. There are many plasmids, promoters, packaging cell lines, and pseudotypes for investigators to choose from. Using stable producer cell lines provides a consistent vector source vector with reproducible titer that can be produced inexpensively. The extensive published experience with transduction conditions provides a solid framework for developing gene transfer protocols for most cell types. As these vectors have been moved into the clinical arena they have shown great promise, but have also identified significant risks, most notably insertional mutagenesis. Since a large body of information regarding tumor development is associated with retroviral insertion, strategies to overcome the limitations of these vectors are now being actively pursued. As is true in the development of all new therapeutic interventions, refinement in current vector design will lead to improved efficacy and safety, and retroviral vectors are likely to remain an important gene transfer tool when integration of transgene sequences is required for therapeutic effect.

Acknowledgments

The author is supported in part by the Indiana Genomics Initiative (INGEN) and grants from the National Institutes of Health (NCRR U42 RR11148 and NHLBI PPG 1 P01 HL53586).

REFERENCES

1. Miller AD, Eckner RJ, Jolly DJ, Friedmann T, Verma IM. Expression of a retrovirus encoding human HPRT in mice. *Science*. 1984;230:1395–1398.

2. Williams DA, Orkin SH, Mulligan RC. Retrovirus-mediated transfer of human adenosine deaminase gene sequences into cells in culture and into murine hematopoietic cells in vivo. *Proc Natl Acad Sci U S A*. 1986;83:2566–2570.

3. Eglitis MA, Kantoff P, Gilboa E, Anderson WF. Gene expression in mice after high efficiency retroviral-mediated gene transfer. *Science*. 1985;230:1395–1398.

4. Rosenberg SA, Aebersold PM, Cornetta K, et al. Gene transfer into humans: immunotherapy of patients with advanced melanoma, using tumor infiltrating lymphocytes modified by retroviral gene transduction. *N Engl J Med*. 1990;323:570–578.

5. Coffin JM, Hughes SH, Varmus HE. *Retroviruses at the National Center for Biotechnology Information*. Wordbury, NY: Cold Spring Harbor Laboratory Press; 1997.

6. Armentano D, Yu SF, Kantoff PW, von Ruden T, Anderson WF, Gilboa E. Effect of internal viral sequences on the utility of retroviral vectors. *J Virol*. 1987;61:1647–1650.

7. Jahner D, Stuhlmann H, Stewart CL, Harbers K, Lohler J, Simon I, Jaenisch R. De novo methylation and expression of retroviral genomes during mouse embryogenesis. *Nature*. 1982;298:623–628.

8. Challita PM, Kohn DB. Lack of expression from a retroviral vector after transduction of murine hematopoietic stem cells is associated with methylation in vivo. *Proc Natl Acad Sci U S A*. 1994;91:2567–2671.

9. Pannell D, Ellis J. Silencing of gene expression: implications for design of retrovirus vectors. *Rev Med Virol*. 2001;11:205–217.

10. Hawley RG. Progress towards vector design for hematopoietic stem cell gene therapy. *Curr Gene Ther*. 2001;1:1–17.

11. Cavazzana-Calvo M, Hacein-Bey S, de Saint Basile G, et al. Gene therapy of human severe combined immunodeficiency (SCID)-X1 disease. *Science*. 2000;288:669–672.

12. Hacein-Bey-Abina S, von Kalle C, Schmidt M, et al. A serious adverse event after successful gene therapy for X-linked severe combined immunodeficiency. *N Engl J Med*. 2003;348:255–256.

13. Hacein-Bey-Abina S, von Kalle C, Schmidt M, et al. LMO2-associated clonal T cell proliferation in two patients after gene therapy for SCID-X1. *Science*. 2003;302:415–419. [Erratum: *Science*. 2003;302:568].

14. Hacein-Bey-Abina S, Le Deist F, Carlier F, et al. Sustained correction of X-linked severe combined immunodeficiency by ex vivo gene therapy. *N Engl J Med*. 2002;346:1185–1193.

15. Yu SF, von Ruden T, Kantoff PW, et al. Self-inactivating retroviral vectors designed for transfer of whole genes into mammalian cells. *Proc Natl Acad Sci U S A.* 1986;83:3194–3198.

16. Kraunus J, Schaumann DHS, Meyer J, et al. Self-inactivating retroviral vectors with improved RNA processing. *Gene Ther.* 2004;11:1568–1578.

17. Hatzoglou M, Hodgson CP, Mularo F, Hanson RW. Efficient packaging of a specific VL30 retroelement by psi 2 cells which produce MoMLV recombinant retroviruses. *Hum Gene Ther.* 1990;1:385–397.

18. Cosset F, Takeuchi Y, Battini J, Weiss RA, Collins MKL. High-titer packaging cells producing recombinant retroviruses resistant to human serum. *J Virol.* 1995;69:7430–7436.

19. Sanburn N, Cornetta K. Rapid titer determination using quantitative real-time PCR. *Gene Ther.* 1999;6:1340–1345.

20. Pyra H, Boni J, Schupbach J. Ultrasensitive retrovirus detection by a reverse transcriptase assay based on product enhancement. *Proc Natl Acad Sci U S A.* 1994;191:1544–1548.

21. Sastry L, Xu Y, Marsh J, Cornetta K. Product enhanced reverse transcriptase (PERT) assay for detection of RCL associated with HIV-1 vectors. *Hum Gene Ther.* 2005;16:1227–1236.

22. Cornetta K, Anderson WF. Protamine sulfate as an effective alternative to polybrene in retroviral-mediated gene transfer: implications for human gene therapy. *J Virol Methods.* 1989;23:187–194.

23. Bodine DM, Karlsson S, Nienhuis AW. Combination of interleukin-3 and 6 preserves stem cell function in culture and enhances retrovirus-mediated gene transfer into hematopoietic stem cells. *Proc Natl Acad Sci U S A.* 1989;86:8897–8901.

24. Nolta JA, Kohn DB. Comparison of the effects of growth factors on retroviral vector–mediated gene transfer and the proliferative status of human hematopoietic progenitor cells. *Hum Gene Ther.* 1990;1:257–268.

25. Luskey BD, Rosenblatt M, Zsebo K, Williams DA. Stem cell factor, IL-3 and IL-6 promote retroviral-mediated gene transfer into murine hematopoietic stem cells. *Blood.* 1992;80:396–402.

26. Bodine DM, McDonagh KT, Seidel NE, Nienhuis AW. Survival and retrovirus infection of murine hematopoietic stem cells in vitro: effects of 5-FU and method of infection. *Exp Hematol.* 1991;19:206–212.

27. Moritz T, Patel VP, Williams DA. Bone marrow extracellular matrix molecules improved gene tranfer into human hematopoietic cells via retroviral vectors. *J Clin Invest.* 1994;93:1451–1457.

28. Hanenberg H, Xiao XL, Dilloo D, Hashino K, Kato I, Williams DA. Colocalization of retrovirus and target cells on specific fibronectin fragments increases genetic transduction of mammalian cells. *Nat Med.* 1996;2:1–6.

29. Tonks A, Tonks AJ, Pearn L, Mohamad Z, Burnett AK, Darley RL. Optimized retroviral transduction protocol which preserves the primitive subpopulation of human hematopoietic cells. *Biotechnol Prog.* 2005;21:953–8.

30. Fehse B, Kustikova OS, Bubenheim M, Baum C. Pois(s)on: It's a question of dose. *Gene Ther.* 2004;11:879–881.

31. Markowitz D, Goff S, Bank A. A safe packaging line for gene transfer: seperating viral genes on two different plasmids. *J Virol.* 1988;62:1120–1124.

32. Miller AD, Buttimore C. Redesign of retrovirus packaging cell lines to avoid recombination leading to helper virus production. *Mol Cell Biol.* 1986;6:2895–2902.

33. Markowitz D, Goff S, Bank A. Construction and use of a safe and efficient amphotropic packaging cell line. *Virology.* 1988;167:400–406.

34. Miller AD, Garcia JV, Von Suhr N, Lynch CM, Wilson C, Eiden MV. Construction and properties of retrovirus packaging cells based on gibbon ape leukemia virus. *J Virol.* 1991;65:2220–2224.

35. Neff T, Peterson LJ, Morris JC, et al. Efficient gene transfer to hematopoietic repopulating cells using concentrated RD114-pseudotyped vectors produced in human packaging cells. *Mol Ther.* 2004;9:157–159.

3 Lentivirus Vectors

GWENDOLYN K. BINDER
Abramson Family Cancer Research Institute, School of Medicine,
University of Pennsylvania, Philadelphia, Pennsylvania

BORO DROPULIC
Lentigen Corporation,, Baltimore, Maryland

The field of lentiviral vectors is a rapidly expanding and dynamic area of leading-edge science. The year 2006 marks the tenth anniversary of the first report of successful application of lentiviral vectors for gene transfer in the laboratory.[1] Within six years, in 2003, the first lentiviral vector clinical trial had been opened for enrollment, and at the time this book went to press, nine trials have been opened. This chapter is designed to provide an overview of the evolution of lentiviral vector technology over the past 10 years (Figure 3.1), to set the stage for more-in-depth chapters. To support a comprehensive understanding of the field and its potential applications, an overview of vector elements and constructs is given first, followed by examples of therapeutic applications for lentiviral vectors, and finally, some perspectives on the future directions of the field.

BIOSAFETY THROUGH THE GENERATIONS

Lentiviral vectors have evolved over the past decade from the first generation to the current third-generation vector systems. The generation refers primarily to sequential reductions in the number of virus-specific genes in the packaging system for improved biosafety in respect to reversion to a replication-competent lentivirus (RCL). The foundational first-generation lentiviral vectors were derived from HIV, the production system included a heterologous envelope on a single plasmid, and the packaging construct expressed *gag/pol tat/rev, nef*, and *vif*. The transfer vector retained the full 5′ and 3′ long terminal repeats (LTRs), the packaging signal, the *rev* response element (RRE), and an expression cassette for cytomegalovirus (CMV) expression of a marker gene downstream of the splice acceptor site.[1] Separation of constructs to three plasmids is a classic method for prevention of recombination to replication-competent virus. However, due

Concepts in Genetic Medicine, Edited by Boro Dropulic and Barrie Carter
Copyright © 2008 John Wiley & Sons, Inc.

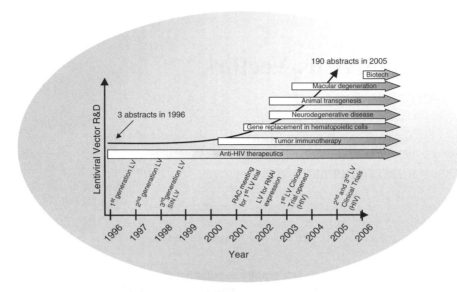

Figure 3.1   Overview of lentiviral research, 1996 to 2006.

to the pathogenic potential of lentiviral vectors in humans, additional steps to reduce the chances of recombination to wild type were warranted. Removal of virulence genes from HIV significantly attenuate the virus[2]; therefore, a logical next step for improved biosafety of vector production systems was to remove these genes to reduce the chance of recombination to a virulent human pathogen. The resulting vectors are known as second-generation vectors.[3,4]

First- and second-generation transfer vectors retained the native LTR promoter, which requires expression of tat in the packaging system in order to drive sufficient expression of transfer vector for packaging. To remove the requirement for tat, the third generation of vectors modified the U3 region of the LTR to express instead a heterologous promoter for constitutive expression during packaging. Since upon reverse transcription, the 3′ LTR would be copied to the 5′ end, the resulting transduction unit would retain the full 5′ and 3′ LTRs, like the first- and second-generation vectors. The dependence on Rev could not be removed efficiently; alternative export elements to RRE were tested but were not efficient. Therefore, Rev was moved to a third packaging plasmid, resulting in a four-plasmid production system.[5]

Transduction units with full 5′ and 3′ LTR sequences are capable of being packaged and spread (mobilized) subsequently in the presence of an RCL, such as wild-type HIV infection. Mobilization would be limited by the envelope provided; nevertheless, unintentional spread of transfer vectors poses an additional biosafety concern in most settings (it may be beneficial for HIV gene therapy). Therefore, third-generation vectors were further modified with a deletion in the 3′ LTR, so that both LTRs would not be functional in the transduction unit. These vectors are commonly known as self-inactivating (SIN) vectors.[6,7]

Interestingly, the first lentiviral vector to be used in the clinic was completely independent of the generational and SIN vectors, in large part because its application was for treatment of HIV. This vector was a conditionally replicating HIV vector expressing its payload (antisense) under the control of the LTR, which was produced using a two-plasmid system that had been designed to prevent recombination.[8] The advantage of the two-plasmid system was reportedly that higher titers were achieved during production, which is currently still performed using transient transfection. Also, nonintegrating vector systems are also recently in development, although it is challenging to achieve efficient titers.

VECTOR SPECIES

Lentiviral vectors are most commonly referred to as primate or nonprimate vectors, due to the perception that nonprimate vectors are less likely to become pathogenic if an RCL occurs. Lentiviruses exhibit strong host specificity, and therefore the perception that nonprimate vectors could be safer is not unfounded.[9] However, the extensive modifications made to current-day third-generation vectors make the possibility of an RCL so remote that it merits renewed consideration whether safety distinctions between primate and nonprimate vectors remain relevant. Primate vectors include human immunodeficiency virus type 1 and 2 (HIV-1 and HIV-2)[1,10,11] and simian immunodeficiency virus (SIV)-derived vectors.[12,13] Nonprimate vectors include primarily those derived from the feline immunodeficiency virus (FIV),[14,15] equine infectious anemia virus (EIAV),[16,17] and more recently, vectors from bovine immunodeficiency virus (BIV).[18,19] Vectors derived from the rare Jembrana disease virus (JDV), maedi/visna virus (MVV), and caprine arthritis/encephalitis virus (CAEV) have also been described, but these vectors have not been developed extensively, due to low efficiencies of transduction.[20-22] Some attempts have also been made at mixing elements from non-HIV lentiviruses with the HIV-1 transfer vector to further reduce the chance of an RCL.[23]

The host-restrictive nature of lentiviruses transfers somewhat to the transduction efficiencies of the vectors that are derived from them. In many cases, HIV is more efficient than other lentiviral vectors in transduction or expression in human cells.[24-26] Nevertheless, some human cells, such as neurons and retinal pigmented epithelial cells or corneal cells in the eye, are efficiently transduced, by nonprimate lentiviral vectors, with genes that express well.[27,28] These and other data suggest that host cell restrictions are also cell specific, although the mechanism of restriction is still understood superficially. Restrictions are linked to several factors: transcriptional blocks, RNA instability, postentry inhibition, and gene silencing.[24,25,29] As more is learned about the mechanisms for species specificity, vector modifications could be made to overcome them. For example, to improve RNA stability, different polyadenylation sequences can be added; or for postentry blocks, the *gag* protein of the lentivirus can be modified to avoid interaction with the TRIM5α family of inhibitors.[30] SIV-derived vectors are inefficient in human cells, as are HIV-derived vectors in simian cells, and therefore

SIV vectors have been derived primarily for development of nonhuman primate modeling for lentiviral vector applications.

Amid safety concerns, human application of HIV-derived vectors was discussed publicly at the Recombinant Advisory Committee (RAC) of the NIH and the Biological Response Modifiers Advisory Committee (BRMAC) of the U.S. Food and Drug Administration (FDA) in 2001 prior to initiation of the first clinical trial evaluating a lentiviral vector. The vector used in this trial was an HIV-1-derived vector for inhibition of HIV.[8] Use of an HIV-derived vector first in HIV-infected persons helped to move clinical application forward since the risk/benefit ratio in these patients is more favorable. Presently, all clinical trials using lentiviral vectors are in the setting of HIV, although plans are in place to start broadening out into other applications, such as cancer. First clinical applications of nonprimate lentiviral vectors is most likely to be for diseases of the central nervous system (CNS) or the eye.

TOOLS

The molecular "toolbox" has come a long way for lentiviral vectors and has received important contributions from the lessons of retroviral vectors[31-35] (and references therein). The goals for vector modification are typically to increase titers, heighten biosafety, improve transduction efficiency, and promote high and durable gene expression. These goals have been addressed primarily through the inclusion of *cis*-acting sequences, degeneration and minimization of vector sequences whenever possible, pseudotyping with appropriate envelopes, and application of efficient promoters. As the field progresses, vectors have evolved to exhibit new characteristics, such as efficient dual-gene expression, tissue or cell specificity, episomal gene expression (nonintegrating vectors), or RNA-only expression.

Promoters

The earliest lentiviral vectors used either the native LTR promoter region or an internal CMV promoter to drive gene expression. Advances in the use of promoters has been pursued to reduce gene silencing, to allow for tissue-specific gene expression, or to permit inducible expression. Early on it was found that promoters could afford differential expression in tissues.[36] Since then, various promoters have been described for expression in CD4 cells,[37] B cells,[38] antigen-presenting cells,[39] erythroid cells,[40] prostate cells,[41] and endothelial cells,[42] among others. Notably, restriction of gene expression by silencer elements can be as important as cell-specific promoter elements for tissue-specific expression,[37] and promoter interference between the U3 region of the LTR and internal promoters has been shown, providing an explanation for previously confusing data between different vectors using the same internal promoter.[43]

Silencing of nonhuman promoters is also an issue, in particular with CMV, which can be silenced as quickly as two weeks posttransduction.[44] Replacing the CMV promoter with alternative virus promoters or tissue promoters can overcome the silencing problem.[44,45] In some cases, constitutive expression, even in a cell-type-specific manner, is not optimal, and therefore inducible expression is warranted. This can be achieved using well-known drug-inducible systems such as the tetracycline or ecdysone system.[46–49] Pol III promoters that can be used for expression of siRNA can be drug inducible as well.[48,50] A less conventional but elegant alternative application of inducible expression is to use promoters sensitive to the disease state, as exemplified in glial cells and neurons during brain lesion.[51]

Multiple Gene Expression

Expression of one or more genes can be therapeutically necessary in many situations. As examples, dual- or triple-expression cassettes are helpful where a disease gene needs to be knocked down in order for the replacement gene to work properly,[52] where expression of multiple sequences is necessary to ensure a sustained therapeutic effect,[53,54] in situations where a drug selection gene or suicide gene is required,[55] or when a marker gene is useful in conjunction with the transgene to be expressed. Recently, several approaches for multigene expression have arisen, the first and still most common of which is use of the viral internal ribosome entry site (IRES) for expression of multiple proteins from a single RNA transcript.[56] The IRES has been used successfully for sustained expression of up to three genes from a single transcript.[54] Although expression levels from IRES are typically lower than expression of the gene closest to the promoter, levels of expression can be high enough to allow functional expression as demonstrated in an in vivo model for drug-mediated selection of stem cells by an IRES-driven O^6-methylguanine–DNA methyltransferase (MGMT) gene.[57] Alternative splicing using the lentivirus splicing sequences can also help to regulation expression of two genes, and is about as efficient as IRES if Rev is removed from the system.[58] Multiple internal promoters can also be used; although it is generally known that multiple promoters may interfere with each other, this approach has been reported to be successful, and interference could be reduced by the addition of insulators if necessary.[59] Linked bidirectional promoters also work well and express genes more equivalently than IRES can.[60] Another alternative to the IRES is the use of self-cleaving 2A cleavage factors, which are derived from various picornaviruses. The cleavage factor results in a polyprotein that self-cleaves, resulting in predictable stoichiometry of both proteins.[61] Improved efficiency of cleavage can be obtained by including the proper linker between the protein and the cleavage factor, and at lower copy numbers the cleavage factor appears to be somewhat more efficient than the IRES.[62]

Important cis-Acting Elements

In addition to promoters, the packaging signal (ψ), integration signals (attL and attR), primer binding site and splice donor, and in most cases, splice acceptor sites (SD and SA) are required elements. The length of the packaging signal, which is located within the *gag* gene, can be minimized[63] or to further reduce homologies with the packaging constructs, it could be replaced with an RNA with high affinity for capsid, although this has not been regularly put into practice.[64] RNA transport elements are also required, except in certain cell types when the SA/SD are removed from the vector.[65] Most often, the rev response element (RRE) is used, which requires incorporation of Rev in the production system. RRE can be replaced with alternative RNA export elements, such as the constitutive transport element (CTE) derived from the beta retroviruses and simian retrovirus type 1 (SRV-1). Until recently, these elements were not as efficient as the RRE, but two reports now show that removal of the RRE from the transfer vector may be possible, which would further improve vector biosafety.[66,67] Additional improvements in biosafety can be made through codon optimization of the *gag* gene, which also improves expression.[68]

Nonrequisite cis-acting sequences are commonly added to improve titers and gene expression from vectors. One significant breakthrough was the discovery that a sequence in the *gag* gene called the central polypurine tract and central termination sequence (CPPT/CTS) was important for efficient reverse transcription and nuclear import.[69] Resulting vector titers and transduction efficiencies were so much better with this sequence that it is now a standard element in all vectors. Improved gene expression was obtained by inclusion of a posttranscription regulatory element in the 3′ untranslated region (UTR) from the human hepatitis virus (HPRE) that aids in efficiently exporting RNA from the nucleus. Later, it was found that the PRE from woodchuck hepatitis virus (WPRE) could be much more efficient in gene expression than the HPRE,[70] and it worked well in retroviral vectors.[71] There is presently some concern about this element, however, as it was linked to oncogenesis after liver delivery in fetal and neonatal mice using a nonprimate lentiviral vector, although the role of the WPRE is not presently conclusive.[72] The WPRE used in that study contains in its C terminus an overlapping promoter for the X-protein of woodchuck hepatitis virus, which in theory could activate neighboring genes leading to oncogenesis. Removal of this promoter sequence reduced the efficiency of the WPRE only minimally, so this may offer a safe way to continue to incorporate the element in lentiviral vectors in the future.[125] PREs isolated from the UTRs of eukaryotic mRNAs have also been shown to exhibit additive gene expression effects when used in conjunction with the WPRE due to improved RNA stability.[73]

Gene Silencing

Retroviral vectors undergo a significant level of silencing that can impede long-term gene expression. It has been proposed that lentiviral vectors may be more resistant to this silencing,[74,75] but this conclusion is not yet definitive and needs to be investigated further.[76] Silencing of vectors occurs in large part via chromatin condensation following methylation. Inclusion of insulator regions can help to reduce methylation and serve as a barrier to condensation by facilitating the acetylation of histones to prevent methylation.[77,78] The use of insulators to improve gene expression is an active area of ongoing research, and they have been shown to standardize expression in some cell types.[79] Due to their size (about 1.2 kb), the use of insulators can be limited by transgene size and the resulting packaging efficiencies of larger vector genomes.

Envelope Proteins

Targeting of lentiviral vectors can be achieved through packaging with heterologous viral envelopes, and a review of the various envelopes tested to date can be found in Cronin et al.[80] The gold standard for lentiviral envelopes is the G protein from vesicular stomatitis virus (VSV-G), since it increases transduction efficiency, results in high titers, and is highly stable during concentration and clinical purification.[81,82] However, the protein is cytotoxic and is a challenge during production. Despite its broad range, VSV-G does not transduce all cells well, the best example of which is airway epithelium, which is better transduced with the envelope protein from filoviruses or Sendai virus.[83,84] Filovirus envelopes are also more efficient at transducing muscle cells.[85] As another example, certain envelopes may be better than VSV-G for enabling retrograde axonal transport, which may allow for less invasive neuronal routes of delivery.[86,87] Table 2 of the Cronin et al. review summarizes nicely the various envelopes for different target organs or cells. Targeting of vectors by pseudotyping remains in the early stages and faces several hurdles, including complement inactivation and production and purification challenges for envelopes less sturdy than VSV-G. Tissue specificity is still addressed primarily through tissue-specific regulation by promoters or other tools, such as micro RNAs.[88] Tissue-specific expression is known to reduce immunogenicity of the transgene, probably through the induction of peripheral tolerance.

APPLICATIONS

Toward Clinical Gene Therapy

The very first clinical application of lentiviral vectors was for treatment of HIV in 2003.[89,90] Since then, at the time of this book going to press, nine more trials for HIV gene therapy using lentiviral vectors have opened (www.wiley.co.uk/genmed/clinical). The safety database accrued from these trials is anticipated to help the general field of clinical application of lentiviral vectors to move forward, and it is anticipated that non-HIV trials will begin soon in some of the areas described next.

Since the first report of lentiviral vectors working successfully in culture,[1] there has been an explosion in use of the vectors for preclinical development of gene therapeutics. In general, these applications take advantage of the durability of the lentiviral vector expression to treat disorders that benefit from long-term survival of cells modified for a lasting therapeutic effect. This may evolve with time to include short-term applications, as future vectors may include integrase-deficient or reverse transcription–deficient vectors for temporary expression of gene products,[91,92] such as zinc-finger endonucleases for gene knockout or growth factors that should not be expressed constitutively.[93,94]

The most prevalent models studied include CNS disorders, infectious disease, ocular gene delivery, and hematopoietic gene replacement studies. Neuronal delivery is an obvious area for lentiviral vectors because of their nondividing nature. Several applications have been investigated and are reviewed in Ralph et al.,[94] and most utilize the EIAV vector as a delivery vehicle. Direct injection of the vector is sometimes used, such as for Parkinson's disease.[54,95] However, an attractive delivery method is intramuscular (IM) delivery, which can work for rabies virus G protein-pseudotyped vectors.[87] There is some nice data showing rabies-pseudotyped vectors injected IM that are subsequently transported up into motor neurons for treatment of motor neuron diseases such as spinal muscular atrophy (SMA) and amyotrophic lateral sclerosis (ALS) that showing at least a partial therapeutic benefit.[96,97]

Therapeutic ocular delivery by lentiviral vectors is another area of rapid advancement because it, too, allows for direct injection of vector into tissue, resulting in efficient gene transfer with controlled biodistribution. There does not appear to be a species restriction in this tissue, as FIV, BIV, EIAV, and HIV-1 and 2 vectors all transduce this tissue efficiently.[28,98–101] Gene delivery of endostatin or angiostatin to this tissue has reversed symptoms of macular degeneration in experimental animal models.[100,102] Gene replacement has also helped to improve eye health in a rat model for retinal degeneration.[103] Direct injection of RNA into the retina for treatment of wet macular degeneration has already made it to the clinic, but it requires multiple injections for sustained benefit. Vector-based delivery systems offer a single-dose alternative that is likely to be highly attractive for ongoing development.

The transduction efficiency of lentiviral vectors offers the hope of successful phenotypic correction after gene replacement. This has been investigated experimentally for such genetic disorders as hemophilia,[104] cystic fibrosis,[83] and β-thalassemia.[105] Diseases where cells can be modified ex vivo, or where vector can be delivered to a restricted area, such as lung, brain, or eye, are more likely to advance to the clinic more quickly since the targeting efficiency of directly injected lentiviral vectors is still at an early stage of research. In utero modification of tissue is an interesting area of research, still in its early stages, that could offer options for delivery of genes to large numbers of cells, such as muscle cells for treatment of Duchenne muscular dystrophy.[85,106] In utero delivery is also attractive because it is likely to avoid issues of immunogenicity of the transgene. A recent elegant use of lentiviral vectors for treatment of sickle cell anemia used a bicistronic cassette for simultaneous knockdown of the diseased gene and expression of a replacement gene to abrogate the dominant negative effect of the endogenous gene and allow functional gene correction.[52]

Another area of preclinical development is the use of lentiviral vectors for cancer gene therapy for breaking immune tolerance to tumors. There are several approaches that have been in development, the furthest along of which is the use of chimeric antibody receptors (CARs) for expression on T cells (T body) for breaking tolerance to the tumor antigen.[107] This has already been tested in a clinical trial for B-cell lymphoma using retroviral vectors,[108] or plasmid transfection,[127] and for treatment of renal cell carcinoma.[128] Greater efficiency of gene transfer by lentiviral vectors may improve any therapeutic effect. A lentiviral vector-based T-body trial is also in preparation and is anticipated to start in 2008. Other approaches use lentiviral vectors to deliver tumor antigens to autologous dendritic cells (DCs) to help educate the immune system to the tumor.[109] Vector-mediated delivery of tumor antigens appears to elicit more potent antitumor immunity than with antigen loading of DCs, perhaps due to the improved MHC-I loading and better TH1 and CTL induction.[110] Delivery of cytokine genes directly to the tumor cells to awaken the immune system, and this principle has shown great promise with the GVAX vaccine now under fast-track approval for metastatic prostate cancer. Tumors are efficiently transduced with lentiviral vectors,[111] but getting to all tumor cells is not feasible, so immune-based approaches are most likely to be successful at the present stage of vector development.

Transgenic Animals

Generation of transgenic mice has been made dramatically more efficient with lentiviral vectors. Formerly, transgenesis was performed by pronuclear injection with DNA, which is tremendously difficult, expensive, and inefficient. Instead, vectors can be added to the single-cell embryo, which while still technically challenging, results in up to an astonishing 80% transgenesis.[75] The first proof of principle used the GFP gene under the control of the ubiquitin promoter for expression in all tissues. Later in the same study, they showed tissue-specific gene expression by transgenesis using a promoter specific for skeletal tissue. Importantly, with lentiviral vector–mediated delivery, gene silencing does not seem to occur,[74] which is contrary to retroviral vectors, which undergo extensive methylation in the embryo and face gene silencing.[112] Lentiviral vectors have also been used to generate transgenic rats,[113] pigs,[114] and cattle,[115] and it has been attempted unsuccessfully in nonhuman primates (although placental expression was achieved).[116] A unique application for this is using murine transgenesis to model promoter tissue specificity, which could help establish the safety profile for directly injected therapeutic vectors.[117]

Biotechnology and Proteomics

Lentiviral vectors are useful tools for determining gene function and for protein production as a result of their integrating nature and gene transfer efficiency. Overexpression of a gene of interest can be achieved, and the level of expression can be modulated by the promoter used or the copy number, which can easily be titrated up or down with these vectors.[118] Gene knockdown can be achieved easily using the ubiquitous RNAi mechanism induced by small hairpin RNAs delivered by lentiviral vectors.[119] Gene expression and knockdown can be controlled using conditional gene expression of either the RNAi or the transgene by conditional promoters.[48,50] Dual vector systems offer more stringent methods for expression control, and allow for inducible RNAi expression through the cre-lox system[120] or via targeting of the transgene 3' UTR by simian RNAs.[121] In these cases, expression control is limited by transduction of the cells with the second vector, or alternatively, the second vector can be controlled under an inducible promoter, thus providing a tiered approach to regulation.

Inducible expression systems are also useful for protein production in biotechnology. Constitutive high levels of protein expression can reduce the fitness of producer cells, which is particularly important if the protein being expressed is toxic to the producer cells, such as VSV-G during lentiviral vector production.[122,123] Protein manufacture can therefore be enhanced if protein expression can be limited to the period of production. The efficiency, stability, and long-term gene expression of lentiviral vectors makes them a very useful tool for this area of biotechnology. For example, difficult to manufacture proteins such as factor VIII could be produced more cost-effectively by using lentiviral vectors both to decrease the time to generate high-expressing cell clones and to increase protein yield. Recent studies showing a lack of tumorgenicity of lentiviral vectors in highly sensitive animal models makes these vectors highly appropriate for biopharmaceutical manufacturing purposes.[126]

PERSPECTIVES: LENTIVIRAL VECTORS AND TRANSLATIONAL MEDICINE

The explosion of research application of lentiviral vectors speaks volumes for the broad and flexible utility of the lentiviral vector system. Scaling up from the bench to clinical applications, and then to biopharmaceutical-driven drug development, is, however, presently as real a challenge as the original technological development itself has been. With the first lentiviral vector clinical trial completed and several more under way, the initial hurdle of gaining scientific consensus for adequate safety in vector construction, production, and patient monitoring has been traversed. With this achievement, it is expected that the clinical application of lentiviral vectors will begin to catch up to the flurry of research-based application that has been seen over the past 10 years. The roadblock for the past few years has been a source for adequate GMP (good manufacturing practice) manufacture of lentiviral vector for clinical trials, and this may be reaching a turning point after several years of intense focus on this problem in the academic and biotech sectors; however at the time of this chapter going to press, the National Gene Vector Laboratories is unfortunately no longer providing academic funding for GMP lentivival vector manufacture. Manufacturing of lentiviral vectors is costly and is much more challenging than production of adenoviral vectors, for example, since lentiviral vectors are enveloped and can lose titer easily. As different envelopes are used for tissue-specific delivery or for reduced immunogenicity, this will provide a new challenge to high-titer GMP production.

There remains a serious concern for the safety of lentiviral vectors in terms of insertional oncogenesis, as that risk has now been realized in a clinical trial utilizing murine-derived retroviral vectors. Due to this concern, it will take establishment of a larger safety database of patient treatment before these vectors will be accepted for clinical application in nonserious diseases. Additional research studies in serial transplantation of stem cells and T cells in immunodeficient mice will help to elucidate the effects of lentiviral integration on clonal dominance, and such studies will help to further establish the safety–risk profile of individual vectors.[124] Lentiviral vectors have not been shown to be oncogenic in nature except for a single study in neonatal mice involving direct injection for liver delivery.[72] The oncogenesis in this study may be associated with a vector element that can be modified to reduce such a risk,[125] and it may also be unique to the animal model used in that study. It is notable that T-cell leukemia is not a recognized side effect of HIV infection, although a high proportion of proviruses are defective and therefore would not mask a leukemic event. More recently, studies have shown that lentiviral vectors demonstrate low genotoxicity after integration in a tumor-prone mouse model, providing further evidence for the lack of oncogenic potential for this vector class.[126]

Finally, a roadblock to large-scale biopharmaceutical development of a licensed first in class lentiviral vector-based genetic therapy is the complex landscape for intellectual property. The tendency to mix various elements together to optimize a vector, such as a SIN vector with a CPPT/CTS, RNAi, and VSV-G as a simple example, creates a technology licensing challenge that could impede commercial development. Although clinical trials in the United States are exempt from patent infringement under a *Code of Federal Regulations* exemption (271e), commercial development will still have to face these issues until the patent terms for these elements run out. The first commercial success for lentiviral gene therapy, or gene therapy in general, is likely to propel the clinical development field forward, as it will stimulate greater biopharmacuetical investment into clinical trials. Therefore, continued affordable nonexclusive inlicensing of intellectual property is needed to help continue advancement in the field.

Overall, the field of lentiviral vectors has been advancing at an accelerated pace. In under a decade from the original laboratory proof of principle, these vectors were applied in the clinic. The potential benefits from successful therapeutic development of these vectors is entertaining to envision and provides a great deal of hope to many with otherwise incurable disease.

REFERENCES

1. Naldini L, Blomer U, Gallay P, et al. In vivo gene delivery and stable transduction of nondividing cells by a lentiviral vector. *Science*. 1996;272:263–267.

2. Desrosiers RC. HIV with multiple gene deletions as a live attenuated vaccine for AIDS. *AIDS Res Hum Retrovirus*. 1992;8:411–421.

3. Zufferey R, Nagy D, Mandel RJ, Naldini L, Trono D. Multiply attenuated lentiviral vector achieves efficient gene delivery in vivo. *Nat Biotechnol*. 1997;15:871–875.

4. Kim VN, Mitrophanous K, Kingsman SM, Kingsman AJ. Minimal requirement for a lentivirus vector based on human immunodeficiency virus type 1. *J Virol*. 1998;72:811–816.

5. Dull T, Zufferey R, Kelly M, et al. A third–generation lentivirus vector with a conditional packaging system. *J Virol*. 1998;72:8463–8471.
6. Miyoshi H, Blomer U, Takahashi M, Gage FH, Verma IM. Development of a self-inactivating lentivirus vector. *J Virol*. 1998;72:8150–8157.
7. Zufferey R, Dull T, Mandel RJ, et al. Self-inactivating lentivirus vector for safe and efficient in vivo gene delivery. *J Virol*. 1998;72:9873–9880.
8. Lu X, Humeau L, Slepushkin V, et al. Safe two-plasmid production for the first clinical lentivirus vector that achieves >99% transduction in primary cells using a one-step protocol. *J Gene Med*. 2004;6:963–973.
9. Desrosiers RC. Nonhuman lentiviruses. In: Knipe DM, Howeley PM, eds. *Fields Virology*. Philadelphia, PA: Lippincott Williams & Wilkins; 2001:2095–2121.
10. Arya SK, Zamani M, Kundra P. Human immunodeficiency virus type 2 lentivirus vectors for gene transfer: expression and potential for helper virus-free packaging. *Hum Gene Ther*. 1998;9:1371–1380.
11. Poeschla E, Corbeau P, Wong-Staal F. Development of HIV vectors for anti-HIV genetherapy. *Proc Natl Acad Sci U S A*. 1996;93:11395–11399.
12. Stitz J, Muhlebach MD, Blomer U, et al. A novel lentivirus vector derived from apathogenic simian immunodeficiency virus. *Virology*. 2001;291:191–197.
13. Pandya S, Boris-Lawrie K, Leung NJ, Akkina R, Planelles V. Development of an *rev*-independent, minimal simian immunodeficiency virus-derived vector system. *Hum Gene Ther*. 2001;12:847–857.
14. Johnston JC, Gasmi M, Lim LE, et al. Minimum requirements for efficient transduction of dividing and nondividing cells by feline immunodeficiency virus vectors. *J Virol*. 1999;73:4991–5000.
15. Poeschla EM, Wong-Staal F, Looney DJ. Efficient transduction of nondividing human cells by feline immunodeficiency virus lentiviral vectors. *Nat Med*. 1998;4:354–357.
16. Olsen JC. Gene transfer vectors derived from equine infectious anemia virus. *Gene Ther*. 1998;5:1481–1487.
17. Mitrophanous KA, Yoon S, Rohll JB, et al. Stable gene transfer to the nervous system using a non-primate lentiviral vector. *Gene Ther*. 1999;6:1808–1818.
18. Molina RP, Matukonis M, Paszkiet B, et al. Mapping of the bovine immunodeficiency virus packaging signal and RRE and incorporation into a minimal gene transfer vector. *Virology*. 2002;304:10–23.
19. Matukonis M, Li M, Molina RP, et al. Development of second- and third-generation bovine immunodeficiency virus-based gene transfer systems. *Hum Gene Ther*. 2002;13:1293–1303.
20. Metharom P, Takyar S, Xia HH, et al. Novel bovine lentiviral vectors based on Jembrana disease virus. *J Gene Med*. 2000;2:176–185.
21. Mselli-Lakhal L, Favier C, Teixeira MFD, et al. Defective RNA packaging is responsible for low transduction efficiency of CAEV-based vectors. *Arch Virol*. 1998;143:681–695.
22. Berkowitz RD, Ilves H, Plavec I, Veres G. Gene transfer systems derived from visna virus: analysis of virus production and infectivity. *Virology*. 2001;279:116–129.
23. White SM, Renda M, Nam NY, et al. Lentivirus vectors using human and simian immunodeficiency virus elements. *J Virol*. 1999;73:2832–2840.

24. O'Rourke JP, Newbound GC, Kohn DB, Olsen JC, Bunnell BA. Comparison of gene transfer efficiencies and gene expression levels achieved with equine infectious anemia virus–and human immunodeficiency virus type 1–derived lentivirus vectors. *J Virol*. 2002;76:1510–1515.

25. Price MA, Case SS, Carbonaro DA, et al. Expression from second-generation feline immunodeficiency virus vectors is impaired in human hematopoietic cells. *Mol Ther*. 2002;6:645–652.

26. Dupuy FP, Mouly E, Mesel-Lemoine M, et al. Lentiviral transduction of human hematopoietic cells by HIV-1- and SIV-based vectors containing a bicistronic cassette driven by various internal promoters. *J Gene Med*. 2005;7:1158–1171.

27. Beutelspacher SC, Ardjomand N, Tan PH, et al. Comparison of HIV-1 and EIAV-based lentiviral vectors in corneal transduction. *Exp Eye Res*. 2005;80: 787–794.

28. Takahashi K, Luo T, Saishin Y, et al. Sustained transduction of ocular cells with a bovine immunodeficiency viral vector. *Hum Gene Ther*. 2002;13:1305–1316.

29. Ikeda Y, Ylinen LMJ, Kahar-Bador M, Towers GJ. Influence of *gag* on human immunodeficiency virus type 1 species-specific tropism. *J Virol*. 2004;78: 11816–11822.

30. Kootstra NA, Munk C, Tonnu N, Landau NR, Verma IM. Abrogation of postentry restriction of HIV-1-based lentiviral vector transduction in simian cells. *Proc Natl Acad Sci U S A*. 2003;100:1298–1303.

31. Trono D. *Lentiviral Vectors*. New York: Springer-Verlag; 2002.

32. Pages JC, Bru T. Toolbox for retrovectorologists. *J Gene Med*. 2004;6:S67–S82.

33. Delenda C. Lentiviral vectors: optimization of packaging, transduction and gene expression. *J Gene Med*. 2004;6:S125–S138.

34. Baum C, Schambach A, Bohne J, Galla M. Retrovirus vectors: toward the plentivirus? *Mol Ther*. 2006;13(6):1050–1063.

35. Sinn PL, Sauter SL, McCray PL. Gene therapy progress and prospects: development of improved lentiviral and retroviral vectors—design, biosafety, and production. *Gene Ther*. 2005;12:1089–1098.

36. Couture LA, Mullen CA, Morgan RA. Retroviral vectors containing chimeric promoter/enhancer elements exhibit cell-type-specific gene-expression. *Hum Gene Ther*. 1994;5:667–677.

37. Marodon G, Mouly E, Blair EJ, et al. Specific transgene expression in human and mouse CD4(+) cells using lentiviral vectors with regulatory sequences from the CD4 gene. *Blood*. 2003;101:3416–3423.

38. Werner M, Kraunas K, Baum C, Brocker T. B-cell-specific transgene expression using a self-inactivating retroviral vector with human CD 19 promoter and viral post-transcriptional regulatory element. *Gene Ther*. 2004;11:992–1000.

39. Cui Y, Golob J, Kelleher E, Pardoll D, Cheng LZ. Targeting transgene expression to antigen presenting cells (APC) differentiated in vivo from lentiviral transduced, engrafting human and mouse hematopoetic stem/progenitor cells. *Blood*. 2001;98:214A.

40. Richard E, Mendez M, Mazurier F, et al. Gene therapy of a mouse model of protoporphyria with a self-inactivating erythroid-specific lentiviral vector without preselection. *Mol Ther*. 2001;4:331–338.

41. Yu D, Chen DL, Chiu C, et al. Prostate-specific targeting using PSA promoter-based lentiviral vectors. *Cancer Gene Ther.* 2001;8:628–635.

42. De Palma M, Venneri MA, Naldini L. In vivo targeting of tumor endothelial cells by systemic delivery of lentiviral vectors. *Hum Gene Ther.* 2003;14:1193–1206.

43. Ginn SL, Fleming J, Rowe PB, Alexander IE. Promoter interference mediated by the U3 region in early-generation HIV-1-derived lentivirus vectors can influence detection of transgene expression in a cell-type and species-specific manner. *Hum Gene Ther.* 2003;14:1127–1137.

44. Gerolami R, Uch R, Jordier F, et al. Gene transfer to hepatocellular carcinoma: transduction efficacy and transgene expression kinetics by using retroviral and lentiviral vectors. *Cancer Gene Ther.* 2000;7:1286–1292.

45. Demaison C, Parsley K, Brouns G, et al. High-level transduction and gene expression in hematopoietic repopulating cells using a human imunodeficiency virus type 1-based lentiviral vector containing an internal spleen focus forming virus promoter. *Hum Gene Ther.* 2002;13:803–813.

46. Vaillancourt P, Felts KA. Retroviral delivery of the ecdysone-regulatable gene expression system. *Biotechnol Prog.* 2003;19:1750–1755.

47. Koponen JK, Kankkonen H, Kannasto J, et al. Doxycycline-regulated lentiviral vector system with a novel reverse transactivator rtTA2(S)-M2 shows a tight control of gene expression in vitro and in vivo. *Gene Ther.* 2003;10:459–466.

48. Szulc J, Wiznerowicz M, Sauvain MO, Trono D, Aebischer P. A versatile tool for conditional gene expression and knockdown. *Nat Methods.* 2006;3:109–116.

49. Paulus W, Baur I, Boyce FM, Breakefield XO, Reeves SA. Self-contained, tetracycline-regulated retroviral vector system for gene delivery to mammalian cells. *J Virol.* 1996;70:62–67.

50. Amar L, Desclaux M, Faucon-Biguet N, Mallet J, Vogel R. Control of small inhibitory RNA levels and RNA interference by doxycycline induced activation of a minimal RNA polymerase III promoter. *Nucl Acids Res.* 2006;34:e37.

51. Jakobsson J, Rosenqvist N, Marild K, Agoston V, Lundberg C. Evidence for disease-regulated transgene expression in the brain with use of lentiviral vectors. *J Neurosci Res.* Epub: May 8, 2006.

52. Samakoglu S, Lisowski L, Budak-Alpdogan T, et al. A genetic strategy to treat sickle cell anemia by coregulating globin transgene expression and RNA interference. *Nat Biotechnol.* 2006;24:89–94.

53. Li MJ, Kim J, Li S, et al. Long-term inhibition of HIV-1 infection in primary hematopoietic cells by lentiviral vector delivery of a triple combination of anti-HIV shRNA, anti-CCR5 ribozyme, and a nucleolar-localizing TAR decoy. *Mol Ther.* 2005;12:900–909.

54. Azzouz M, Martin-Rendon E, Barber RD, et al. Multicistronic lentiviral vector-mediated striatal gene transfer of aromatic L-amino acid decarboxylase, tyrosine hydroxylase, and GTP cyclohydrolase I induces sustained transgene expression, dopamine production, and functional improvement in a rat model of Parkinson's disease. *J Neurosci.* 2002;22:10302–10312.

55. Neff T, Horn PA, Peterson LJ, et al. Methylguanine methyltransferase–mediated in vivo selection and chemoprotection of allogeneic stem cells in a large-animal model. *J Clin Invest.* 2003;112:1581–1588.

56. Martinez-Salas E. Internal ribosome entry site biology and its use in expression vectors. *Curr Opin Biotechnol*. 1999;10:458–464.

57. Davis BM, Humeau L, Dropulic B. In vivo selection for human and murine hematopoietic cells transduced with a therapeutic MGMT lentiviral vector that inhibits HIV replication. *Mol Ther*. 2004;9:160–172.

58. Zhu Y, Feuer G, Day SL, Wrzesinski S, Planelles V. Multigene lentiviral vectors based on differential splicing and translational control. *Mol Ther*. 2001;4:375–382.

59. Yu XB, Zhan XC, D'Costa J, et al. Lentiviral vectors with two independent internal promoters transfer high-level expression of multiple transgenes to human hematopoietic stem-progenitor cells. *Mol Ther*. 2003;7:827–838.

60. Amendola M, Venneri MA, Biffi A, Vigna E, Naldini L. Coordinate dual-gene transgenesis by lentiviral vectors carrying synthetic bidirectional promoters. *Nat Biotechnol*. 2005;23:108–116.

61. Szymczak AL, Workman CJ, Wang Y, et al. Correction of multi-gene deficiency in vivo using a single 'self-cleaving' 2A peptide-based retroviral vector. *Nat Biotechnol*. 2004;22:589–594.

62. Chinnasamy D, Milsom MD, Shaffer J, et al. Multicistronic lentiviral vectors containing the FMDV 2A cleavage factor demonstrate robust expression of encoded genes at limiting MOI. *Virol J*. 2006;3(1):14–16.

63. Browning MT, Mustafa F, Schmidt RD, Lew KA, Rizvi TA. Sequences within the *gag* gene of feline immunodeficiency virus (FIV) are important for efficient RNA encapsidation. *Virus Res*. 2003;93:199–209.

64. Clever JL, Taplitz RA, Lochrie MA, Polisky B, Parslow TG. A Heterologous, high-affinity RNA ligand for human immunodeficiency virus *gag* protein has RNA packaging activity. *J Virol*. 2000;74:541–546.

65. Cui Y, Iwakuma T, Chang LJ. Contributions of viral splice sites and cis-regulatory elements to lentivirus vector function. *J Virol*. 1999;73:6171–6176.

66. Mautino MR, Keiser N, Morgan RA. Improved titers of HIV-based lentiviral vectors using the SRV-1 constitutive transport element. *Gene Ther*. 2000;7:1421–1424.

67. Wodrich H, Bohne J, Gumz E, Welker R, Krausslich HG. A new RNA element located in the coding region of a murine endogenous retrovirus can functionally replace the *rev/rev*-responsive element system in human immunodeficiency virus type 1 *gag* expression. *J Virol*. 2001;75:10670–10682.

68. Wagner R, Graf M, Bieler K, et al. *Rev*-independent expression of synthetic *gag–pol* genes of human immunodeficiency virus type 1 and simian immunodeficiency virus: implications for the safety of lentiviral vectors. *Hum Gene Ther*. 2000;11:2403–2413.

69. Sirven A, Pflumio F, Zennou V, et al. The human immunodeficiency virus type-1 central DNA flap is a crucial determinant for lentiviral vector nuclear import and gene transduction of human hematopoietic stem cells. *Blood*. 2000;96:4103–4110.

70. Donello JE, Loeb JE, Hope TJ. Woodchuck hepatitis virus contains a tripartite posttranscriptional regulatory element. *J Virol*. 1998;72:5085–5092.

71. Zufferey R, Donello JE, Trono D, Hope TJ. Woodchuck hepatitis virus posttranscriptional regulatory element enhances expression of transgenes delivered by retroviral vectors. *J Virol*. 1999;73:2886–2892.

72. Themis M, Waddington SN, Schmidt M, et al. Oncogenesis following delivery of a nonprimate lentiviral gene therapy vector to fetal and neonatal mice. *Mol Ther.* 2005;12:763–771.

73. Brun S, Faucon-Biguet N, Mallet J. Optimization of transgene expression at the posttranscriptional level in neural cells: implications for gene therapy. *Mol Ther.* 2003;7:782–789.

74. Pfeifer A, Ikawa M, Dayn Y, Verma IM. Transgenesis by lentiviral vectors: lack of gene silencing in mammalian embryonic stem cells and preimplantation embryos. *Proc Natl Acad Sci U S A.* 2002;99:2140–2145.

75. Lois C, Hong EJ, Pease S, Brown EJ, Baltimore D. Germline transmission and tissue-specific expression of transgenes delivered by lentiviral vectors. *Science.* 2002;295:868–872.

76. Ellis J. Silencing and variegation of gammaretrovirus and lentivirus vectors. *Hum Gene Ther.* 2005;16:1241–1246.

77. Burgess-Beusse B, Farrell C, Gaszner M, et al. The insulation of genes from external enhancers and silencing chromatin. *Proc Natl Acad Sci U S A.* 2002;99:16433–16437.

78. West AG, Huang S, Gaszner M, Litt MD, Felsenfeld G. Recruitment of histone modifications by USF proteins at a vertebrate barrier element. *Mol Cell.* 2004;16:453–463.

79. Ramezani A, Hawley TS, Hawley RG. Performance- and safety-enhanced lentiviral vectors containing the human interferon-β scaffold attachment region and the chicken β-globin insulator. *Blood.* 2003;101:4717–4724.

80. Cronin J, Zhang XY, Reiser J. Altering the tropism of lentiviral vectors through pseudotyping. *Curr Gene Ther.* 2005;5:387–398.

81. Burns JC, Friedmann T, Driever W, Burrascano M, Yee J. Vesicular stomatitis virus G glycoprotein pseudotyped retroviral vectors: concentration to very high titer and efficient gene transfer into mammalian and nonmammalian cells. *Proc Natl Acad Sci U S A.* 1993;90:8033–8037.

82. Slepushkin V, Chang N, Cohen R, et al. Large-scale purification of a lentiviral vecor by size exclusion chromatography or mustang Q ion exchange capsule. *Bioprocess J.* 2003;2:89–95.

83. Fe Medina M, Kobinger GP, Rux J, et al. Lentiviral vectors pseudotyped with minimal filovirus envelopes increased gene transfer in murine lung. *Mol Ther.* 2003;8:777–789.

84. Griesenbach U, Mitomo K, Inoue M, et al. Lentivirus pseudotyped with envelope proteins F and HN from Sendai virus transduce airway epithelium efficiently and persistently [abstract]. *Mol Ther.* 2006;13:S139–S140.

85. MacKenzie TC, Kobinger GP, Kootstra NA, et al. Efficient transduction of liver and muscle after in utero injection of lentiviral vectors with different pseudotypes. *Mol Ther.* 2002;6:349–358.

86. Mazarakis ND, Azzouz M, Rohll JB, et al. Rabies virus glycoprotein pseudotyping of lentiviral vectors enables retrograde axonal transport and access to the nervous system after peripheral delivery. *Hum Mol Genet.* 2001;10:2109–2121.

87. Wong LF, Azzouz M, Walmsley LE, et al. Transduction patterns of pseudotyped lentiviral vectors in the nervous system. *Mol Ther.* 2004;9:101–111.

88. Brown B, Venneri MA, Zingale A, Sergi LS, & Naldini L. Endogenous microRNA regulation suppresses transgene expression in hematopoietic lineages and enables stable gene transfer [abstract]. *Mol Ther.* 2006;13:S311.

89. Manilla P, Rebello T, Afable C, et al. Regulatory considerations for novel gene therapy products: a review of the process leading to the first clinical lentiviral vector. *Hum Gene Ther.* 2005;16:17–25.

90. Humeau LM, Binder GK, Lu X, et al. Efficient lentiviral vector-mediated control of HIV-1 replication in CD4 lymphocytes from diverse HIV+ infected patients grouped according to CD4 count and viral load. *Mol Ther.* 2004;9:902–913.

91. Galla M, Will E, Kraunus J, Chen L, Baum C. Retroviral pseudotransduction for targeted cell manipulation. *Mol Cell.* 2004;16:309–315.

92. Saenz DT, Loewen N, Peretz M, et al. Unintegrated lentivirus DNA persistence and accessibility to expression in nondividing cells: analysis with class I integrase mutants. *J Virol.* 2004;78:2906–2920.

93. Urnov FD, Miller JC, Lee YL, et al. Highly efficient endogenous human gene correction using designed zinc-finger nucleases. *Nature.* 2005;435:646–651.

94. Ralph GS, Binley K, Wong LF, Azzouz M, Mazarakis ND. Gene therapy for neurodegenerative and ocular diseases using lentiviral vectors. *Clin Sci.* 2006;110:37–46.

95. Dowd E, Monville C, Torres EM, et al. Lentivector-mediated delivery of GDNF protects complex motor functions relevant to human Parkinsonism in a rat lesion model. *Eur J Neurosci.* 2005;22:2587–2595.

96. Azzouz M, Le T, Ralph GS, et al. Lentivector-mediated SMN replacement in a mouse model of spinal muscular atrophy. *J Clin Invest.* 2004;114:1726–1731.

97. Azzouz M, Ralph GS, Storkebaum E, et al. VEGF delivery with retrogradely transported lentivector prolongs survival in a mouse ALS model. *Nature.* 2004;429:413–417.

98. Cheng L, Chaidhawangul S, Wong-Staal F, et al. Human immunodeficiency virus type 2 (HIV-2) vector-mediated in vivo gene transfer into adult rabbit retina. *Curr Eye Res.* 2002;24:196–201.

99. Cheng L, Toyoguchi M, Looney DJ, et al. Efficient gene transfer to retinal pigment epithelium cells with long-term expression [abstract]. *Retina.* 2006;25:193–201.

100. Balaggan KS, Binley K, Esapa M, et al. EIAV vector-mediated delivery of endostatin or angiostatin inhibits angiogenesis and vascular hyperpermeability in experimental CNV. *Gene Ther.* 2006;13:1153–1165.

101. Bainbridge JWB, Stephens C, Parsley K, et al. In vivo gene transfer to the mouse eye using an HIV–based lentiviral vector; efficient long-term transduction of corneal endothelium and retinal pigment epithelium. *Gene Ther.* 2001;8:1665–1668.

102. Takahashi K, Saishin Y, Saishin Y, et al. Intraocular expression of endostatin reduces VEGF-induced retinal vascular permeability, neovascularization, and retinal detachment. *FASEB J.* 2003; 02-0824fje.

103. Tschernutter M, Schlichtenbrede FC, Howe S, et al. Long-term preservation of retinal function in the RCS rat model of retinitis pigmentosa following lentivirus-mediated gene therapy. *Gene Ther.* 2005;12:694–701.

104. Kang Y, Xie L, Tran DT, et al. Persistent expression of factor VIII in vivo following nonprimate lentiviral gene transfer. *Blood.* 2005;106:1552–1558.

105. Hanawa H, Hargrove PW, Kepes S, et al. Extended β-globin locus control region elements promote consistent therapeutic expression of a γ-globin lentiviral vector in murine β-thalassemia. *Blood*. 2004;104:2281–2290.

106. Gregory LG, Waddington SN, Holder MV, et al. Highly efficient EIAV-mediated in utero gene transfer and expression in the major muscle groups affected by Duchenne muscular dystrophy. *Gene Ther*. 2004;11:1117–1125.

107. Sadelain M, Riviere I, Brentjens R. Targeting tumours with genetically enhanced T lymphocytes. *Nat Rev Cancer*. 2003;3:35–45.

108. Press O, Wang J, Lindgren CG, et al. Preliminary results of a pilot phase I clinical trial of adoptive immunotherapy for B cell lymphoma using CD8+ T cells genetically modified to express a chimeric T cell receptor recognizing CD20. [abstract]. *Mol Ther*. 2006;13:S22–S23.

109. Breckpot K, Dullaers M, Bonehill A, et al. Lentivirally transduced dendritic cells as a tool for cancer immunotherapy. *J Gene Med*. 2003;5:654–667.

110. He Y, Zhang J, Mi Z, Robbins P, Falo LD Jr. Immunization with lentiviral vector–transduced dendritic cells induces strong and long-lasting T cell responses and therapeutic immunity. *J Immunol*. 2005;174:3808–3817.

111. Pellinen R, Hakkarainen T, Wahlfors T, et al. Cancer cells as targets for lentivirus-mediated gene transfer and gene therapy [abstract]. *Intl J Oncol*. 2006;25: 1753–1762.

112. Jahner D, Stuhlmann H, Stewart CL, et al. Denovo methylation and expression of retroviral genomes during mouse embryogenesis. *Nature*. 1982;298:623–628.

113. Hamra FK, Gatlin J, Chapman KM, et al. Production of transgenic rats by lentiviral transduction of male germ-line stem cells. *Proc Natl Acad Sci U S A*. 2002;99:14931–14936.

114. Hofmann A, Kessler B, Ewerling S, et al. Efficient transgenesis in farm animals by lentiviral vectors. *EMBO Rep*. 2003;4:1054–1060.

115. Hofmann A, Zakhartchenko V, Weppert M, et al. Generation of transgenic cattle by lentiviral gene transfer into oocytes. *Biol Reprod*. 2004;71:405–409.

116. Wolfgang MJ, Eisele SG, Browne MA, et al. Rhesus monkey placental transgene expression after lentiviral gene transfer into preimplantation embryos. *Proc Natl Acad Sci U S A*. 2001;98:10728–10732.

117. Ikawa M, Tanaka N, Kao WWY, Verma IM. Generation of transgenic mice using lentiviral vectors: a novel preclinical assessment of lentiviral vectors for gene therapy. *Mol Ther*. 2003;8:666–673.

118. Zhang B, Metharom P, Jullie H, et al. The significance of controlled conditions in lentiviral vector titration and in the use of multiplicity of infection (MOI) for predicting gene transfer events. *Genet Vaccines Ther*. 2004;2:6.

119. Abbas-Terki T, Blanco-Bose W, Deglon N, Pralong W, Aebischer P. Lentiviral-mediated RNA interference. *Hum Gene Ther*. 2002;13:2197–2201.

120. Tiscornia G, Tergaonkar V, Galimi F, Verma IM. From the cover: CRE recombinase-inducible RNA interference mediated by lentiviral vectors. *Proc Natl Acad Sci U S A*. 2004;101:7347–7351.

121. Mangeot PE, Cosset FL, Colas P, Mikaelian I. A universal transgene silencing method based on RNA interference. *Nucl Acids Res*. 2004;32:e102.

122. Klages N, Zufferey R, Trono D. A stable system for the high-titer production of multiply attenuated lentiviral vectors. *Mol Ther*. 2000;2:170–176.

123. Ni YJ, Sun SS, Oparaocha T, et al. Generation of a packaging cell line for pro-longed large-scale production of high-titer HIV-1-based lentiviral vector. *J Gene Med.* 2005;7:818–834.

124. Kustikova O, Fehse B, Modlich U, et al. Clonal dominance of hematopoietic stem cells triggered by retroviral gene marking. *Science.* 2005;308:1171–1174.

125. Schambach A, Bohne J, Baum C, et al. Woodchuck hepatitis virus posttranscrip-tional regulatory element deleted from X protein and promoter sequences enhances retroviral vector titer and expression. *Gene Ther.* 2006;13:641–645.

126. Montini E, Cesana D, Schmidt M, et al., Hematopoietic stem cell gene transfer in a tumor-prone mouse model uncovers low genotoxicity of lentiviral vector integration. *Nat Biotechnol.* 2006;24:687–696.

127. Press O, Wang J, Lindgren CG, et al. Preliminary results of a pilot phase I clinical trial of adoptive immunotherapy for B cell lymphoma using CD8+T cells geneti-cally modified to express a chimeric T cell receptor recognizing CD20. *Mol Ther.* 2006;13(S1);S22–S23.

128. Lamers CIIJ, Sleijfer S, Vulto AG, et al. Treatment of metastatic renal cell carcinoma with autologous T-lymphocytes genetically retargeted agains carbonic anhydrase IX: first clinical experience. *J Clin Oncol.* 2006;24(13):e20–e22.

4 Adenoviral Vectors: History and Perspective

DOUGLAS J. JOLLY
Advantagene, Inc., Encinitas, California

ESTUARDO AGUILAR-CORDOVA and LAURA K. AGUILAR
Advantagene, Inc., Waban, Massachusetts

Adenoviruses have been characterized extensively and make attractive vectors for gene transfer because of their relatively benign clinical risk, their ease of manipulation and production, the availability of physical and characterization standards, their ability to transduce dividing and quiescent cells, and their broad range of target tissues. However, they are not ideal vectors for all indications. Current data indicate that adenoviral vectors are most applicable for indications such as cancer and vaccines, where local delivery and short-term expression are desired.

ADENOVIRUS BACKGROUND

Adenoviruses are relatively well-characterized and well-understood infectious human agents. Some strains have served as critical tools for understanding DNA replication, RNA processing, and viral life cycles. Adenoviruses were first isolated in 1953 from tonsils and adenoidal tissue of children: thus the name [1]. They form their own family, Adenoviridae [2], characterized by having a linear double-stranded DNA genome encapsidated in an icosohedral protein shell measuring 70 to 90 nm in diameter. Adenovirus virions contain 13% DNA and 87% protein, with a genome approximately 36 kb in length (Figure 4.1). Human adenoviruses belong to the genus *Mastadenovirus*, which is composed of six subgenera (groups A, B, C, D, E, and F) with more than 50 serotypes. As discussed below, a combination of properties have made vectors based on adenoviruses popular for gene transfer applications.

Adenoviruses are highly prevalent in human populations, with relatively benign consequences. They are primarily an etiologic agent of respiratory infections with coldlike symptoms. Adenoviruses can also infect other tissues, such as eyes,

Concepts in Genetic Medicine, Edited by Boro Dropulic and Barrie Carter
Copyright © 2008 John Wiley & Sons, Inc.

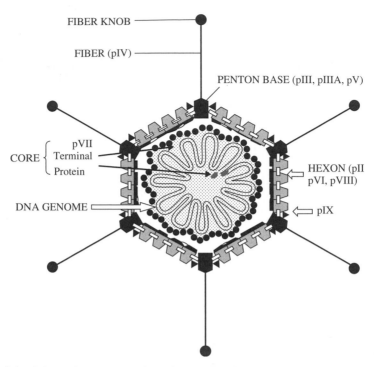

Figure 4.1   Schematic representation of an adenoviral virion. The Ad capsid consists of 252 subunits called capsomeres, 240 hexon proteins and 12 penton bases. On each of 12 capsid verties there is a penton base surrounded by 5 hexons. Fibers (trimers of pIV) protrude from the penton base located at each of the vertices of the capsid. The fiber contains three domains: an N-terminus that noncovalently binds fiber to penton base, a C-terminus which forms a globular "knob" which is responsible for binding to a receptor and a rod-like shaft whose length depends on virus serotype. Other capsid proteins, such as pIX, are thought to be involved in the cementing of the virion structure. Inside the capsid the core is composed of the terminal protein, which is covalently linked to the double-stranded DNA genome, and the basic polypeptides pV, pVII, and pX (also known as μ). Polypeptide pVII is the major core protein that binds the viral genome to form a compact nucleoprotein complex. (Modified with permission from http://www.micro.msb.le.ac.uk/3035/Adenoviruses.html.)

gastrointestinal and urinary tracts, brain, heart, kidney, and liver, but generally pose minor health risks. In normal individuals, most infections are self-limiting without significant clinical sequelae. However, immunocompromised persons may suffer more severe conditions, often associated with uncommon variants, such as group B, serotype 35 [3]. In addition, adenoviral DNA is not usually incorporated into host cell chromosomes, minimizing concerns about insertional mutagenesis or potential germ line effects. The natural clinical mildness of adenoviruses, which is probably related to their immunogenicity, has contributed to their popularity as gene transfer vectors. However, because of their immunogenicity, these viruses are not generally useful as vectors for applications that require long-term expression, such as genetic diseases.

ADENOVIRUSES AND THE IMMUNE SYSTEM

Adenoviral immunogenicity comes from the antigens contained in the inoculated particles as well as from the antigens expressed from the viral genome. Host immune systems have evolved to recognize viral particles as foreign and dangerous. The initial recognition is innate and happens without the adaptive branch of the immune system. It results in the release of danger signals, including heat shock proteins, cytokines, and chemokines, with the consequent recruitment of neutrophils, natural killer (NK) cells, and maturation of antigen presenting cells (APCs) [4,5]. This, in turn, precipitates death of the infected or transduced cells. The local APCs scavenge and present viral antigens in the context of class I and class II major histocompatibility complexes (MHCs), leading to B- and T-cell-mediated antiviral adaptive immune responses [6].

For gene transfer, a key consideration with respect to the immune reaction to the virus or vector is the potential for readministration. It is clear that activation of the innate immune system predisposes the induction of the acquired immune response [7] and around 80% of people in the United States and Europe test seropositive for Ad5 [8]. Yet, although most of us have been exposed to adenoviruses, symptomatic reinfections occur. This is probably due to the variability in levels of neutralizing antibodies [9,10]. However, it is also clear that preexisting humoral immunity makes the intravascular vector administration route problematic [11]. In addition, the administered capsid proteins by themselves, without viral protein synthesis, are capable of inducing both humoral responses [12] and cytotoxic T-cell responses that can lead to elimination of transduced cells [13]. This means that intravascular administration of vector to seropositive individuals or readministration probably need to be either carefully timed, given in conjunction with transient immune suppression [14], or given with vectors to which there is no immunity, such as vectors derived from other human or animal strains of adenovirus [15]. However, local intratumoral readministration has been effective in animal models and human clinical trials [16–18]. Thus, the immunological consequences of adenoviruses pose significant drawbacks for their use in long-term expression or systemic delivery applications, but are either inconsequential or positive for their use as vectors for cancer and possibly vaccine indications.

MOLECULAR UNDERSTANDING OF THE GENOME AND VIRAL LIFE CYCLE

A basic understanding of the biology of adenovirus is critical to a discussion of adenoviral vectors. Although a thorough examination of this point is beyond the scope of this chapter, a brief overview is given below. For readers wishing more detail, there are many good reviews of the viral life cycle that describe in detail the sequence of cellular and molecular events after viral infection [2,19,20].

Viral Attachment and Entry

The conventional receptor binding structure is the knob at the end of the fiber protein that sticks out from the capsid (Figure 4.1). The primary receptor for most adenoviruses (except those from group B) is the coxsackie–adenovirus receptor (CAR). Recent data demonstrate that other molecules, including MHC class I and heparin sulfate glycosaminoglycans, can also serve as receptors for adenoviruses [21,22]. CD46, a ubiquitously expressed complement regulatory protein, serves as a receptor for group B adenoviruses [23]. After this initial attachment, the RGD peptide on the penton base interacts with integrins on the cell surface, triggering virus internalization by clathrin-dependent, receptor-mediated endocytosis. The acidic environment of the endosome induces the escape of virions into the cytoplasm, although this process is not well understood. Subsequently, dynein mediates trafficking of virions along microtubules in the cytoplasm, which then enter the nucleus through the nuclear pore complex and release viral DNA in the process. This relatively simple story does not necessarily reflect what happens in vivo with vectors. For example, in animal models, most vector delivered to the bloodstream ends up in the liver by a CAR independent mechanism [24].

Adenoviral Genome Transcription and Replication

Like that of many viruses, the adenoviral genome is transcribed from both chains, divided by temporal expression, either early, before virus replication, or late, following virus replication. Coding sequences are flanked by two inverted terminal repeats (ITRs), situated at each end of the linear genome (Figure 4.2). The genome is naturally found in the nucleus of infected cells as a circular episome held together by the interaction of proteins covalently linked to each of the $5'$ ends of the linear genome. First to be transcribed is the immediate early (*E1A*) gene, which leads to transcription of the other early genes (*E1B, E2A, E2B, E3, E4*). These regulate viral and cellular gene transcription, translation, and transport, to maximize virus yields. For example, *E1A* and *E1B*, in addition to transcriptional regulation, also inhibit cellular Rb- and p53-mediated apoptotic pathways, respectively; *E2* encodes DNA polymerase, preterminal protein, and single-stranded DNA binding protein involved in replication of the viral genome; the *E3* gp19 interacts with class I MHC molecules, causing their retention in the endoplasmic reticulum and thus protecting infected cells from quick immune clearance by inhibiting the presentation of viral epitopes on the cell surface; and *E4* encodes proteins influencing cell cycle control and transformation. Viral DNA synthesis triggers initiation of late gene expression. Unlike early genes, which are expressed from six promoters, most late gene expression starts from the major late promoter (MLP), resulting in a very large primary transcript that is processed to five families (L1 through L5) of mRNA molecules by using five different polyadenylation signals and alternative splice sites (Figure 4.2) [25].

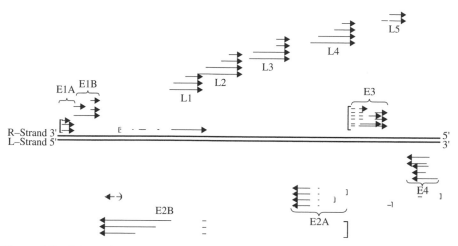

Figure 4.2 Schematic representation of the AdV-5 genome. Arrows indicate the location and orientation of transcribed genes and the various polypeptides derived from them. The ITR sequences and the packaging domain are located at both ends of the genome. The genes expressed early during infection are designated E1A and E1B, E2A and E2B, E3 and E4. For the most part they encode proteins involved in AdV and host gene regulation and DNA replication. The late gene products (L1–L5) are encoded in a very long pre-mRNA transcript from the major late promoter (MLP). These transcript encodes most of the structural components by alternative splicing and differential polyadenylation. (Used with permission from http://www-micro.msb.le.ac.uk/3035/Adenoviruses.html.)

These encode the viral structural proteins, including hexon, penton base, fiber, pIIIa, pV, pVI, pVII, pVIII, and μ, which together with pIX and the viral genome, make up an infections particle (Figure 4.1). A single infected cell can produce over 10^5 new particles in 24 to 48 hours.

PROPERTIES OF ADENOVIRAL VECTORS THAT HAVE ATTRACTED WIDESPREAD USE

Although different vector systems have always been recognized as having different sets of strengths and weaknesses, adenoviral vectors are widely used (see Table 4.1 and Figure 4.3). It seems worth looking at possible reasons for the wide use of adenoviral vectors and to ask how this knowledge might guide further development.

There seem to be several factors explaining why adenoviral-based vectors are used so commonly and increasingly successfully. These include a well-developed molecular understanding of the genome and viral life cycle, including the ability to work with viral genomes as plasmids, facilitating molecular manipulations. Another advantage is the high transgene capacity, with the ability to package up to 105% of the total genome size (38 kb) with the only required adenovirus

TABLE 4.1 Current Publicly Acknowledged Pharmaceutical and Biotechnology Company Programs Using Adenoviral Vectors

Company	Vector[a]	Gene(s)[b]	Target	Product Name[e]	Clinical Stage
Merck & Co., West Point, PA /HIV VTN/NIH	Ad5 G1	HIV-1 gag-pol-nef	AIDS vaccine[c]	N.A.	3000 patients, phase II [94] NCT00095576
Eli Lilly, Indianpolis, IN	Ad5 G1	PlGF, binds VEGF receptor	Coronary or peripheral artery disease	N.A.	Preclinical [95]
Schering Plough, Kenilworth, NJ	Ad5 G1	Alpha interferon	Bladder cancer	N.A.[f]	Preclinical [96]
Biogen-Idec, Boston, MA	Ad5 G1	Beta interferon	Colorectal cancer	N.A.	Phase I
Genzyme, Cambridge, MA	Ad5 G1	HIF-1α	Heart bypass; peripheral artery disease	N.A.	In phases I and II
Shenzen SiBiono Genetech, Shenzen, China	Ad5 G1	p53 tumor suppressor	Head and neck cancer	Gendicine[g]	Market in China [91,92]
Berlex, Seattle, WA	Ad5 G1	FGF-4	Myocardial ischemia	AGT-MI[h]	Phase II complete [97]
Barr Labs, VA	Ad 4,7 (rep.)	None	Oral vaccine for U.S. army	N.A.	In phases II and III
Introgen, TX	Ad5 G1	p53 tumor suppressor	Head and neck cancer	Advexin[g]	In two phase III trials
GenVec, MD	Ad5 G2	PEDF	Wet macular degeneration	N.A.	Phase I
		Tumor necrosis factor-α	Pancreatic cancer	TNFerade	Phase II [98]
		VEGF-121	Coronary artery disease	BIOBYPASS	Phase IIB

Company	Vector[a]	Gene[b]	Indication	Product	Phase
Cell Genesys, CA	Ad 5 (rep.)	GM-CSF	Bladder cancer	CG0070	Phase I
		Prostate specific antigen promoter	Prostate cancer	CG7870	Phases I and II
Transgene SA, France	Ad5 G1	Gamma-interferon	Cutaneous T-cell lymphoma	N.A.	In phase II
Ark Therapeutics, UK	Ad5 G1	Herpes thymidine kinase	Malignant glioma	Cerepro[i]	Phase III
Advantagene, MA	Ad5 G1	Herpes thymidine kinase	Prostate cancer	ProstAtak	Phase II
			Glioma	GliAtak	Phase IB
Shanghai Sunway Biotech, China	Ad 5 (rep.)	None	Head and neck, NSCLC[d], osteosarcoma	H101[j] (Onyx-015)	Market in China [60]
Tissue Repair Company, San Diego, CA[k]	Ad5 G1	PDGF-β	Diabetic ulcers	N.A.	Phase I

Source: Information is from scientific articles where referenced, conference presentations, company Web sites, and press releases.

[a] Ad5 G1, first-generation adenoviral vector based on adenovirus 5; Ad5 G2, second-generation adenoviral vector based on adenovirus 5; Ad5 (rep.), replicating adenovirus derived from adenovirus 5.

[b] PIGF, placental growth factor; VEGF, vascular endothelial growth factor; HIF, hypoxia inducible factor; FGF, fibroblast growth factor; PEDF, pigmented epithelium derived growth factor; GM-CSF, granulocyte macrophage colony stimulating factor; PDGF, platelet derived growth factor.

[c] Merck vaccine studies show that preexisting immunity may have no significant effect at moderate (2×10^{10} vector particle) doses.

[d] NSCLC, non-small cell lung cancer.

[e] N.A., not available.

[f] This product was developed at Canji, the Schering site in San Diego that Schering has closed. A clinical trial is pending.

[g] The Shenzen Bio product appears to be very similar to the Introgen product.

[h] Currently being developed by Cardium Therapeutics in San Diego.

[i] Ark Therapeutics has filed an MAA (marketing authority application) in Europe with the European Medicines Agency for Cerepro.

[j] Sunway licensed this product (then Onyx-015) from Onyx Pharmaceuticals (Emeryville, CA) in January 2005 and altered it slightly, calling the new agent H101; Onyx took it as far as phase II in the United States.

[k] Tissue Repair Company has been acquired by Cardium Therapeutics.

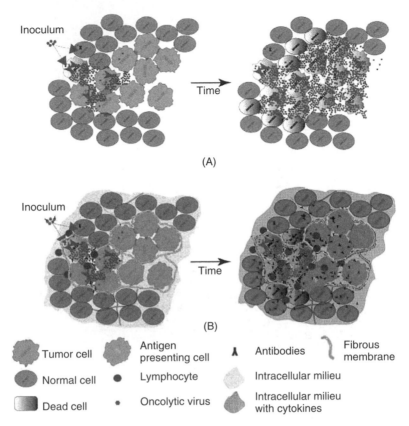

Figure 4.3 In vivo barriers to oncolytic virus theory and models. (A) The theory behind the system and in vitro model for oncolytic viruses. A virus is engineered to preferentially replicate in tumor cells by targeted infection to tumor cell receptors or by tissue-specific promoters. The virus finds tumor cells, replicates and lyses, releasing thousands more virions that can repeat the cycle until all the tumor cells are exhausted. Normal cells are spared since infection of normal cells is a dead end for the virus. (B) Added in vivo complexities. Host immune and in vivo microenvironment conditions can hinder virus cytopathic effects. These effects include: tumor connective or fibrotic tissue preventing free-flow of the produced viruses; host innate immunity protection against the viral infection; existing or acquired cellular and antibody response to the virus infection, potentially compromising follow-up treatments; and tumor necrosis preventing viral spread. These in vivo conditions can slow or abolish the response to an oncolytic virus

sequences being the small packaging signal and ITR (<300 bp), facilitating manipulations to decrease the incidence of replication-competent recombinants and allowing transduction of relatively large portions of DNA. Additional benefits are the relatively simple and reliable manufacturing methods, high expression in a variety of replicating and nonreplicating tissues, known toxicity profile, understanding of the effect of the route of administration on vector genome uptake, and finally, an increasing understanding of the interaction of the vectors with the immune system.

RELATIVELY SIMPLE AND RELIABLE MANUFACTURING METHODS

A major advantage to the clinical application of adenoviral vectors has been that they are relatively straightforward to manufacture and characterize. A well-characterized standard [26] for infectious and vector particle measurements was developed by an international academic, regulatory, and industry consortium (available from ATCC catalog no. VR-1516). Clinical vector manufacturing has been performed at many of the companies listed in Table 4.1, academic institutions, and contract manufacturers. With yields of up to $1 \times 10^{11}/1 \times 10^6$ cells, thousands of patient doses can be produced with relatively small-scale processes. The yield is dependent on the specific construct. Typically, around 10^{15} vector particles (vp) can be generated from about 10 L. Vector lots can be produced in serum-free medium and in suspension [27], so that scale-up, if necessary, is relatively straightforward. With clinical doses in the range of 10^{10} to 10^{12} vp, a 10 L scale can make 1000 to 100,000 doses. The particles are harvested and can be processed by column chromatography or high-performance liquid chromatography and concentrated to give final formulated vector at up to 10^{13} vp/mL, although it is usually advisable to keep it below 10^{12} vp/mL to avoid potential particle precipitation. A good deal of effort has gone into standardizing vector titer measurements, and this is now routinely given as vp/mL. The vector particles are quite stable and there are formulations where less than 10% loss of activity has been observed over 24 months at $4°C$ [28]. There are many publications describing methods of fermentation, purification, and formulation [29,30].

EVOLUTION OF ADENOVIRAL VECTORS

The first-generation clinical vectors were based on deletions of the *E1* region to make the vectors replication deficient and to add capacity, up to 5 kb, for the transgene expression cassette. These vectors also usually have *E3* deletions, which are inconsequential for in vitro growth, for an added 3 kb of transgene capacity. The canonical cell line for vector manufacture has been the human embryonic kidney–derived 293 cell line. This cell line has 11% of the left end of the adenoviral genome (nucleotides 1 through 4344) and thus significant sequence overlap with conventional vectors. Hence, homologous recombination between the vector and the adenoviral sequences in the cell can generate replication-competent adenovirus (RCA) recombinants during the amplification process. The U.S. Food and Drug Administration currently requires less than one RCA per 3×10^{10} vector particles. Other cell lines, such as PER.C6 [31] and SL003 [32], have been designed to avoid the overlap and minimize RCA risk, but 293 remains commonly used to prepare clinical vectors.

During the first decade of adenoviral vector use, many groups spent significant effort in developing vector systems with further deletions in the *E2* or *E4* regions (second-generation vectors) and matching complementing cell lines [33] in an effort to decrease immunogenicity and potential toxicity from first-generation vectors. This was complicated by the toxicity of early viral genes to producer cells. Propagation of vector constructs deleted in multiple regions is less likely to generate RCAs but also results in lower yields. However, it was not production difficulties that limited use of these multiply-deleted vectors, but rather, the limited effect on immunogenicity from the multiple deletions that led to the general loss of enthusiasm for using adenoviral vectors for applications requiring low immunogenicity and long-term expression [34–36]. Long-term expression and added safety from multiple deleted adenoviral vectors were not achieved.

However, recent data suggest that long-term expression may be possible with vectors with all viral genes removed. These vectors, devoid of all viral genes, have a cloning capacity for >37 kb and reduced immunogenic potential, allowing for a longer expression of the transgene [37,38]. Although these vectors would still elicit the immune reaction to the inoculated virions, early data suggest a potential for long-term expression. However, until recently, these vectors, variously referred to as "gutless," "helper dependent," or "high capacity," have been difficult to produce in high enough quantities, and without significant helper contamination, for widespread clinical analysis. Recent advances should help overcome these hurdles [39].

In more recent years, efforts for newer generations of adenoviral vectors switched from multiple deletions to focus on targeting. The rationale has been to expand potentially limiting tropisms, to address potential toxicity from overexpression in undesired tissues and as a potential way to improve the probability of systemic delivery. There are two principal approaches to adenoviral targeting: engineering the virion to transduce desired cells, or using gene regulation to limit transgene expression to specific tissues. The former can be accomplished by genetic modifications of the fiber-knob component or by covalently binding a "bridging" molecule to the virion [40–47]. The possibilities for modifications are endless, from de novo peptide additions, hybrid fiber-knob combinations with other human and nonhuman adenoviruses, common receptor ligands, RGD motifs, and so on, or any combination thereof. For example, Borovjagin et al. [48] used a strategy they called *complex mosaicism*, which is a combination of an RGD-4 C peptide in the HI-loop at the carboxy terminus, or both locales of the Ad3 knob in the context of Ad5/3 vector. This vector was targeted simultaneously to integrins and Ad3 receptors. In their in vitro assay with bladder cancer cell lines, it showed up to a 55-fold increase in gene transfer. Capsid modifications have yielded other in vitro examples of improved transduction of Ad5- or Ad2-resistant targets [49]; however, there are also potential concomitant decreases in gene expression [50]. The *bridging molecule* approach has the potential advantage of an innumerable number of antibodies and ligands that can be used to form bispecific (adenovirus and target), bridging molecules. However, a huge disadvantage is that since each bispecific molecule and virion combination may have unique efficacy, distribution, and toxicity characteristics, each would have to be characterized individually and as a component of a complex biological drug for clinical use, with the requisite preclinical and clinical data. The advantage of Ad35 (group B) fiber vectors in transducing hematopoietic derived cells in vitro has been demonstrated convincingly; however, additional in vivo clinical advantages for tropism-retargeted vectors remains to be seen. Another use for retargeted or distinct serotype vectors is to bypass antivector memory immune responses that could overwhelm antitransgene responses in vaccine applications. Promising preclinical results with canine and nonhuman primate adenoviruses have been reported [15,51,52].

Transcriptional targeting is accomplished by placing the gene of interest under the control of a tissue- or tumor-specific promoter. This could be particularly important for applications where long-term gene expression may be desired, where even small levels of expression in a nontargeted cell could significantly impact effectiveness or toxicity, or when large-scale transduction of nontarget cells with a potentially deleterious gene is expected. One of the earliest examples in cancer was use of the carcinoembryonic antigen promoter (CEA) to drive expression of the herpes simplex thymidine kinase gene in a human lung cancer cell line [53]. Since then many similar examples with different promoters have been reported [54,55]. Transcriptional targeting has shown potential efficacy with theoretical added safety; however, clinical benefits have not yet been demonstrated.

Another area of vector development that has received significant effort in recent years is conditionally replicating adenoviruses (CRAds). The basis for CRAds is that most of the cancers have mutations in p53 or Rb genes. The original designs did not carry a transgene but rather, relied on the cytotoxic effects of the viruses. The prototype for this approach was Onyx-015 (originally known as dl1520) [56]. This virus has a mutant E1B protein that does not bind to p53. In the absence of this binding, the infected cell can undergo p53-mediated apoptosis in response to the viral infection and does not enter the S phase of mitosis, necessary for virus replication. However, since many tumors have nonfunctional mutated p53s, Onyx-015 would be able to replicate on those cells. Later results showed the system was much more complex and that Onyx-015 could also replicate in p53-normal cells [57]. Trials with this vector showed clinical safety of a replication-competent agent. A trial in head and neck tumors, where direct injection of Onyx-015 into tumors was combined with classical chemotherapy, led to tumor regression in 63% of treated patients, 27% with complete responses and 36% with regressions of up to 50% in tumor volume [58]. Six months after treatment, there was no evidence of new tumors or regrowth of treated ones. In contrast, Onyx-015 showed no durable responses in treatment of metastases [59]. In November 2005, a slightly modified version of Onyx-015, H101 from Shanghai Sunway Biotech, received market approval in China as a treatment for head and neck cancer [60]. Details of supporting clinical studies are not yet available.

The early CRAds were followed by many designed constructs that placed early viral genes under control of tissue- or cancer-specific promoters such as cyclo-oxygenase, prostate-specific antigen, telomerase, and many others [61–67]. These were followed by more elaborate and efficient strategies to improve selectivity and efficacy of replication [68–70] (see also http://www.oncolyticvirus.org/). The success of the *oncolytic virus* concept is contingent on two variables: (1) tumor cell specificity and (2) viral cytopathicity. Specificity confers safety, and this has mostly been achieved. The extent of viral cytopathicity confers treatment efficacy. This requires overcoming natural barriers to infection from the host, such as antibodies, cytokines, and cellular immunity, in addition to physical barriers to viral spread, such as connective tissue and tumor matrix, all of which may limit the spread of virus. Although CRAds have in vitro cytopathicities comparable to those of wild-type viruses, in vivo issues still pose large barriers that may be difficult to overcome, especially for systemic dissemination (Figure 4.3) [71]. However, even with limited replication capacity, CRAds may provide vectors with in vivo transgene amplification potential. Many of the CRAd strategies discussed above are now being used as "armed" CRAds for delivery of transgenes [72]. Two such constructs, one with an HSV-tk/CD fusion gene and one with a GM-CSF cytokine gene, have entered clinical trials for prostate and bladder cancer, respectively [73,74].

TOXICITY PROFILE OF ADENOVIRAL VECTORS IN RELATION TO DOSE AND ROUTE OF DELIVERY

There is a wealth of data about toxicity in animals and humans, in terms of both dose and mechanism of action [75] based on the long history of the wild-type virus and knowledge of its pathology, its use as a vaccine, the extensive general use of this vector type, and the after-effects of the highly publicized fatal event in an adenoviral vector trial. These data allow for more informed decisions in planning for safe and efficacious clinical trials. It contrasts with most other vector systems, where, in general, it has not been possible to make sufficient vector to administer and observe acute toxicities. The potential toxicity of intravascular delivery of adenoviral vectors was highlighted by the death of a patient in 1999 in a clinical trial where a large dose of vector was delivered into the hepatic artery of a patient with partial ornithine transcarbamylase (OTC) deficiency, who had concurrent liver dysfunction [76]. This unfortunate event prompted a thorough analysis of adenoviral trials across the board and development of a well-characterized adenovirus standard to calibrate measurements from individual laboratories [75,77,78]. The investigators attributed the toxicity to "a systemic, Ad vector-induced shock syndrome, due to a cytokine cascade that led to disseminated intravascular coagulation, acute respiratory distress, and multi-organ failure" and concluded that "the high dose of Ad vector, delivered by infusion directly to the liver, quickly saturated available receptors for the vector . . . then spilled into the circulatory and other organ systems, including the bone marrow, thus inducing the systemic immune response." This appears broadly correct, but more information on the likely mechanisms of adenoviral overdosing is now available.

Toxicity in the OTC trial appeared at a dose of 6×10^{11} vp/kg (approximately 3×10^{13} total vp), in a patient with compromised liver function. Subsequent studies in several types of animal models, including nonhuman primates, suggested that for healthy animals, toxicity appeared above about 0.5 to 1×10^{12} vp/kg [75], a range similar to that seen in the human trial. There appear to be two kinds of toxicity that are potentially linked. The first and most discussed is the induction of a disseminated intravascular coagulopathy (DIC)-like syndrome with transient thrombocytopenia and leukocytopenia, plus liver damage, that are linked to an inflammatory response initiated by the innate immune system. This leads to the appearance of cytokines in the blood and in a way that is still not fully understood, to coagulopathy, organ failure, and potentially, death. The vector interacts with the reticuloendothelial system and induces release of pro-inflammatory cytokines, including IL-1, IL-6, IL8, IL10, TNFα, and IFNγ. Based on animal models, it appears that the virus is first taken up in a saturable, CAR-independent, nonproductive fashion by nonparenchymal Kuppfer cells in the liver, and that this is also associated with the toxicity, although direct interaction with blood cells and platelets can also occur [79]. The second type of toxicity is associated with acute cardiovascular events [78,80], including bradychardia, drop in blood pressure, and hypothermia. These toxicities appear at about the same dose and are probably linked.

Dose-limiting toxicities (DLT) have also been observed after local delivery of adenovirus vectors. In nonhuman primates, dose-limiting toxicity was observed after delivery directly into the brain parenchyma of 1.5×10^9 pfu. These studies were done prior to standardization of vector titers, so exact correlations to today's standards are not possible; however, we estimate the vp titer to have been in the range of 1.5×10^{11} to 1.5×10^{12} vp [81]. In a follow-up clinical trial with direct injection into recurrent malignant brain tumors, DLT was observed at 2×10^{12} vp/injection [82]. A ten-fold higher dose delivered intraperitoneally had no deleterious effects, emphasizing the importance of the delivery site [83]. Hundreds of patients have received intratumoral delivery of adenoviral vectors in the range 10^{11} to 10^{12} vp without toxicity.

POTENTIAL FOR SYSTEMIC DELIVERY OF ADENOVIRAL VECTORS

The discussion above would indicate that systemic adenoviral delivery has not been effective. However, great effort has and continues to be spent in attempting to make adenoviral vectors a systemic drug delivery platform. In general, the theory is that vector administered intravascularly leads to the most widespread distribution of the vectors. Injection in most other sites (intramuscular, intratumor, etc.) leads to most vector staying at the injection site, with some spillage that is consistent with leakage into the vasculature. One of the puzzles about intravascular administration of adenoviral vector has been the rapid removal of the vector from the circulation—the half-life is less than 2 minutes [84] Another puzzle has been that the biodistribution of the vector bears no resemblance to occurrence of the canonical CAR receptor in animals [24,85]. When vector is administered intravascularly and the fate of the genome tracked by polymerase chain reaction at times between about 6 and 72 hours, the liver is the organ with the largest uptake, followed by the spleen, but vector DNA appears in most tissues, including gonads [86]. In rodents the liver preference is clear, whereas in larger animals this preference is less pronounced. At longer time points the vector genome persists mainly in liver and spleen and decays more quickly in other tissues [87]. As was noted above, liver uptake, at least in animal models, appears to be initially in liver Kuppfer cells without leading to vector expression, and independent of CAR interaction. This uptake is essentially a sink that must be filled or removed before significant uptake into other tissue, such as hepatocytes, can occur. The Kuppfer cell "sink" can be avoided, at least partially, in animal models by rapid repeat redosing, by temporary chemical alteration of the Kuppfer cells, or by elimination of the binding sites on the vector for CAR, for heparin sulfate proteoglycan, and for the alpha$_v$ beta 3/5 integrin [88]. In addition, while antiadenovirus humoral responses may be overcome by routes of administration such as intramuscular or intratumoral [16], it is clear that preexisting humoral immunity makes the intravascular route problematic [11]. Current approaches include vector given in conjunction with transient immune suppression or given with vectors to which there is no preexisting immunity, such as vectors derived from other human or animal strains of adenovirus [15,51,52]. Viral "sink" distribution, and the native and adaptive immune responses, must be overcome for systemic vector delivery to make sense.

EARLY CLINICAL APPLICATIONS

The first clinical uses of adenovirus began shortly after their discovery with the use of formalin-inactivated virions as vaccines. Wyeth-Ayerst subsequently made live oral vaccines of Ad4 and Ad7 [89] (subfamilies E and B, respectively) for the U.S. army from 1971 to 1996. This vaccine is now being made by Barr Labs, after technology transfer from Wyeth, and it is undergoing clinical testing to requalify it for human use. Full licensure is expected for 2008. The adenoviral strains were developed as replicating vectors for hepatitis B vaccines [90] by a team led by Paul Hung at Wyeth-Ayerst in the late 1980s. However, these were never used commercially.

CURRENT USE OF ADENOVIRAL VECTORS

The adenoviral vectors most often used for gene transfer belong to the subgenus C, serotypes 2 or 5 (Ad2 or Ad5). These serotypes include the first approved gene therapy product (Gendicine for Head&Neck Cancer [91]) in China and are the basis of about 25% of all worldwide and U.S. gene transfer trials. They are also the backbones of most vectors being investigated as potential clinical agents by pharmaceutical and biotechnology companies and academic investigators (Table 4.1). From public databases, one can estimate that over 3500 subjects have received adenoviral vectors in clinical trials. In addition, it has been reported that the Genedicine product has been given as an approved product to over 3500 patients in China [92]. Such widespread use provides a high general level of comfort about the safe use of adenoviral vectors despite early misuse in monogenic diseases and the skepticism induced by the 1999 fatal incident.

NEXT STEPS

The most anticipated next step is for products based on adenoviral vectors to be licensed in other parts of the world, as has already happened in China. Potential candidates are listed in Table 4.1. In terms of the science, it seems likely that there will be further investigation in helper-dependent adenoviruses for applications where the strengths of the adenoviral platform are required but longer-term expression is desired. Additional efforts will also be focused on other adenovirus serotypes for applications where preexisting immunity to the vector is a major obstacle, most likely for prophylactic vaccines, and on armed CRAds for applications where in vivo tissue penetration or transgene amplification may be necessary. However, there is no guarantee that for most applications any of these will significantly improve on the first-generation system. Early-generation adenoviral vector systems are well suited for applications where high-level expression for 15 to 30 days is sufficient or desirable and where some degree of inflammation is helpful rather than a problem. Clearly, this description fits vaccine and cancer indications very well but may also be beneficial in other disease indications, such as some forms of cardiovascular disease.

CONCLUSIONS

The biology of the wild-type virus and its interaction with the host drive the potential use for a vector system. Adenoviruses are promiscuous infectious agents and easy to manufacture; thus, they provide an enticing vector choice. They are also transient and immunogenic, thus are probably most appropriate for indications where these characteristics are beneficial, or at least not detrimental. In 1995, the Orkin–Motulsky report [93] on why there was a delay in implementation of gene therapy methods to treat human disease came to the unsurprising conclusion that "major difficulties at the basic level include shortcomings in all current gene transfer vectors and an inadequate understanding of the biological interaction of these vectors with the host," but then went on to recommend "greater focus on basic aspects of gene transfer, and gene expression within the context of gene transfer approaches." Although the diagnosis seems correct, the report was taken by many to mean that new or improved vector systems should be developed prior to going forward with clinical products. This could lead to a never-ending chase for the ideal or next better vector. Another valid reaction to the conclusion would be to work on available systems, using the existing knowledge base, in order to understand how to use them better. This is in fact what has happened for the first-generation adenoviral system, and the level of use and activity suggests that the current database provides the confidence and general background needed for the development of agents that can benefit large numbers of people.

REFERENCES

1. Rowe WP, Huebner RJ, Gilmore LK, Parrott RH, Ward TG., Isolation of a cytopathogenic agent from human adenoids undergoing spontaneous degeneration in tissue culture. *Proc Soc Exp Biol Med.* 1953;84:570–573.
2. Shenk T. In: Howley PM, Griffin DE, Martin MA, Roizman B, Straus SE, Knipe DM, eds. *Fields Virology.* 4th Ed. Philadelphia, PA: Lippincott Williams & Wilkins; 2001:2265–2300.
3. Kojaoghlanian T, Flomenberg P, Horwitz MS. The impact of adenovirus infection on the immunocompromised host. *Rev Med Virol.* 2003;13:155–171.
4. Adesanya MR, Redman RS, Baum BJ, O'Connell BC. Immediate inflammatory responses to adenovirus-mediated gene transfer in rat salivary glands. *Hum Gene Ther.* 1996;7:1085–1093.
5. Worgall S, Wolff G, Falck-Pedersen E, Crystal RG. Innate immune mechanisms dominate elimination of adenoviral vectors following in vivo administration. *Hum Gene Ther.* 1997;8:37–44.
6. Brown BD, Lillicrap D. Dangerous liaisons: the role of "danger" signals in the immune response to gene therapy. *Blood.* 2002;100:1133–1139.
7. Bangari DS, Mittal SK. Current strategies and future directions for eluding adenoviral vector immunity. *Curr Gene Ther.* 2006;6:215–226.
8. Heemskerk B, Louise A, Veltrop-Duits LA, van Vreeswijk T, ten Dam MM, et al. Extensive cross-reactivity of CD4 adenovirus-specific T cells: implications for immunotherapy and gene therapy. *J. Virol.* 2003;77:6562–6566.
9. Harvey BG, Hackett NR, El-Sawy T, et al. Variability of human systemic humoral immune responses to adenovirus gene transfer vectors administered to different organs. *J Virol.* 1999;73:6729–6742.
10. van der Linden RR, Haagmans BL, Mongiat-Artus P, et al. Virus specific immune responses after human neoadjuvant adenovirus-mediated suicide gene therapy for prostate cancer. *Eur Urol.* 2005;48:153–161.
11. Nunes FA, Furth EE, Wilson JM, Raper SE. Gene transfer into the liver of nonhuman primates with *E1*-deleted recombinant adenoviral vectors: safety of readministration. *Hum. Gene Ther.* 1999;10:2515–2526.
12. Gahery-Segard H, Juillard V, Gaston J, et al. Humoral immune response to the capsid components of recombinant adenoviruses: routes of immunization modulate virus-induced Ig subclass shifts. *Eur J Immunol.* 1997;27:653–659.
13. Kafri T, Morgan D, Krahl T, Sarvetnick N, Sherman L, Verma I. Cellular immune response to adenoviral vector infected cells does not require de novo viral gene expression: implications for gene therapy *Proc Natl Acad Sci USA.* 1998;95:11377–11382.

14. Kuzmin AI, Galenko O, Eisensmith RC. An immunomodulatory procedure that stabilizes transgene expression and permits readministration of *E1*-deleted adenovirus vectors. *Mol Ther.* 2001;3:293–301.

15. Bangari DS, Mittal SK. Development of nonhuman adenoviruses as vaccine vectors. *Vaccine.* 2006;24:849–862.

16. Vlachaki MT, Hernandez-Garcia A, Ittmann M, et al. Impact of preimmunization on adenoviral vector expression and toxicity in a subcutaneous mouse cancer model. *Mol Ther.* 2002;6:342–348

17. Shalev M, Kadmon D, Teh BS, et al. Suicide gene therapy toxicity after multiple and repeat injections in patients with localized prostate cancer. *J Urol.* 2000;163(6):1747–1750.

18. Miles BJ, Shalev M, Aguilar-Cordova E, et al. Prostate-specific antigen response and systemic T cell activation after in situ gene therapy in prostate cancer patients failing radiotherapy. *Hum Gene Ther.* 2001;12:1955 1967.

19. McConnel MJ, Imperiale MJ. Biology of adenovirus and its use as a vector for gene therapy. *Hum Gene Ther.* 2004;15:1022–1033.

20. Volpers C. and Kochanek S. Adenoviral vectors for gene transfer and therapy. *J Gene Med.* 2004;6:S164–S171.

21. Dechecchi, MC, Melotti P, Bonizzato A, Santacatterina M, Chilosi M, Cabrini G, Heparin sulfate glycosaminoglycans are receptors sufficient to mediate the initial binding of adenovirus types 2 and 5. *J Virol.* 2001;75, 8772–8780.

22. Hong SS, Karayan L, Tournier J, Curiel DT, Boulanger PA, Adenovirus type 5 fiber knob binds to MHC class I alpha2 domain at the surface of human epithelial and B lymphoblastoid cells. *EMBO J.* 1997;16:2294–2306.

23. Gaggar A, Shayakhmetov DM, Lieber A. CD46 is a cellular receptor for group B adenoviruses. *Nat Med.* 2003;9:1408–1412.

24. Shayakhmetov DM, Li ZY, Ni S, Lieber A. Analysis of adenovirus sequestration in the liver, transduction of hepatic cells, and innate toxicity after injection of fiber-modified vectors. *J Virol.* 2004;78(10):5368–5381.

25. Shaw AR, Ziff EB. Transcripts from the adenovirus-2 major late promoter yield a single early family of 30 coterminal mRNAs and five late families. *Cell.* 1980;22:905–916.

26. https://www.atcc.org/documents/pdf/VR-1516text2.pdf.

27. Cote J, Bourget L, Garnier A, Kamen A. Study of adenovirus production in serum-free 293SF suspension culture by GFP-expression monitoring. *Biotechnol Prog.* 1997;13:709–714.

28. Evans RK, Nawrocki DK, Isopi LA, et al. Development of stable liquid formulations for adenovirus-based vaccines. *J Pharm Sci.* 2004;93:2458–2475.

29. Kamen A, Olivier HO. Development and optimization of an adenovirus production process. *J Gene Med.* 2004;6:S184–S192.

30. Nedim E, Altaras NE, Aunins JG, et al. Production and formulation of adenovirus vectors. *Adv Biochem Eng Biotechnol.* 2005;99:193–260.

31. Fallaux FJ, Bout A, van der Velde I, et al. New helper cells and matched early region 1-deleted adenovirus vectors prevent generation of replication-competent adenoviruses. *Hum Gene Ther.* 1998;9:1909–1917.

32. Howe JA, Pelka P, Antelman D, et al. Matching complementing functions of transformed cells with stable expression of selected viral genes for production of *E1*-deleted adenovirus vectors. *Virology.* 2006;345:220–230.

33. Brough DE, Lizonova A, Hsu C, Kulesa VA, Kovesdi I. A gene transfer vector-cell line system for complete functional complementation of adenovirus early regions E1 and E4. *J Virol*. 1996;70:6497–6501.

34. O'Neal WK, Zhou H, Morral N, et al. Toxicological comparison of *E2a*-deleted and first-generation adenoviral vectors expressing alpha1-antitrypsin after systemic delivery. *Hum Gene Ther*. 1998;9:1587–1598.

35. Lusky M, Christ M, Rittner K, et al. In vitro and in vivo biology of recombinant adenovirus vectors with *E1, E1/E2A*, or *E1/E4* deleted. *J Virol*. 1998;72:2022–2032.

36. Morral N, O'Neal WK, Rice K, et al. Lethal toxicity, severe endothelial injury, and a threshold effect with high doses of an adenoviral vector in baboons. *Hum Gene Ther*. 2002;13:143–154.

37. Morsy MA, Gu M, Motzel S, et al. An adenoviral vector deleted for all viral coding sequences results in enhanced safety and extended expression of a leptin transgene. *Proc Natl Acad Sci USA*. 1998;95:7866–7871.

38. Kochanek S, Clemens PR, Mitani K, Chen HH, Chan S, Caskey CT. A new adenoviral vector: replacement of all viral coding sequences with 28kb of DNA independently expressing both full-length dystrophin and beta-galactosidase. *Proc Natl Acad Sci USA*. 1996;93:5731–5736.

39. Palmer DJ, Ng P. Helper-dependent adenoviral vectors for gene therapy. *Hum Gene Ther*. 2005;16:1–16.

40. Barnett BG, Crews CJ, Douglas JT. Targeted adenoviral vectors. *Biochim Biophys Acta*. 2002;1575:1–14.

41. Everts M, Curiel DT. Transductional targeting of adenoviral cancer gene therapy. *Curr Gene Ther*. 2004;4:337–346.

42. Krasnykh VN, Douglas JT, van Beusechem VW. Genetic targeting of adenoviral vectors. *Mol Ther*. 2000;1(5 Pt 1):391–405

43. Wickham TJ. Targeting adenovirus. *Gene Ther*. 2000;7:110–4

44. Dmitriev I, Krasnykh V, Miller CR, et al. An adenovirus vector with genetically modified fibers demonstrates expanded tropism via utilization of a coxsackievirus and adenovirus receptor-independent cell entry mechanism. *J Virol*. 1998;72:9706–9713.

45. van Beusechem VW, van Rijswijk AL, van Es HH, et al. Recombinant adenovirus vectors with knobless fibers for targeted gene transfer. *Gene Ther*. 2000;7:1940–1946.

46. Xia H, Anderson B, Mao Q, et al. Recombinant human adenovirus: targeting to the human transferrin receptor improves gene transfer to brain microcapillary endothelium. *J Virol*. 2000;74:11359–11366

47. Henning P, Andersson KM, Frykholm K, et al. Tumor cell targeted gene delivery by adenovirus 5 vectors carrying knobless fibers with antibody-binding domains. *Gene Ther*. 2005;12:211–224.

48. Borovjagin AV, Krendelchtchikov A, Ramesh N, Yu DC, Douglas JT, Curiel DT. Complex mosaicism is a novel approach to infectivity enhancement of adenovirus type 5-based vectors. *Cancer Gene Ther*. 2005;12:475–486.

49. Shinozaki K, Suominen E, Carrick F, et al. Efficient infection of tumor endothelial cells by a capsid-modified adenovirus. *Gene Ther*. 2006;13:52–59.

50. Shayakhmetov DM, Li ZY, Ternovoi V, Gaggar A, Gharwan H, Lieber A. The interaction between the fiber knob domain and the cellular attachment receptor determines the intracellular trafficking route of adenoviruses. *J. Virol*. 2003;77:3712–3723.

51. Kremer EJ. CAR chasing: canine adenovirus vectors—all bite and no bark? *J Gene Med.* 2004;6(Suppl 1):S1.

52. Tatsis N, Tesema L, Robinson ER, et al. Chimpanzee-origin adenovirus vectors as vaccine carriers. *Gene Ther.* 2006;13:421–429.

53. Osaki T, Tanio Y, Tachibana I, et al. Gene therapy for carcinoembryonic antigen-producing human lung cancer cells by cell type-specific expression of herpes simplex virus thymidine kinase gene. *Cancer Res.* 1994;54:5258–5261.

54. Ambriovi'c A, Adam M, Monteil M, Paulin D, Eloit M. Efficacy of replication-defective adenovirus-vectored vaccines: protection following intramuscular injection is linked to promoter efficiency in muscle representative cells. *Virology.* 1997;238:327–335.

55. Barker SD, Coolidge CJ, Kanerva A, et al. The secretory leukoprotease inhibitor (SLPI) promoter for ovarian cancer gene therapy. *J Gene Med.* 2003;5:300–310.

56. Bischoff JR, Kirn DH, Williams A, et al. An adenovirus mutant that replicates selectively in p53-deficient human tumor cells. *Science.* 1996;274:373–376.

57. Edwards SJ, Dix BR, Myers CJ, et al. Evidence that replication of the antitumor adenovirus Onyx-015 is not controlled by the p53 and p14(ARF) tumor suppressor genes. *J Virol.* 2002;76:12483–12490.

58. Khuri FR, Nemunaitis J, Ganly I, et al. A controlled trial of intratumoral Onyx-015, a selectively-replicating adenovirus, in combination with cisplatin and 5-fluorouracil in patients with recurrent head and neck cancer. *Nat Med.* 2000;6:879–885.

59. Hamid O, Varterasian ML, Wadler S, et al. Phase II trial of intravenous CI-1042 in patients with metastatic colorectal cancer. *J Clin Oncol.* 2003;21:1498–1504.

60. Garber K. China approves world's first oncolytic virus therapy for cancer treatment. *J Nat Cancer Inst.* 2005;98:298–300.

61. Wildner O. Comparison of replication-selective, oncolytic viruses for the treatment of human cancers. *Curr Opin Mol Ther.* 2003;5:351–361.

62. Rodriguez R, Schuur ER, Lim HY, Henderson GA, Simons JW, Henderson DR. Prostate attenuated replication competent adenovirus (ARCA) CN706: a selective cytotoxic for prostate-specific antigen-positive prostate cancer cells. *Cancer Res.* 1997;57:2559–2563.

63. Cheng WS, Kraaij R, Nilsson B, et al. A novel TARP-promoter-based adenovirus against hormone-dependent and hormone-refractory prostate cancer. *Mol Ther.* 2004;10:355–364.

64. Shirakawa T, Hamada K, Zhang Z, et al. A Cox-2 promoter–based replication-selective adenoviral vector to target the Cox-2–expressing human bladder cancer cells. *Clin Cancer Res.* 2004;10:4342–4348.

65. Huang TG, Savontaus MJ, Shinozaki K, Sauter BV, Woo SL. Telomerase-dependent oncolytic adenovirus for cancer treatment. *Gene Ther.* 2003;10:1241–1247

66. DeWeese TL, van der Poel H, Li S, et al. A phase I trial of CV706, a replication-competent, PSA selective oncolytic adenovirus, for the treatment of locally recurrent prostate cancer following radiation therapy. *Cancer Res.* 2001;61:7464–7472.

67. Fueyo J, Gomez-Manzano C, Alemany R, et al. A mutant oncolytic adenovirus targeting the Rb pathway produces anti-glioma effect in vivo. *Oncogene.* 2000;19:2–12.

68. Ramachandra M, Rahman A, Zou A, et al. Re-engineering adenovirus regulatory pathways to enhance oncolytic specificity and efficacy. *Nat Biotechnol.* 2001;19:1035–1041.

69. Liu TC, Wang Y, Hallden G, et al. Functional interactions of antiapoptotic proteins and tumor necrosis factor in the context of a replication-competent adenovirus. *Gene Ther.* 2005;12:1333–1346.

70. Ahmed A, Thompson J, Emiliusen L, et al. A conditionally replicating adenovirus targeted to tumor cells through activated RAS/P-MAPK-selective mRNA stabilization. *Nat Biotechnol.* 2003;21(7):771–777.

71. Aguilar-Cordova E. Vectorology recapitulates virology—will it capitulate oncology? *Nat Biotechnol.* 2003;21:756–757.

72. Hermiston TW, Kuhn I. Armed therapeutic viruses: strategies and challenges to arming oncolytic viruses with therapeutic genes. *Cancer Gene Ther.* 2002;9:1022–1035.

73. Freytag SO, Khil M, Stricker H, et al. Phase I study of replication-competent adenovirus-mediated double suicide gene therapy for the treatment of locally recurrent prostate cancer. *Cancer Res.* 2002;62:4968–4976.

74. Ramesh N, Ge Y, Ennist DL, et al. CG0070, a conditionally replicating granulocyte macrophage colony-stimulating factor—armed oncolytic adenovirus for the treatment of bladder cancer. *Clin Cancer Res.* 2006;12:305–313.

75. NIH Recombinant DNA Advisory Committee. Assessment of adenoviral vector safety: report of the National Institutes of Health Recombinant DNA Advisory Committee. *Hum Gene Ther.* 2001;13:3–31.

76. Raper SE, Chirmule N, Lee FS, et al. Fatal systemic inflammatory response syndrome in an ornithine transcarbamylase deficient patient following adenoviral gene transfer. *Mol Genet Metab.* 2003;80:148–158.

77. St George JA. Gene therapy progress and prospects: adenoviral vectors. *Gene Ther.* 2003;10:1135–1141.

78. Reid T, Warren R, Kirn D. Intravascular adenoviral agents in cancer patients: lessons from clinical trials. *Cancer Gene Ther.* 2002;9:979–986.

79. Wolins N, Lozier J, Eggerman TL, Jones E, Aguilar-Cordova E, Vostal JG. Intravenous administration of replication-incompetent adenovirus to rhesus monkeys induces thrombocytopenia by increasing in vivo platelet clearance. *Br J. Haematol.* 2003;123:903–905.

80. Machemer T, Engler T, Tsai V, et al. Characterization of hemodynamic events following intravascular infusion of recombinant adenovirus reveals possible solutions for mitigating cardiovascular responses. *Mol Ther.* 2005;12:254–263.

81. Goodman JC, Trask TW, Chen SH, et al. Adenoviral-mediated thymidine kinase gene transfer into the primate brain followed by systemic ganciclovir: pathologic, radiologic, and molecular studies. *Hum Gene Ther.* 1996;7:1241–1250.

82. Trask TW, Trask RP, Aguilar-Cordova, E, Phase I study of adenoviral delivery of the *HSV*-tk gene and ganciclovir administration in patients with recurrent malignant brain tumors. *Mol Ther.* 2000;1:195–203.

83. Hasenburg A, Tong XW, Fischer DC. Adenovirus-mediated thymidine kinase gene therapy in combination with topotecan for patients with recurrent ovarian cancer: 2.5-year follow-up. *Gynecol Oncol.* 2001;83:549–554.

84. Alemany R, Suzuki K, Curiel DT. Blood clearance rates of adenovirus type 5 in mice. *J Gen Virol.* 2000;81:2605–2609.

85. Fechner AH, Haack A, Wang H, et al. Expression of coxsackie adenovirus receptor and alpha-integrin does not correlate with adenovector targeting in vivo indicating anatomical vector barriers. *Gene Ther.* 1999;6:1520–1535.

86. Morral N, O'Neal WK, Rice K, et al. Lethal toxicity, severe endothelial injury, and a threshold effect with high doses of an adenoviral vector in baboons. *Hum Gene Ther.* 2002;13:143–154.

87. Smith TAG, Idamakanti N, Marshall-Neff J, et al. Receptor interactions involved in adenoviral-mediated gene delivery after systemic administration in non-human primates. *Hum Gene Ther.* 2003;14:1595–1604.

88. Liu Q, Zaiss AK, Colarusso P, et al. The role of capsid–endothelial interactions in the innate immune response to adenovirus vectors. *Hum Gene Ther.* 2003;14:627–643.

89. Top FH Jr. Control of adenovirus acute respiratory disease in U.S. Army trainees. *Yale J Biol Med.* 1975;48:185-195.

90. Lubeck MD, Davis AR, Chengalvala M, et al. Immunogenicity and testing in chimpanzees of an oral hepatitis B vaccine based on live recombinant adenovirus. *Proc Natl Acad Sci USA.* 1989;86:6763-6767.

91. Peng Z. Current status of gendicine in China: recombinant human Ad-p53 agent for treatment of cancers. *Hum Gene Ther.* 2005;16:1016–1027.

92. Jia H. Controversial Chinese gene-therapy drug entering unfamiliar territory *Nat Rev Drug Discov.* 2006;5:269–270.

93. http://www4.od.nih.gov/oba/rac/panelrep.htm

94. Shiver J. Presentation at the Phacilitate Cell and Gene Therapy Forum, Washington, DC, January 2005.

95. Singh J. Presentation at the Phacilitate Cell and Gene Therapy Forum, Washington, DC, January 2005.

96. Benedict WF, Tao Z, Kim CS, et al. Intravesical Ad-IFNα causes marked regression of human bladder cancer growing orthotopically in nude mice and overcomes resistance to IFN-α protein. *Mol Ther.* 10:525–532.

97. Grines CL, Watkins MW, Helmer G, et al. Angiogenic gene therapy (AGENT) trial in patients with stable angina pectoris. *Circulation.* 2002;105:1291–1297.

98. Senzer N, Mani S, Rosemurgy A, et al. TNFerade biologic, an adenovector with a radiation-inducible promoter, carrying the human tumor necrosis factor alpha gene: a phase I study in patients with solid tumors. *J Clin Oncol.* 2004;22:592–601.

5 Adeno-Associated Virus Vectors

BARRIE J. CARTER
Targeted Genetics Corporation, Seattle, Washington

Gene delivery vectors based on adeno-associated virus (AAV) were first described in 1984 (Carter, 2004). AAV vectors are very simple in design and are now relatively straightforward to manufacture and to scale up in GMP (good manufacturing practice) mode for use in clinical trials (see Chapter 20, this volume). AAV vectors can persist in vivo for very long periods mostly as episomes and thus are particularly attractive for therapies for chronic diseases. In the last two decades, a large expansion of studies on AAV vectors has led to at least 13 different AAV vectors being introduced into clinical trials (Carter, 2005). These phase I and II trials have been conducted over nine years and have enrolled several hundred subjects, including patients afflicted with several diseases and normal healthy volunteers. These vectors, all of which have been based on AAV serotype 2, have shown an impressive safety profile when administered by several routes of delivery, including inhaled aerosol to the airway, intramuscular, intravenous via hepatic artery, and intracranially by stereotactic injection. The development of AAV vectors has also spurred significant advances in studies of many AAV serotypes and increased understanding of many aspects of AAV vector biology. This will probably lead to increased sophistication in the design and application of AAV vectors in the future. Consequently, AAV vectors represent one of the most promising gene delivery systems.

AAV VECTOR GENOME DESIGN

AAV vectors have many advantages. The parental virus does not cause disease. The vectors transduce nondividing cells in vivo and persist long term. They contain no viral genes and generally do not elicit innate or cellular immune responses. Thus, AAV vectors can mediate impressive long-term gene expression in vivo and can easily be purified and concentrated. AAV vectors are limited in payload capacity to about 4.5 kb, and host antibody responses to the viral capsid might present some limitations for certain applications. AAV vectors are described more extensively elsewhere (Carter et al., 2004).

Adeno-associated viruses are DNA-containing, replication-defective parvoviruses that replicate only in the nucleus of cells coinfected by a helper virus, generally an adenovirus or some herpesviruses (Flotte and Berns, 2005). Infection of cells in vitro by AAV in the absence of helper functions results in the persistence of AAV as a latent provirus integrated into the host cell genome at a preferred site on human chromosome 19. This process is mediated by the AAV rep protein, but integrated AAV proviruses have not been demonstrated in humans. AAV vectors are deleted for the *rep* gene and persist mainly in vivo as episomes. AAV has not been associated with the cause of any disease but has been isolated from humans (Blacklow, 1988) and many other animal species. Initially, at least five serotypes of AAV were identified, but a much more extended clade structure is now being defined (Gao et al., 2004).

AAV are nonenveloped 25-nm particles comprised of a protein capsid enclosing a linear single-stranded DNA genome. AAV DNA genomes are about 4700 nucleotides long with one copy of an inverted terminal repeat (ITR) at each end and a unique sequence region that contains two main open reading frames for the *rep* and *cap* genes (Figure 1A). For AAV2, the ITR is 145 nucleotides and the unique region is 4381 nucleotides. The ITR sequences act in *cis* as origins of replication and signals for encapsidation. The *rep* and *cap* genes provide *trans*-acting functions for replication and encapsidation of viral genomes, respectively (Carter et al., 2004; Flotte and Berns, 2005).

The generation of AAV vectors is based on molecular cloning of double-stranded AAV DNA in bacterial plasmids (see Chapter 20, this volume). AAV vectors are constructed by substituting all of the AAV coding sequence with foreign DNA to generate a vector plasmid. The only AAV DNA sequences that need to be retained in the vector genome are the ITRs (Figure 1B). One effect of the capsid structure is to limit the size of DNA genome that can be packaged in an AAV vector particle to about 5 kb. Otherwise, there are no obvious limitations on the design of gene cassettes in AAV vectors. Cell-specific promoters retain specificity, introns function and may enhance expression, more than one promoter and gene cassette can be inserted in the same vector, and transcription from AAV vectors does not seem to be susceptible to in vivo silencing (Carter et al., 2004). The ITRs can function as weak transcription promoters (Flotte et al., 1993) but do not interfere with other promoters.

After uncoating in the host cell nucleus, the vector genome must be converted to a duplex to enable transcription. This conversion may be inefficient in some cells but can be overcome by utilizing self-complementary vectors based on a property of AAV DNA replication (McCarty et al., 2001; Carter, 2003). If the vector genome is not more that one-half unit length (i.e., about 2.3 kb), duplex-replicating forms can be packaged, but upon uncoating, immediately form (snap back) into a duplex genome. Such self-complementary vectors have only half the payload capacity of the usual AAV vectors, but cDNAs of many genes can easily be accommodated.

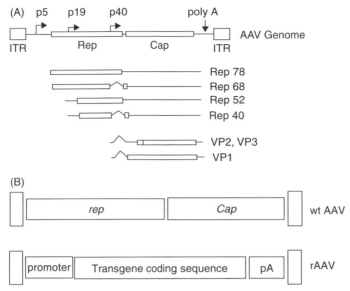

Figure 5.1 (A) AAV genome structure. The structure of the AAV serotype 2 genome is shown schematically. The linear single-stranded DNA genome is 4681 nucleotides long. The 145 nucleotides at either end represented by the open boxes are the inverted-terminal repeats (ITRs). The first 125 nucleotides of the ITR can form a T-shaped, base-paired hairpin structure that acts as the DNA replication of origin. Two coding regions for the *rep* and *cap* genes are contained in the left and right halves of the genome. The three transcription promoters p5, p19, and p40 lead to expression of three families of mRNA, all of which are terminated at the same polyA site. Splicing of the p5 and p19 mRNAs in the region immediately downstream of the p40 promoter leads to expression of four rep proteins that have a common internal coding sequence but differ at the amino- and carboxyl-terminal regions, as shown by the open rectangles. Alternate splicing of the p40 mRNA leads to expression of three capsid proteins, VP3, VP2, and VP1, such that all contain the same VP3 polypeptide sequence but VP2 and VP1 have larger *n*-terminal extensions. (B) AAV vector design. The wild-type AAV2 genome is shown schematically with the ITR regions folded into a T-shaped hairpin conformation. For generation of AAV vectors, all of the coding region for the *rep* and *cap* genes is deleted and replaced by the transgene coding sequence and an appropriate transcription promoter and polyA site.

The payload capacity of AAV vector can be extended to nearly 10 kb using a dual AAV vector system (Yan et al., 2005). In nondividing cells, in vivo AAV vector genomes generally are converted to circular duplexes and then to head-to-tail concatemeric duplexes by intermolecular recombination. Consequently, two different vector genomes can be recombined into a single unit after infection and uncoating. Thus, a gene or expression cassette can be divided into two parts, each not more that about 4.5 kb, and the single intact transcription unit will be recreated in vivo by the concatemerization process.

ELEMENTS OF AAV STRUCTURE AND BIOLOGY THAT INFLUENCE VECTOR PROPERTIES

The AAV vector genome design is important for arrangement of the expression cassettes and for its persistence as an unintegrated episome. The episomal persistence of the genome in nondividing cells is very important in determining the general applications of AAV vectors. However, the AAV capsid plays an important role in determining the efficiency of transduction of AAV vectors in particular cell targets.

The structure of the capsid mediates the efficiency of vector interaction and cellular uptake and capsids of individual serotypes bind different cellular receptors and coreceptors. This differential receptor binding affects the efficiency with which AAV vectors enter various cells and thus may have a very large impact on the efficiency of transduction by vectors. The best characterized AAV, serotype 2, binds heparin sulfate proteoglycan and is then internalized using either an $\alpha_v\beta_5$ integrin or an FGF receptor. Most other serotypes do not bind heparin sulfate. For instance, AAV5 binds sialic acid and uses a PDGF (platelet-derived growth factor) receptor for internalization. The structures of AAV capsids are being resolved by physical techniques such as x-ray crystallography (Xie et al., 2002) and cryoelectronmicroscopy (Padron et al., 2005). In addition, site-specific mutagenesis of the capsid protein reveals the location of receptor and coreceptor binding sites. By using capsids of different serotypes to encapsidate a genome having AAV2 ITRs (a process known as *pseudotyping*) it has become clear that the relative transduction efficiency of an AAV vector for a particular cell type is dictated largely by the capsid structure. As the structure of each serotype is resolved and mutagenesis studies identify the functional roles of each residue in the capsid, it is likely that more sophisticated capsids can be designed by generation of mutant or chimeric capsids (Muzyczka and Warrington, 2005).

The transduction efficiency as determined by the capsid structure partially reflects the cellular receptor binding and internalization process, but additional biological insights have also emerged with respect to cellular trafficking of the vectors from the cell membrane to the cell nucleus (Vihinen-Ranta et al., 2004). For instance, AAV particles interact with the proteosome pathway, and ultimately this may be important for successful transport into the nucleus. However, AAV vectors may be held up in this pathway, and use of proteosome inhibitors can dramatically increase the transduction efficiency (Yan et al., 2004). Thus, adjunct treatments, perhaps involving design of small molecules, could be a fruitful approach to enhancing AAV vector efficiency (Zhang et al., 2004).

The capsid structure may also play a role in the process by which the AAV genome is transported across the nuclear membrane and unpackaged, but the biochemistry of this is still unclear. Nevertheless, the study of AAV vector structure and cellular trafficking, in addition to paying dividends in AAV vector development, is becoming a very exciting area of cellular biology.

AAV VECTOR PERSISTENCE, SAFETY, AND CLINICAL APPLICATIONS

Because AAV vectors persist in vivo as unintegrated episomes, they are ideally suited for transduction of nondividing cells, such as in muscle, brain, retina, or liver, or in cells that turn over relatively slowly, such as airway epithelial cells. AAV vectors have shown excellent safety profiles in extensive preclinical studies in many animal models when administered by various routes, including inhaled aerosols, intramuscular or intraarticular injection, and intracranial stereotactic injection as well as by intravenous and subretinal locations (Carter et al., 2004; Flotte, 2004). Most of these routes of delivery have been utilized in 17 clinical trials of 13 different AAV2 vectors involving over 260 subjects (Carter, 2005). This includes delivery to the airways of 140 cystic fibrosis patients with follow-up over seven to eight years, and more recently by intramuscular injection in more than 50 normal subjects (in the context of testing an AAV vector as a potential HIV vaccine). In general, the preclinical safety profile of AAV vectors has been recapitulated in the clinical trials, and no dose-limiting toxicities or maximum-tolerated doses have been observed in either context. All of the clinical trials so far have utilized AAV2 vectors, but several pseudotyped vectors with capsids of other serotypes will probably enter clinical trials in the next several years. The excellent safety profiles of the AAV vectors reflect the general absence of significant inflammatory responses, and AAV does not appear to induce either significant innate immune responses or cellular immunity (Flotte, 2004; Carter, 2005). The AAV capsid can induce an antibody response, but this is dependent on dose and route of delivery, and where there has been direct comparison, the response in clinical trials has reflected that in preclinical studies. For instance, in the lung, the immune response is relatively blunted, and even if a serum IgG response is generated at high doses, it does not appear to directly affect transduction in the lung (see Chapter 12, this volume).

The other important feature of AAV vectors is the ability to persist primarily as an episome, because this reduces the frequency of integration (McCarty et al., 2004). However, even though in the absence of the AAV *rep* gene the integration is very much lower, any integration that might occur is probably not specific for the chromosome 19 site. Any integration events carry the possibility of a resulting mutant phenotypes as sequelae, so it was particularly important for studies aimed at developing AAV as a potential HIV vaccine (Johnson et al., 2005) to determine the possible integration frequency. A series of very extensive studies in rodents and rabbits after intramuscular injection of AAV2 vectors has been conducted (Munson et al., 2003; Schnepp et al., 2003a,b). The biodistribution to various tissues for up to six months after administration was assessed, and persisting vector genomes were tested for integration using a highly sensitive and carefully calibrated and controlled genome-wide polymerase chain reaction assay. These studies revealed no integration events and placed an upper limit on the integration frequency as being at least several orders of magnitude below the spontaneous rate of mutation for human genes (Cole and Skopek, 1994).

Similar studies have been performed with plasmid DNA or adenovirus vectors administered intramuscularly, with similar results. Thus, AAV vectors administered intramuscularly do not integrate with any higher frequency than adenovirus or plasmid genomes, even though the latter do not persist. These studies are important for enhancing the safety profile of AAV vectors and will be important for regulatory considerations in determining the relative need and extent of long-term follow-up of subjects who are administered gene therapy vectors (Nyberg et al., 2004).

Overall, the development of AAV vectors is proceeding at a remarkable pace. There are dramatic advances in the basic biology research and advancing development of AAV vectors in the clinic. This provides an exciting environment to expand basic science and to apply this technology to the goal of providing therapeutic solutions to unmet medical needs.

REFERENCES

Backlow NR (1988). Adeno-associated viruses of humans. In: Pattison JR, ed. *Parvoviruses and Human Disease*. Boca Raton, FL: CRC Press; 165–174.

Carter BJ (2003). Metabolically activated recombinant adeno-associated virus vectors and methods for their preparation and use. US patent 6,596,535, issued July 22.

Carter BJ (2004). Adeno-associated virus and the development of adeno-Associated virus vectors: a historical perspective. *Mol Ther.* 10:981–989.

Carter BJ (2005). Adeno-associated virus vectors in clinical trials. *Hum Gene Ther.* 16:541–550.

Carter BJ, Burstein HB, Peluso RW (2004). AAV vectors for gene therapy. In: Templeton-Smith N, ed. *Gene and Cell Therapy: Therapeutic Mechanisms and Strategies*. 2nd ed. New York: Marcel Dekker; 53–101.

Cole J, Skopek TR (1994). International Commission for Protection Against Environmental Mutagens and Carcinogens. Working paper 3. Somatic mutant frequency, mutation rates and mutational spectra in the human population in vivo. *Mutat Res.* 304:33–105.

Flotte TR (2004). Immune responses to recombinant adeno-associated virus vectors: putting preclinical findings into perspective. *Hum Gene Ther.* 15:716–717.

Flotte TR, Berns KI (2005). Adeno-associated virus: a ubiquitous commensal of mammals. *Hum Gene Ther.* 16:401–407.

Flotte TR, Zeitlin PL, Solow R, et al. (1993). Expression of the cystic fibrosis transmembrane conductance regulator from a novel adeno-associated virus promoter. *J Biol Chem.* 268:3781–3790.

Gao G, Vandenberghe LH, Alvira MR, et al. (2004). Clades of adeno-associated viruses are widely disseminated in human tissues. *J Virol.* 78:6381–6388.

Johnson PR, Schnepp BC, Connell MJ, et al. (2005). Novel adeno-associated virus vector vaccine restricts replication of simian immunodeficiency virus in macaques. *J Virol.* 79:955–965.

McCarty DM, Monahan PE, Samulski RJ (2001). Self-complementary recombinant adeno-associated virus (scAAV) vectors promote efficient transduction independently of DNA synthesis. *Gene Ther.* 8:1248–1254.

McCarty DM, Young SM, Samulski RJ (2004). Integration of adeno-associated virus (AAV) and recombinant AAV vectors. *Annu Rev Genet.* 38:819–845.

Munson K, Kelly EJ, Allen T, et al. (2003). Safety, local tolerability and biodistribution of AAV2-gag-PR-RT. *Mol Ther.* 7:S267.

Muzyczka N, Warrington KH (2005). Custom adeno-associated virus capsids: the next generation of recombinant vectors with novel tropism. *Hum Gene Ther.* 16:408–416.

Nyberg K, Carter BJ, Chen T, et al. (2004). Long-term follow-up of participants in human gene transfer research. *Mol Ther.* 10:976–980.

Padron E, Bowman V, Kaludov N, et al. (2005). Structure of adeno-associated virus type 4. *J Virol.* 79:5047–5058.

Schnepp BC, Clark KR, Klemanski DL, Pacak CA, Johnson PR (2003a). Genetic fate of recombinant adeno-associated virus vector genomes in muscle. *J Virol.* 77:3495–3504.

Schnepp BC, Soult MC, Kelly E, Munson K, Clark KR, Johnson PR (2003b). Genome-wide amplification for the detection of integrated AV2 vector DNA in rabbit tissue. *Mol Ther.* 7:S160.

Vihinen-Ranta M, Suikkanen S, Parrish CR (2004). Pathways of cell infection by parvoviruses and adeno-associated virus. *J Virol.* 78:6709–6714.

Xie Q, Bu W, Bhatia S, Hare J, et al. (2002). The atomic structure of adeno-associated virus (AAV-2), a vector for human gene therapy. *Proc Natl Acad Sci U S A.* 99: 10405–10410.

Yan Z, Zak R, Zhang Y, et al. (2004). Distinct classes of proteosome-modulating agents cooperatively augment recombinant adeno-associated virus type 2 and type 5-mediated transduction from the apical surfaces of human airway epithelia. *J Virol.* 78:2863–2874.

Yan Z, Zak R, Zhang Y, Engelhardt JF (2005). Inverted terminal repeat sequences are important for intermolecular recombination and circularization of adeno-associated virus genomes. *J Virol.* 79:364–379.

Zhang LN, Karp P, Gerard CJ, et al. (2004). Dual therapeutic utility of proteasome modulating agents or pharmaco-gene therapy of the cystic fibrosis airway. *Mol Ther.* 10:990–1002.

6 SV40 Virus–Derived Vectors

DAVID S. STRAYER

Department of Pathology and Cell Biology,
Jefferson Medical College, Philadelphia, Pennsylvania

The goal of gene therapy is to prevent and treat disease: to mitigate human suffering. Gene transfer occurs via vehicles: that is, vectors. As currently constructed, vectors determine most key parameters of gene delivery: what cells will be transduced; how long transgene expression will last; what dose can be administered; whether daughter cells will express a transgene delivered to cycling parent or progenitor cells; whether readministration is possible; and so on. The diversity of therapeutic goals calls for many different responses to these questions, which in turn demands corresponding heterogeneity among delivery vehicles.

Although some early gene transfer studies applied reengineered simian virus 40s (SV40s) (Muzycka, 1980; Gething and Sambrook, 1981), this virus was largely ignored until relatively recently. The work of a number of laboratories suggests that the characteristics of this vector as a gene transfer vehicle may be advantageous for several important gene therapy applications (Sandalon et al., 1997; Naeger et al., 1999; Kimchi-Sarfati et al., 2002; DeFillippis et al., 2003; Vera and Fortes 2004; Vera et al., 2004; Arad et al., 2005).

NATURE OF SV40-BASED VECTORS

Wild-type (wt) SV40 is a nonenveloped virus in the polyoma family that has a 5.25-kb circular double-stranded DNA genome. It can be rendered replication incompetent—and so suitable to use as a vector—by replacing some or all of the SV40 genes with one or more transgenes, additional constitutive or conditional pol II or pol III promoters, transcriptional stop signals, and so on.

Production of these vectors is illustrated in Figure 6.1. Briefly, the 2.5-kb DNA encoding large and small T antigen genes (*Tag* and *tag*, respectively), which overlap in sequence and are both driven by the SV40 early promoter (SV40-EP), may be replaced by a polylinker, often with a second promoter, such as the cytomegalovirus immediate early promoter (CMV-IEP) (Strayer, 1999).

SV40-EP overlaps the origin of replication (ori) and so cannot be removed (Fried and Prives, 1986; Cole and Conzen, 2001).

Larger inserts may require removing SV40 capsid genes (see Figure 6.1). In that event, 0.7 kb of essential SV40 sequences (encapsidation sequences, ori, etc.) is kept. Using this approach, we routinely express inserts up to 5 kb (Strayer, 1999a).

Vectors are produced by excising rSV40 DNA from its carrier plasmid, re-circularizing it, then transfecting into packaging cells (Strayer, 1999; Strayer et al., 2001). COS7 cells carry wtSV40 genomes deficient at the ori (Gluzman et al., 1980; Gluzman, 1981), and package rSV40 genomes into virions directly. Even "gutless" vectors lacking all SV40 genes are encapsidated by COS7 cells. Vectors are amplified by *infecting* COS7 cells with recombinant virus. No helper virus or additional transfection is required (Strayer et al., 2001).

Vectors are band-purified on discontinuous sucrose or cesium chloride gradients (Rosenberg et al., 1981; Strayer et al., 2001) and titered using quantitative (real time) polymerase chain reaction (PCR) (QPCR) or in situ PCR (Strayer et al., 1997a). Generally, rSV40 titers are between 10^9 and 10^{11} infectious units (IU)/mL.

EXPRESSION CONSTRUCTS THAT HAVE BEEN EFFECTIVELY DELIVERED USING rSV40s

rSV40s have been used with numerous constitutive and conditional pol II promoters to express proteins or untranslated transcripts (BouHamdan et al., 2001; Jayan et al., 2001; Cordelier et al., 2003a; Matskevich et al., 2003; Matskevich and Strayer, 2003; Strayer et al., 2005a). Pol III promoters may also be used to drive transcription of untranslated transcripts (e.g., RNA interference, antisense, ribozymes) (Zern et al., 1999; Cordelier et al., 2003b). SV40-EP must be present (it overlaps the ori; see above), so if a pol III or conditional pol II promoter is used, the EP constitutive promoter function should be blocked by inserting a polyadenylation signal.

APPLICATIONS FOR WHICH SV40-DERIVED VECTORS MAY BE ADVANTAGEOUS

Transduction Efficiency

rSV40 vectors are generally highly efficient gene delivery vehicles. In vitro, at virus/cell ratios ≥ 10, they deliver their genes to virtually every susceptible target cell (Strayer et al., 2002a), without selection. The efficiency of gene transfer is high both in vitro and in vivo, whether target cells are cycling or quiescent.

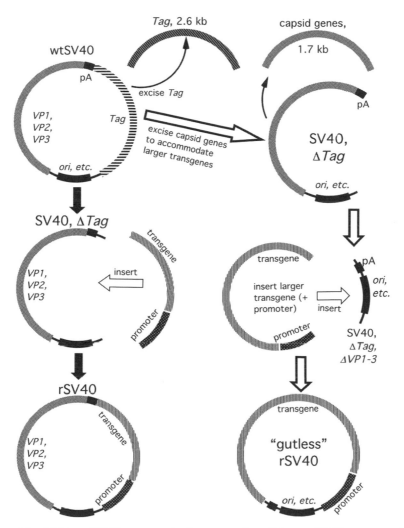

Figure 6.1 Making rSV40 vectors. At the outset, the wild-type SV40 genome, cloned in a carrier plasmid (not shown), is modified by excising the *Tag* and *tag* genes (2.6 kb). The result, shown in the left panel, is a viral genome containing the SV40 capsid genes, polyadenylation signal (pA), *ori*, encapsidation signal (*ses*), enhancer, and early promoter (which overlaps the *ori*, and so cannot be excised). This construct, shown on the left, is then made into a gene delivery vehicle genome by inserting the desired DNA (transgene, promoter, etc.), as shown in the left panels. To accommodate larger DNA inserts (e.g., larger transgenes, more than one transgene, multiple promoters, insulators, etc.), this *Tag*-deleted genome can be modified further by excising the capsid genes (1.7 kb), as shown in the right panels. In this case, the only remaining SV40 sequences are the *ori*, *ses*, early promoter, and pA (middle, right). Resulting recombinant SV40 vectors lack both SV40 early genes and SV40 capsid genes. All these vectors are replication incompetent in cells that lack *Tag*. The latter, gutless, vectors also require packaging cells to supply the capsid genes in trans.

As a practical matter, to transduce high percentages of cells in vivo, repeated administration may be useful, but effectiveness in gene transfer may be as high as 80 to 90% of cells (Sauter et al., 2000; Strayer et al., 2002b; Liu et al., 2005).

In one series of studies, we compared the effectiveness of rSV40 transduction of lymphocytes to that of murine leukemia virus (MuLV). Both vectors carried the same combination of promoter + transgene and delivered the same therapeutic effect. However, retroviral gene delivery was effective only when transduced cells were first selected, to ensure adequate numbers of transgene-expressing cells. rSV40 vectors did not require selection (BouHamdan et al., 1999). In addition, rSV40-delivered transgene expression was detected many months after the initial transduction (Strayer et al., 2002b).

To date, rSV40 gene delivery is the only approach to demonstrate in vivo protection from HIV. An rSV40 carrying an antibody versus. HIV-1 integrase was injected into human thymus that had been implanted into SCID (severe combined immunodeficiency) mice. Implants were then challenged by direct injection of a clinical isolate of HIV-1. By immunostaining, 80% of implant cells expressed the transgene. HIV replication was reduced by approximately 85% in anti-IN transduced grafts compared to mock- or control-transduced grafts. This is the only reported demonstration that in vivo gene delivery can protect from in vivo challenge with immunosuppressive lentivirus (e.g., HIV or SIV) (Goldstein et al., 2002).

Combination Genetic Therapy

Such efficient transduction can be exploited to deliver different genes in sequence to the same cells. Transduction with one rSV40 carrying a transgene targeting HIV-1 integrase, for example, may be followed by a different rSV40 gene delivery using another anti-HIV transgene targeting HIV-1 protease, for example. Cells that are multiply transduced resist HIV challenge better than do singly transduced cells (Strayer et al., 2002c).

Combinatorial therapeutics is well established in conventional pharmacotherapy: Several drugs that act differently against a disease target may improve protection without necessarily increasing toxicity (Ho, 1998). Although non-SV40 vectors can be used to deliver more than one gene, generally either two vectors must be given simultaneously (Putzer et al., 1998) or a new vector must be produced for each different transgene combination (Krisky et al., 1998; Mobley et al., 1998; Moriuchi et al., 2005; Tai et al., 2003). The high efficiency of rSV40 transduction allows sequential treatment with different transgenes, for better flexibility in devising combinations than is possible if new vectors must be made for each new combination.

Target Cell Types

Experiments done in vitro and in vivo have allowed us to determine the cell types to which rSV40 vectors deliver genes best. Most cell types of the hematopoietic system, including lympocytes, monocytes, and their derivatives, and the most primitive defined precursors, CD34 + cells, are very effectively transduced by rSV40 vectors. Epithelial cells of many organs, including the liver and lung, are also good targets for rSV40 gene transfer. When these vectors were tested for comparative transduction of resting and actively cycling cells (lymphocytes or CD34 + cells), both appeared to be transduced with similar efficiency (Strayer et al., 1997b; 2000). Neurons, the quintessential postmitotic G0 cell, are readily transduced by rSV40 vectors (Cordelier et al., 2003c; Louboutin et al., 2007). It should be emphasized that several of these cell types have been particularly difficult targets for gene delivery using other vectors, especially neurons and unstimulated hematopoietic progenitor cells (Strayer and Milano, 1996; Cordelier et al., 2003c).

Some cell types are not transduced, or are transduced very inefficiently, by these vectors. Among these are striated and smooth muscle and germ line cells (ova and sperm). A summary of the types of cells that have been tested for trans-ducibility with SV40-derived vectors and the results of those studies is presented in Table 6.1.

Injecting virus directly into an organ or an organ's blood supply, preferentially delivers vector to that organ but does not give total organ specificity. Thus, administering rSV40s into the hepatic portal vein provides excellent transgene

TABLE 6.1   Cell Types Tested for Transduction by rSV40s, in Vitro and in Vivo[a]

	Test Conditions
Cell Types Efficiently Transduced	
Hepatocytes	In vitro and in vivo by direct injection into hepatic portal vein
Bone marrow CD34 + cells	In vitro with and without stimulation, ex vivo with reimplantation, and in vivo by direct injection into bone marrow
Lymphocytes (B and T)	In vitro with and without stimulation and in vivo
Monocytes, macrophages, and dendritic cells	In vitro (in the case of macrophages and dendritic cells, monocytes were differentiated into these cell types by cytokine treatments)
Neurons	In vitro and by direct intracerebral injection In vivo
Microglia	In vitro and In vivo by direct intracerebral inoculation
Vascular endothelium	In vivo by intravenous (IV) inoculation
Renal tubular epithelium	In vivo by IV inoculation
Keratinocytes	In vivo by subcutaneous inoculation
Lung: alveolar type II cells and airway lining cells	In vitro and In vivo by intratracheal instillation
Cell Types Not Efficiently Transduced	
Striated muscle (normal)	In vivo by direct intramuscular injection
Cardiac muscle (normal)	In vivo by IV injection
Ova	In vitro
Astrocytes (brain)	In vitro and by direct intracerebral injection In vivo

[a]Cell types not mentioned specifically were not examined.

expression in hepatocytes, but cells in some other organs may also be transduced (J. R. Chowdhury and D. S. Strayer, unpublished).

SV40-Derived Vectors Do Not Elicit Detectable Immune Responses

Discussions of vector immunogenicity (i.e., whether they elicit immune responses) usually focus on whether transduced cells are recognized and eliminated by the T-cell arm of the immune system (Bennett, 2003). This type of immunity usually reflects activation of viral capsid genes in trans by cell transcription factors, with subsequent presentation of those proteins at transduced cell membranes, immune recognition, then cellular elimination by T-cell-mediated immunity, and has greatly limited the effectiveness, particularly of adenoviral vectors (Yang et al., 1995). Gene transfer with rSV40 vectors does not lead to elimination of transduced cells by this mechanism.

There is another type of immune reactivity, however, that is rarely mentioned: each virion is a particulate antigen in its own right. As such, it can be phagocytosed by professional antigen-presenting cells. Its capsid or envelope may then elicit neutralizing antibody, which, in the serum, may bind and inactivate succeeding doses of the virus. Consequently, most vectors can be administered only once or twice (Beck et al., 1999; Moskalenko et al., 2000; Chen et al., 2000; Vincent et al., 2001; Liu and Muruve, 2003).

Virtually all viral vectors currently used for gene transfer (adenovirus, adenoassociated virus, lentiviruses, and oncoretroviruses) elicit neutralizing antibody, whether or not they impart antigenicity to transduced cells. If serial dosing is required, different serotypes of the parent virus must be used to make a new vector for each administration (Rober-Guroff et al., 1998).

SV40 vectors are the exception to this rule. Uniquely, rSV40s can be given many times but do not elicit detectable neutralizing antibodies (Kondo et al., 1998; Sauter et al., 2000; McKee and Strayer, 2002). This observation has been repeated in several laboratories and is a unique feature of this vector system. Therefore, alone among gene delivery vehicles, rSV40s, whether bearing one transgene or different transgenes, can be administered repeatedly. If the initial therapeutic effect does not suffice or the target escapes from protection afforded by one transgene, repeat—and repeated—administration of that vector or an rSV40 bearing a different transgene may be performed weeks or months after the first injection without reduction in transduction efficiency. The explanation for this remarkable and distinctive characteristic of rSV40s probably lies in their entry pathway, which totally bypasses the cell's antigen-processing apparatus (Pelkmans et al., 2001,2002).

Longevity of Transgene Expression

Levels of transgene expression provided by most integrating vectors diminish over time, probably due to promoter methylation and other causes (Chen et al.,

1997; Kalberer et al., 2000; Lung et al., 2000; McInerney et al., 2000; Pannell et al., 2000; Svoboda et al., 2000; Yamano et al., 2000; Pannell and Ellis, 2001; Rosenqvist et al., 2002; Swindle and Klug, 2002; Iba et al., 2003; Swindle et al., 2004; Yao et al., 2004). In contrast, rSV40-delivered transgene expression does not vary: A level of transgene expression, once established, is maintained durably: over one year in vitro and in vivo (Strayer and Milano, 1996; Sauter et al., 2000; Strayer et al., 2002b; Liu et al., 2005).

Integration of Vector DNA

rSV40 DNAs appear to persist by integrating into the cell genome. No uninte-grated vector genome is detectable by one week postinoculation (Strayer et al., 2002a). In addition, as with wtSV40 (Botchan et al., 1976,1980), rSV40 vectors integrate randomly into cellular DNA: All cellular integration sites are different and the circular viral genome opens differently for each integrand (Strayer et al., 2002a).

In work by Strayer et al. 2002a, at an input MOI (multiplicity of infection) value between 10 and 100, an average of three copies of rSV40 genomes were integrated per cell. These integrands were distinct. That is, multiple integrations at one site (i.e., concatamers) were not detected.

Protein Production Delivered by rSV40s

Although it should theoretically be possible to express virtually any gene using viral vectors, this expectation has been frustrated repeatedly. Transgene expres-sion delivered using the various viral vectors has not followed predictable pat-terns. Extrapolations from viral expression of native viral genes do not always apply to viruses reengineered to carry foreign genes.

rSV40s are not exceptions to this generalization. They have been used very effectively with constitutive pol II and pol III promoters as well as several types of conditional pol II promoters. In general, expression of small untranslated RNAs (e.g., siRNAs, ribozymes, antisense), whether using pol II or pol III pro-moters, has been excellent in vitro (e.g., Zern et al., 1999) and in vivo (Duan et al., 2004).

The levels of proteins produced after rSV40 transduction, on the other hand, are usually low compared to the initial levels observed after transduction by some other viral vectors (e.g., adenovirus). Thus, rSV40 gene delivery is unlikely to be used to manufacture high levels of serum proteins, although repeated trans-ductions may increase serum protein levels to the level desired.

Low levels of production of physiologically active molecules may actually be preferable. By the same token, supraphysiological production of some proteins driven by powerful promoters may not necessarily be advantageous (McKee and Strayer, 2003; H.J. McKee, and D.S. Strayer, in preparation).

Transgenes that May Not Be Produced Detectably

Some transgenes are not expressed sufficiently to be useful. With few exceptions, these are nonmammalian, invertebrate, or prokaryotic in origin, and are often used as markers (e.g., *Escherichia coli* β-galactosidase, green fluorescent protein). Likely explanations for this phenomenon involve promoter inactivation during packaging and are independent of the packaging cell lines used. Undoubtedly, low levels of marker protein expression have limited the appeal of this vector system, even though these markers have little or no therapeutic value. Markers employed in the rSV40 system are usually peptide epitopes (e.g., FLAG) attached to termini of carrier proteins (Strayer et al., 2002c; Cordelier et al., 2003c; Liu et al., 2005).

Hardiness of rSV40 Vectors

Many vectors used for gene transfer are very fragile (e.g., they lose infectivity on ultracentrifugation or lyophilization). In contrast, rSV40s survive concentration by ultracentrifugation and can be lyophilized without appreciable loss of infectivity. If stored lyophilized, even at room temperature for several weeks, rSV40s retain up to 20% of their original activity (Strayer et al., 2005b). A summary of the characteristics of rSV40 vectors is presented in Table 6.2.

SAFETY OF SV40-DERIVED VECTORS

The main concerns for the safety of SV40-based vectors are contamination of vector stocks with wt replication-competent SV40, and pathogenetically significant insertional mutagenesis. We have never detected *Tag*+SV40 revertants in our vector stocks, as determined by multiple PCR rounds of 40-cycle amplification. Other reports, using vectors prepared differently or in different sublines of COS7 cells, may differ in this respect (Vera et al., 2004). Further, we have engineered a packaging cell line that does not share sequences with any of our "gutless" rSV40 constructs. These cells package vectors as well as COS7 cells and are extremely unlikely to generate wtSV40 revertants. Thus, to date we have no evidence of such contamination in rSV40 vector preparations.

Parenthetically, we take note of the controversy over whether wtSV40 is pathogenic for humans. Some investigators have claimed that *Tag* may be involved in some human tumors. Others have either failed to repeat some of these findings or failed to find epidemiologic evidence of tumorigenesis related to SV40 (Kirschenstein and Gerber, 1962; Deichman et al., 1978; Mortimer et al., 1981; Perbal et al., 1983; Geissler, 1990; Bergsagel et al., 1992; Pepper et al., 1996; Lednicky et al., 1997; Olin and Giesecke, 1997; Suzuki et al., 1997; Strickler et al., 1998; Center for Disease Control, 2002; Institute of Medicine, 2003; Shah, 2006; Poulin and DeCaprio, 2006). Whatever the resolution of this matter, the lack of wtSV40 and of *Tag* in our vector stocks renders this issue largely moot regarding the SV40-derived vectors described here.

TABLE 6.2   Principal Traits of Recombinant SV40-Derived Vectors

Attribute	Typical rSV40 Characteristics	Consequences
Antigenicity of transduced cells	No detectable inflammatory or immune reaction to rSV40-transduced cells	Transgene expression is not limited by immunity directed against the vector
Virion antigenicity	None detectable	Multiple administrations are possible in vivo without loss of transduction efficiency
Titer	Generally, 10^{10} to 10^{11} and can be further concentrated	Transduction is not usually limited by vector titer
Durability of transgene expression	Long-term transgene expression in vivo (tested through 18 months) and in vitro (tested through six months of continuous culture)	Once a level of transgene expression is established it will be maintained; thus, therapeutic effect is likely to be permanent
Cloning capacity	5 kb	Exogenous DNA, including transgenes, promoters, poly-adenylation signals, etc., up to 5 kb can be packaged efficiently
Host cell range	Some cell types are transduced effectively (although some are not); effective transduction is independent of cell cycle	Both resting and cycling cells can be transduced efficiently
Efficiency	Very high: in vitro, > 98% without selection, at MOI = 10	Effective gene delivery, both in cultured cells and in vivo
Persistence in dividing cells	Integration into cellular DNA	Durable transgene carriage and expression in dividing cells
Robustness	Can be lyophilized and stored for several weeks at temperatures that are above optimal (e.g., room temperatures)	Very hardy
Levels of transgene expression	High levels of expression of untranslated RNAs (RNA interference, etc.). Lower levels of protein production driven by pol II promoters	Excellent gene delivery for small RNAs, especially with pol III promoters; more than adequate for most intracellular proteins Produce and export modest levels of protein to the blood

Vector Integration and Consequent Mutagenesis

SV40 integrates randomly into the cellular genome. In doing so, it may activate or inactivate cellular genes. If a critical gene is disrupted, a cell may cease to function normally, or die. As a practical matter, this has not proven to be a problem in studies, especially clinical trials, using other integrating vectors. A greater concern is insertional activation. This mechanism may explain tumors recently reported in human trials using MuLV vectors (Engel et al., 2003; Hacein-Bey-Abina et al., 2003; Kohn et al., 2003; Marshall, 2003).

Unlike retroviral vectors, which have linear genomes, SV40's circular genome opens differently for each integration event (Strayer et al., 2002a). rSV40 vector integration is thus random relative to both cell and virus genomes. The enhancer functions characteristic of oncoretroviruses are not associated with SV40 integration. Further, promoter-related activation of cellular genes would occur only if the virus integrated just 5′ to the transcriptional start site of a cellular gene and if the viral sequences at the integration site were just 3′ to an active pol II promoter. Insertional activation of a cellular gene may thus occur with rSV40s, but is much less likely than for MuLV vectors.

It should be noted that any DNA entering a cell's nucleus may integrate into the cellular DNA. Gene delivery of all types therefore carries some risk. Like all gene delivery vectors, rSV40 vectors must be used cautiously. To date, there is no indication that rSV40 vectors pose any greater safety concern than that of other gene delivery vehicles.

CONCLUSION

Currently, the properties of viral and nonviral vectors that serve to deliver foreign genetic material to cells and organs that are the targets for such delivery determine many parameters of the outcome of gene transfer. There is not, and probably will never be, a gene delivery vector system that is suitable for all needs. However, SV40-derived vectors have important unique properties that make them particularly suitable for certain gene delivery purposes. If one seeks permanent gene delivery with long-term expression (whether conditional or constitutive) and/or in which repeated administration of one or more vectors is desirable, there is no other vector system currently available that matches the ease with which rSV40s can perform these tasks. These vectors are also especially, if not necessarily uniquely, appropriate for gene delivery to cells of the hematopoietic system, liver, brain (neurons and microglia), and certain other epithelial organs. Additionally, the hardiness of rSV40s makes them particularly attractive in settings in which optimal storage and transportation may not be available. There is great need for additional options in gene delivery vehicles. SV40-derived vectors may have an important contribution to make to gene therapy.

Acknowledgments

The many people who have worked with me in my laboratory over the years have been instrumental in generating the data and, more important, asking the questions, that have moved this vector system forward. They are too numerous to name, but special thanks are due Pierre Cordelier, Dawn Geverd, Charles Ko, Maria Lamothe, Aleksey Matsckevich, Hayley McKee, Joe Milano, Carmen Nichols, Maria Vera, Danlan Wei, and Lev Yurgenev. Many collaborators have been key in advancing our understanding of this system, its strengths, its limitations, and its potential therapeutic applications: J. Roy Chowdhury, Ling-Xun Duan, Harris Goldstein, Roger Pomerantz, Elisabeth Van Bockstaele, John Zaia, and Mark Zern. Work described here was supported by NIH grants AI41399, AI48244, MH69122, and MH70287.

REFERENCES

Arad U, Zeira E, El-Latif MA, et al. (2005). Liver-targeted gene therapy by SV40-based vectors using the hydrodynamic injection method. *Hum Gene Ther*. 16:361–371.

Beck SE, Jones LA, Chesnut K, et al. (1999). Repeated delivery of adeno-associated virus vectors to the rabbit airway. *J Virol*. 73:9446–9455.

Bennett J (2003). Immune response following intraocular delivery of recombinant viral vectors. *Gene Ther*. 10:977–982.

Bergsagel DJ, Finegold MJ, Butel JS, Kupsky WJ, Garcea RL. (1992). DNA sequences similar to those of simian virus 40 in ependymomas and choroid plexus tumors of childhood. *N Engl J Med*. 326:988–993.

Botchan M, Topp W, Sambrook J. (1976). The arrangement of simian virus 40 sequences in the DNA of transformed cells. *Cell*. 9:269–287.

Botchan M, Stringer J, Mitchison T, Sambrook J. (1980). Integration and excision of SV40 DNA from the chromosome of a transformed cell. *Cell*. 20:143–152.

BouHamdan M, Duan L-X, Pomerantz RJ, Strayer DS. (1999). Inhibition of HIV-1 by anti-integrase single-chain variable fragment (SFv): delivery by SV40 provides durable protection against HIV-1 and does not require selection. *Gene Ther*. 6:660–666.

BouHamdan M, Strayer DS, Wei D, et al. (2001). Inhibition of HIV-1 infection by down-regulation of the CXCR4 co-receptor using an intracellular single chain variable fragment against CXCR4. *Gene Ther*. 8:408–418.

Centres for Disease Control (2002). Simian virus 40 (SV40), polio virus vaccine, and cancer. http://www.cdc.gov/nip/vacsafe/concerns/Cancer/default.htm.

Chen WY, Bailey EC, McCune SL, Dong JY, Townes TM (1997). Reactivation of silenced, virally transduced genes by inhibitors of histone deacetylase. *Proc Natl Acad Sci U S A*. 94:5798–5803.

Chen Y, Yu DC, Charlton D, Henderson DR (2000). Pre-existent adenovirus antibody inhibits systemic toxicity and antitumor activity of CN706 in the nude mouse LNCaP xenograft model: implications and proposals for human therapy. *Hum Gene Ther*. 11:1553–1567.

Cole CN, Conzen SD (2001). Polyomavirinae: the viruses and their replication. In: Knipe DM, Howley, PM, eds. *Fields Virology*, Philadelphia, PA: Lippincott Williams & Wilkins; 2141–2174.

Cordelier P, Strayer DS (2003). Conditional expression of α1-antitrypsin delivered by recombinant SV40 vectors protects lymphocytes against HIV. *Gene Ther*. 10: 2153–2156.

Cordelier P, Zern MA, Strayer DS (2003a). HIV-1 proprotein processing as a target for gene therapy. *Gene Ther*. 10:467–477.

Cordelier P, Morse B, Strayer DS (2003b). Targeting CCR5 with siRNAs: using recombinant SV40-derived vectors to protect macrophages and microglia from R5-tropic HIV. *Oligonucleotides*. 13:281–294.

Cordelier P, Van Bockstaele E, Calarota SA, Strayer DS (2003c). Inhibiting AIDS in the central nervous system: gene delivery to protect neurons from HIV. *Mol. Ther*. 7:801–810.

DeFillippis RA, Goodwin EC, Wu L, DiMaio D (2003). Endogenous human papillomavirus *E6* and *E7* proteins differently regulate proliferation senescence, and apoptosis in HeLa cervical carcinoma cells. *J Virol*. 77:151–156.

Deichman G, Kashkina L, Rapp, F (1978). Tumor induction in newborn and adult Syrian hamsters infected with SV40 temperature-sensitive mutants. *Intervirology*. 10: 120–124.

Duan Y-Y, Wu J, Zhu J-L, et al. (2004). Bifunctional gene therapy for human α1-antitrypsin deficiency in an animal model using SV40-derived vectors. *Gastroenterology* 127:1222–1232.

Engel BC, Kohn DB, Podsakoff GM (2003). Update on gene therapy of inherited immune deficiencies. *Curr Opin Mol Ther*. 5:503–507.

Fried M, Prives C (1986). The biology of simian virus 40 and polyomavirus. *Cancer Cells*. 4:1–16.

Geissler E (1990). SV40 and human brain tumors. *Prog Med Virol*. 37:211–222.

Gething MJ, Sambrook J (1981). Cell-surface expression of influenza haemagglutinin from a cloned DNA copy of the RNA gene. *Nature*. 293:620–625.

Gluzman Y (1981). SV40-transformed simian cells support the replication of early SV40 mutants. *Cell*. 23:175–182.

Gluzman Y, Sambrook JF, Frisque RJ (1980). Expression of early genes of origin-defective mutants of simian virus 40. *Proc Natl Acad Sci U S A*. 77:3898–3902.

Goldstein H, Pettoello-Mantovani M, Anderson CM, Cordelier P, Pomerantz RJ, Strayer DS (2002). Gene therapy delivered in vivo using an SV40-derived vector inhibits the development of in vivo HIV-1 infection of *Thy/liv-SCID/hu* mice. *J Infect Dis*. 185:1425–1430.

Hacein-Bey-Abina S, Von Kalle C, Schmidt M, et al. (2003). LMO2-Associated clonal T cell proliferation in two patients after gene therapy for SCID-X1. *Science*. 302: 415–419.

Ho DD (1998). Toward HIV eradication or remission: the tasks ahead. *Science*. 280: 1866–1867.

Iba H, Mizutani T, Ito T (2003). SWI/SNF chromatin remodeling complex and retroviral gene silencing. *Rev Med Virol*. 13:99–110.

Institute of Medicine (2003). *Immunization Safety Review:* SV40 contamination of polio vaccine and cancer. http://www.nap.edu/books/0309086108/html/.

Jayan GC, Cordelier P, Patel C, et al. (2001). SV40-derived vectors provide effective transgene expression and inhibition of HIV-1 using constitutive conditional, and pol III promoters. *Gene Ther.* 8:1033–1042.

Kalberer CP, Pawliuk R, Imren S, et al. (2000). Preselection of retrovirally transduced bone marrow avoids subsequent stem cell gene silencing and age-dependent extinction of expression of human beta-globulin in engrafted mice. *Proc Natl Acad Sci U S A.* 97:5411–5415.

Kimchi-Sarfati C, Ben-Nun-Schaul O, Rund D, Oppenheim A, Gottesman MM (2002). In vitro-packaged SV40 pseudovirions as highly efficient vectors for gene transfer. *Hum Gene Ther.* 13:299–310.

Kirschenstein RL, Gerber P (1962). Ependymomas produced after intracerebral inoculation of SV40 into newborn hamsters. *Nature.* 195:299–300.

Kohn DB, Sadelain M, Glorioso JC (2003). Occurrence of leukaemia following gene therapy of X-linked SCID. *Nat Rev Cancer.* 3:477–488.

Kondo R, Feitelson MA, Strayer DS (1998). Use of SV40 to immunize against hepatitis B surface antigen: implications for the use of SV40 for gene transduction and its use as an immunizing agent. *Gene Ther.* 5:575–582.

Krisky DM, Marconi PC, Oligino TJ, et al. (1998). Development of herpes simplex virus replication-defective multigene vectors for combination gene therapy applications. *Gene Ther.* 5:1517–1530.

Lednicky JA, Stewart AR, Jenkins JJ, Finegold MJ, Butel JS (1997). SV40 DNA in human osteosarcomas shows sequence variation among T-antigen genes. *Int J Cancer.* 72:791–800.

Liu O, Muruve DA (2003). Molecular basis of the inflammatory response to adenovirus vectors. *Gene Ther.* 10:935–940.

Liu B, Daviau J, Nichols CN, Strayer DS (2005). In vivo gene transfer to rat bone marrow progenitor cells using rSV40 viral vectors. *Blood.* 105:2655–2663.

Louboutin JP, Agrawal L, Reyes BAS, et al. (in press). Localized and generalized rSV40 gene delivery of antioxidant enzymes to the brain to protect neurons from oxidant stress by HIV-1 gp120. *Gene Ther.*

Lung HY, Meeus IS, Weinberg RS, Atweh GF (2000). *Blood Cells Mol Dis.* 26:613–619.

Marshall E (2003). Gene therapy: second child in French trial is found to have leukemia. *Science.* 299:320.

Matskevich AA, Strayer DS (2005). Exploiting hepatitis C virus activation of NFκB to deliver HCV-responsive expression of interferons α and γ. *Gene Ther.* 10:1861–1873.

Matskevich AA, Cordelier P, Strayer DS (2003). Conditional expression of interferons α and γ activated by HBV as genetic therapy for hepatitis B. *J Interferon Cytokine Res.* 23:709–721.

McInerney JM, Nawrocki JR, Lowrey CH (2000). Long-term silencing of retroviral vectors is resistant to reversal by tricostatin A and 5-azacytidine. *Gene Ther.* 7:653–663.

McKee HJ, Strayer DS (2002). Immune response against SIV envelope glycoprotein, using recombinant SV40 as a vaccine delivery vector. *Vaccine.* 20:3613–3625.

McKee HJ, Strayer DS (2003). Delivery of SIV gag together with immunostimulatory cytokines by SV40-derived vectors generates very strong antigen-specific immune responses. *Mol Ther*. 7:S262.

Mobley SR, Liu TJ, Hudson JM, Clayman GL (1998). In vitro growth suppression by adenoviral transduction of p21 and p16 in squamous cell carcinoma of the head and neck: a research model for combination gene therapy. *Arch. Otolaryngol. Head Neck Surg*. 124:88–92.

Moriuchi S, Glorioso JC, Maruno M, et al. (2005). Combination gene therapy for glioblastoma involving herpes simplex virus vector-mediated codelivery of mutant IkappaBalpha and kinase. *Cancer Gene Ther*. 12:487–496.

Mortimer EA, Jr, Lepow ML, Gold E, Robbins FC, Burton GJ, Fraumeni JF (1981). Long-term follow-up of persons inadvertently inoculated with SV40 as neonates. *N Engl J Med*. 305:1517–1518.

Moskalenko M, Chen L, van Rooey M, et al. (2000). Epitope mapping of human anti-adeno-associated virus type 2 neutralizing antibodies: implications for gene therapy and virus structure. *J Virol*. 74:1761–1766.

Muzyczka N (1980). Construction of an SV40-derived cloning vector. *Gene*. 11:63–77.

Naeger LK, Goodwin EC, Hwang ES, DeFilippis RA, Zhang H, DiMaio D (1999). Bovine papillomavirus E2 protein activates a complex growth-inhibitory program in p53-negative HT-3 cervical carcinoma cells that includes repression of cyclin A and cdc25A phosphatase genes and accumulation of hypophosphorylated retinoblastoma protein. *Cell Growth Diff*. 10:413–422.

Olin P, Giesecke J (1997). Potential exposure to SV40 in polio vaccines used in Sweden during 1957: no impact on cancer incidence rates 1960 to 1993. *Dev Biol Stand*. 94:227–233.

Pannell D, Ellis J (2001). Silencing of gene expression: implications for design of retrovirus vectors. *Rev Med Virol*. 11:205–217.

Pannell D, Osborne CS, Yao S, et al. (2000). Retrovirus vector silencing is de nova methylase independent and marked by a repressive histone code. *EMBO J*. 19:5884–5894.

Pelkmans L, Kartenbeck J, Helenius, A. (2001). Caveolar endocytosis of simian virus 40 reveals a new two-step vesicular-transport pathway to the ER. *Nat Cell Biol*. 3:473–483.

Pelkmans L, Puntener D, Helenius A (2002). Local actin polymerization and dynamin recruitment in SV40-induced internalization of caveolae. *Science*. 296:535–539.

Pepper C, Jasani B, Navabi H, Wynford-Thomas D, Gibbs AR (1996). Simian virus 40 large T antigen (SV40LTAg) primer specific DNA amplification in human pleural mesothelioma tissue. *Thorax*. 51:1074–1076.

Perbal BV, Linke HK, Fareed GC (1983). *Molecular Biology of Polyomaviruses and Herpesviruses*, John Wiley & Sons, New York.

Poulin DL, DeCaprio JA (2006). Is there a role for SV40 in human cancer? *J Clin Oncol*. 24:4356–4365.

Putzer BM, Bramson JL, Addison CL, et al. (1998). Combination therapy with interleukin-2 and wild-type p53 expressed by adenoviral vectors potentiates tumor regression in a murine model of breast cancer. *Hum Gene Ther*. 9:707–718.

Rober-Guroff M, Kaur H, Patterson LJ, et al. (1998). Vaccine protection against a heterologous, non-syncytium-inducing, primary human immunodeficiency virus. *J Virol*. 72:10275–10280.

Rosenberg BH, Deutsch JF, Ungers GE (1981). Growth and purification of SV40 virus for biochemical studies. *J Virol Methods*. 3:167–176.

Rosenqvist N, Hard AF, Segerstad C, Samuelsson C, Johansen J, Lundberg C (2002). Activation of silenced transgene expression in neural precursor cell lines by inhibitors of histone deacetylation. *J Gene Med*. 4:248–257.

Sandalon Z, Oppenheim A (1997). Self-assembly and protein-protein interactions between the SV40 capsid proteins produced in insect cells. *Virology*. 237:414–421.

Sauter BV, Parashar B, Chowdhury NR, et al. (2000). Gene transfer to the liver using a replication-deficient recombinant SV40 vector results in long-term amelioration of jaundice in Gunn rats. *Gastroenterology*. 119:1348–1357.

Shah KV (2006). SV40 and human cancer: A review of recent data. *Int J Cancer*. 120:215–223.

Strayer DS (1999a). Gene therapy using SV40-derived vectors: What does the future hold? *J Cell Physiol*. 181:375–384.

Strayer DS, Milano J (1996). SV40 mediates stable gene transfer in vivo. *Gene Ther*. 3:581–587.

Strayer DS, Duan L-X, Ozaki I, Milano J, Bobraski LE, Bagasra O (1997a). Titering replication-defective virus for use in gene transfer. *BioTechniques*. 22:447–450.

Strayer DS, Kondo R, Milano J, Duan L-X (1997b). Use of SV40-based vectors to transduce foreign genes to normal human peripheral blood mononuclear cells. *Gene Ther*. 4:219–225.

Strayer DS, Pomerantz RJ, Yu M, et al. (2000). Efficient gene transfer to hematopoietic progenitor cells using SV40-derived vectors. *Gene Ther*. 7:886–895.

Strayer DS, Lamothe M, Wei D, et al. (2001). Generation of recombinant SV40 vectors for gene transfer. In: Raptis L, ed. *SV40 Protocols*. Vol. 165, *Methods in Molecular Biology*. Walker JM, ed Totowa, NJ: Humana Press.

Strayer DS, Branco F, Zern MA, et al. (2002a). Durability of transgene expression and vector integration: recombinant SV40-derived gene therapy vectors. *Mol Ther*. 6: 227–237.

Strayer DS, Zern MA, Chowdhury JR (2002b). What can SV40-derived vectors do for gene therapy? *Curr Opin Mol Ther*. 4:313–323.

Strayer DS, Branco F, Landré J, BouHamdan M, Shaheen F, Pomerantz RJ (2002c). Combination genetic therapy to inhibit HIV-1. *Mol Ther*. 5:33–41.

Strayer DS, Feitelson MA, Sun B, Matskevich AA (2005a). Paradigms for conditional expression of RNAi molecules for use against viral targets. *Methods Enzymol*. 392: 227–241.

Strayer DS, Cordelier P, Kondo R, et al. (2005b). What they are, how they work and why they do what they do: the story of SV40-derived gene therapy vectors and what they have to offer. *Curr Gene Ther*. 5:151–165.

Strickler HD, Rosenberg PS, Devesa SS, Hertel J, Fraumeni JF Jr, Goedert JJ (1998). Contamination of poliovirus vaccines with simian virus 40 (1955–1963) and subsequent cancer rates. *JAMA* 279:292–295.

Suzuki SO, Mizoguchi M, Iwaki T (1997). Dection of SV40 T antigen genome in human gliomas. *Brain Tumor Pathol*. 14:125–129.

Svoboda J, Hejnar J, Geryk J, Elleder D, Vernerova Z (2000). Retrovirus in foreign species and the problem of provirus silencing. *Gene*. 261:181–188.

Swindle CS, Klug CA (2002). Mechanisms that regulate silencing of gene expression from retroviral vectors. *J Hematother Stem Cell Res*. 11:449–456.

Swindle CS, Kim HG, Klug CA (2004). Mutation of CpGs in the murine stem cell virus retroviral vector long terminal repeat represses silencing in embryonic stem cells. *J Biol Chem*. 279:34–41.

Tai KF, Chen PJ, Chen DS, Hwang LH (2003). Concurrent delivery of GM-CSF and endostatin genes by a single adenoviral vector provides a synergistic effect on the treatment of orthotopic liver tumors. *J Gene Med*. 5:386–398.

Vera M, Fortes P (2004). Simian virus-40 as a gene therapy vector. *DNA Cell Biol*. 23:271–282.

Vera M, Prieto J, Strayer DS, Fortes P (2004). Factors influencing the production of recombinant SV40 vectors. *Mol Ther*. 10:780–791.

Vincent T, Harvey BG, Hogan SM, Bailey CJ, Crystal RG, Leopold PL (2001). Rapid assessment of adenovirus serum neutralizing antibody titer based on quantitative, morphometric evaluation of capsid binding and intracellular trafficking: population analysis of adenovirus capsid association with cells is predictive of adenovirus infectivity. *J Virol*. 75:1516–1521.

Yamano T, Ura K, Morishita R, Nakajima H, Monden M, Kaneda Y (2000). Amplification of transgene expression in vitro and in vivo using a novel inhibitor of histone deacetylase. *Mol Ther*. 1:574–580.

Yang Y, Ki Q, Ertl HC, Wilson JM (1995). Cellular and humoral immune responses to viral antigens create barriers to lung-directed gene therapy with recombinant adenoviruses. *J Virol*. 69:2004–2015.

Yao S, Sukonnik T, Bharadwai RR, Pasceri P, Ellis J (2004). Retrovirus silencing variegation, extinction, and memory are controlled by dynamic interplay of multiple epigenetic modifications. *Mol Ther*. 10:27–36.

Zern MA, Ozaki I, Duan L-X, Pomerantz R, Liu S-L, Strayer DS (1999). A novel SV40-based vector successfully transduces and expresses an alpha 1-antitrypsin ribozyme in a human hepatoma-derived cell line. *Gene Ther*. 6:114–120.

7 Herpes Simplex Virus Vectors

ANNA-MARIA ANESTI

Biovex Ltd, The Windeyer Institute, London, UK

ROBERT S. COFFIN

Biovex Advanced Vaccines, Abingdon, Oxford, UK

Herpes simplex virus (HSV) has many unique features that support its development as a vector for the delivery of genes to the nervous system. It is a highly infectious, naturally neurotrophic virus able to establish lifelong latency in neurons, following retrograde transport to the cell bodies. The HSV genome has a high capacity to accept foreign DNA, can be easily manipulated, and the virus can be produced to high titers. In addition, the latent viral genome does not integrate into the host chromosome, thus eliminating the possibility of insertional activation or inactivation of cellular genes. Although these aspects of the virus biology were promising, two main issues required to be resolved for long-term application: the appropriate engineering of the vector genome to create safe, nontoxic vectors, and developing promoters to achieve long-term transgene expression during latency. The biology of HSV-1 and the progress being made in the generation of vectors for neuronal gene delivery are discussed in the following sections.

THE BIOLOGY OF HSV-1

Structure and Viral Entry

The mature HSV-1 virion consists of a DNA core contained in an icosahedral capsid surrounded by a matrix of proteins, referred to as the *tegument,* and a trilaminar lipid envelope, in which are embedded at least 10 virally encoded glycoproteins (Figure 7.1). Initial attachment of the viral particle to the cell surface is mediated through binding of the envelope glycoproteins gC (Tal-Singer et al., 1995) and gB (Herold et al., 1994) to cell surface glycosaminoglycans, primarily heparan sulfate (Shieh et al., 1992). This nonspecific step is followed by attachment of glycoprotein gD to a second cellular receptor. A number of such receptors have been identified, including the herpes virus entry mediator A (HveA) and nectin-1 (HveC), which are members of the TNF-α p75 receptor

Concepts in Genetic Medicine, Edited by Boro Dropulic and Barrie Carter
Copyright © 2008 John Wiley & Sons, Inc.

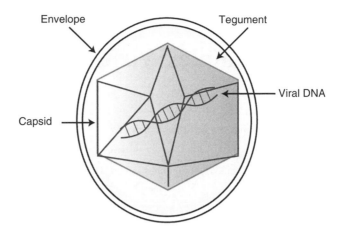

Figure 7.1 The mature HSV-1 virion consists of a lipid envelope, the tegument proteins, which are involved in shutdown of host protein synthesis, induction of vitalgene expression and virion assembly, an icosadeltahedral capsid, and a core of double-standard DNA.

family (Montgomery et al., 1996) and immunoglobulin superfamily (Geraghty et al., 1998), respectively. These molecules are widely expressed, accounting for the broad host range of the virus. HveC, which is thought to be the main entry receptor, is expressed in both neurons and epithelial cells. Entry into the cell is mediated through fusion of the viral envelope with the plasma membrane and release of the nucleocapsid and tegument proteins into the cytoplasm. The nucleocapsid is transported to the nuclear pore in a microtubule-dependent manner and the genome is deposited into the nucleus (Mabit et al., 2002).

HSV-1 Genome

The large HSV-1 genome consists of 152 kb of linear double-stranded DNA arranged as a unique long (U$_L$) and a unique short (U$_S$) region, each flanked by a pair of inverted repeats (IRs) (Figure 7.2). Approximately half of the 84 viral genes expressed are essential for viral replication in vitro. The nonessential genes, which are involved in functions important for virus–host interactions in vivo, such as immune evasion and shutdown of host protein synthesis, can be deleted in the generation of vectors, allowing insertion of large or multiple transgenes (approximately 30 kb can be inserted into the vectors described).

Lytic Infection

Viral gene expression during lytic infection proceeds in a tightly regulated, interdependent cascade in which three classes of viral genes are temporally expressed: immediate early (IE), early (E), and late (L) genes (Honess and Roizman, 1974)

Accessory Genes

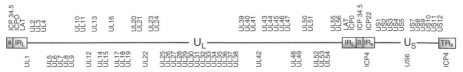

Figure 7.2 The 152-kb-long HSV-1 genome is arranged as unique long (U$_L$ and short (U$_S$) regions flanked by terminal and inverted repeats (TR and IR, respectively). the "a" sequences are required for packaging of the genome into the capsid. The location of the essential and nonessential genes is indicated.

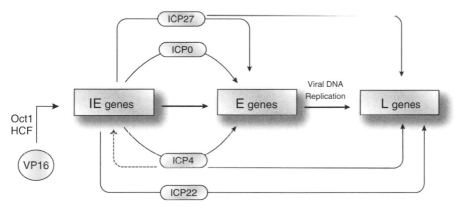

Figure 7.3 HSV-1 gene expression and regulation. The tegument protein VP16 interacts with Oct1 and host cell factor (HCF) to transactive IE gene promotors. Expression of IE genes is followed by expression of E genes, viral DNA replication, and subsequently, expression of L genes. ICP4 and ICP27 regulate expression of both E and L genes. ICP0 and ICP22 regulate E and L gene expression, respectively. ICP4 can also negatively regulate expression of IE genes.

(Figure 7.3). Expression of IE genes begins shortly after the genome arrives in the nucleus in the absence of de novo viral protein synthesis. This is followed by expression of E genes, which mainly encode proteins involved in viral DNA synthesis and replication. Expression of L genes, which mainly encode structural proteins, follows the onset of DNA replication. Viral DNA replication proceeds via a rolling circle mechanism that leads to the production of HSV-1 genome concatemers (Jacob et al., 1979). These are cleaved into genome-length units and packaged into the capsid through recognition of packaging sequences located in the IR.

Expression of IE genes is initiated by the tegument protein VP16 (also called Vmw65), which is a virus structural protein. VP16 activates transcription by binding, in concert with the cellular factors Oct-1 and host cell factor (HCF), to the TAATGARAT elements, which are present in all IE gene promoters

(Preston et al., 1988). The virus encodes five IE proteins, designated infected cell polypeptides (ICPs) 0, 4, 22, 27, and 47. With the exception of ICP47, these nuclear phosphoproteins are known to regulate the coordinated expression of the HSV genome. ICP4 and ICP27 are essential for virus replication. ICP4 acts as a repressor or activator of transcription (DeLuca and Schaffer, 1985) and is necessary for the transition from the IE to the E phase of viral gene expression (Dixon and Schaffer, 1980). ICP27 regulates the processing of viral and cellular mRNAs (Hardy and Sandri-Goldin, 1994), contributes to efficient early- and late-gene expression (Samaniego et al., 1995; Sacks et al., 1985), and may also modulate ICP0 and ICP4 activity (Sekulovich et al., 1988). ICP0 facilitates reactivation from latency in the mouse model (Gordon et al., 1990), is a transactivator of most viral and cellular promoters in transient assays (Everett, 1984; O'Hare and Hayward, 1985), and enhances viral gene expression and growth both in vitro and in vivo (Cai and Schaffer, 1992). Viruses lacking ICP0 function are replication competent, but grow very poorly and reactivate at lower levels than do wild-type viruses. ICP22 is not essential for growth in many cell types, but promotes efficient late-gene expression in a cell-type-specific manner (Sears et al., 1985). It is also involved in the production of a novel phosphorylated form of RNA polymerase II (Rice et al., 1995) and regulates the stability and splicing of ICP0 mRNA (Carter and Roizman, 1996). Finally, ICP47 blocks the presentation of antigenic peptides to CD8+ cells and therefore helps the virus to escape immune surveillance (York et al., 1994).

Life Cycle in Vivo

The life cycle of HSV-1 in vivo begins in epithelial cells of the skin or mucous membrane. Following lytic replication in the infected epithelia, progeny virions enter sensory nerve terminals, innervating the infection site, and the nucleocapsid and tegument proteins undergo retrograde axonal transport to the cell bodies in the spinal ganglia (Marchand and Schwab, 1986) (Figure 7.4). This provides a means of delivering genes to neurons distal from the site of inoculation in regions of the nervous system that are inaccessible by surgical techniques. Although other viral vectors such as adenovirus, adenoassociated virus, and lentivirus can infect neurons, none has evolved to be efficiently transported to neuronal cell bodies in vivo. Upon arrival at the cell body, HSV-1 either initiates lytic expression or enters latency. Reactivation of viral infection can occur and results in the production of progeny virions that are anterogradely transported back to the nerve terminals.

HSV-1 Latency

During latency, the viral genome is maintained in a stable episomal form and sometimes persists for the lifetime of the host in the absence of detectable infection (Mellerick and Fraser, 1987). Although most viral gene expression is silenced, a single region within the long repeat remains transcriptionally active,

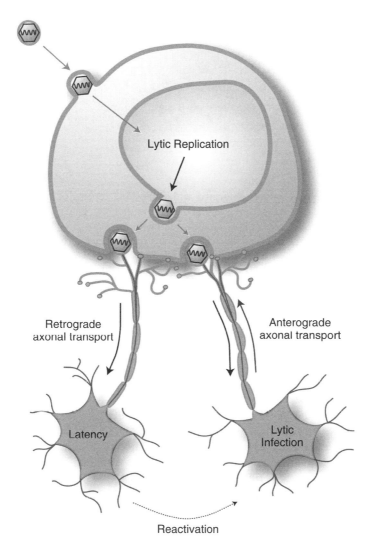

Figure 7.4   Life cycle of HSV-1 in vivo. Entry into epithelial cells is mediated through fusion of the viral envelope with the plasma membrane and release of the nucleocapsid and tegument proteins into the cytoplasm. The capsid is transported to the nucleus in a microtubule-dependent manner and the genome is deposited into the nucleus. Following lytic replication in the infected epithelia, progeny virions are retrogradely transported to the cell bodies of sensory neurons innervating the infection site. Upon arrival at the cell body, the virus either initiates lytic expression or enters latency. Latency allows the virus to persist within the host in the presence of an immune response. Periodic reactivation can occur in response to a wide variety of stimuli and results in the production of progeny virions that are anterogradely transported back to the nerve terminals.

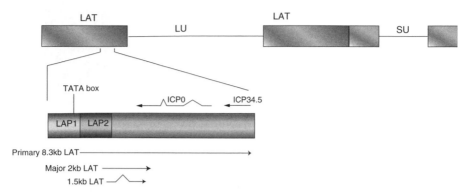

Figure 7.5   The LAT region is located within the long repeats of the HSV-1 genome and is the only region transcriptionally active during latency, generating a population of RNA species. The 2- and 1.5-kb LATs are the most abundant. The LATs are transcibed antisense and the last 723 bp of the 2-kb LAT are complementary to the 3′ end of ICPO. LAT expression is driven by LAP1 and LAP2. The LAP1 TATA box is located 736 bp upstream of the 5′ end the 2-kb LAT. LAP2 lies directly 3′ to LAP1 and is located 750 bp upstream of the 2-kb LAT.

generating a population of RNA species designated latency-associated transcripts (LATs) (Stevens et al., 1987) (Figure 7.5). The 8.3-kb polyadenylated primary LAT transcribed from this region is spliced to give a nonpolyadenylated 2-kb LAT, which can be further spliced to produce smaller LATs (Wechsler et al., 1988). The 2- and 1.5-kb LATs are abundant and accumulate in the nucleus as stable lariat introns (Farrell et al., 1991). Although the functions of LATs remain unknown, it is clear that they are not essential for the establishment and maintenance of latency, or reactivation from latency (Ho and Mocarski, 1989). They have, however, been suggested to regulate the efficiency of these processes (Thompson and Sawtell, 1997; Perng et al., 1999) and to play a role in the prevention of apoptosis in infected neurons (Perng et al., 2000) as well as the antisense regulation of IE gene expression (Chen et al., 1997; Mador et al., 1998).

LAT expression is driven by two promoters, referred to as latency active promoters 1 (LAP1) and 2 (LAP2). LAP1 contains a TATA box, which directs transcription starting 736 bp upstream of the 5′ end of the 2-kb LAT (Zwaagstra et al., 1991). LAP2 lies directly 3′ to LAP1, approximately 750 bp upstream of the 2-kb LAT, and is a GC-rich promoter homologous to mammalian housekeeping gene promoters (Goins et al., 1994). Deletion analysis suggests that LAP1 is primarily responsible for LAT expression during latency, whereas LAP2 is primarily responsible for LAT expression during lytic infection (Chen et al., 1995). Since LATs are not essential for the establishment or maintenance of latency, it is possible to insert genes within the LAT loci that allow the LAT promoters to drive expression during latency.

The mechanisms controlling the repression of viral lytic gene expression and the selective transcription of LATs during latency are poorly understood. In vitro studies have revealed that when sympathetic or sensory neurons are infected with HSV-1 in the presence of acyclovir to prevent virus replication, latency is established provided that nerve growth factor is present in the medium (Wilcox and Johnson, 1988). In other studies, when human fibroblasts are infected with mutants lacking VP16 and/or ICP0, the majority of viral genomes are retained in a quiescent state that resembles latency, and this state depends on the presence of ICP0 (Preston and Nicholl, 1997; Samaniego et al., 1998).

TYPES OF HSV-1 VECTORS

HSV-1 vectors engineered for gene delivery to the nervous system are either amplicons or replication-defective vectors.

Amplicon Vectors

Amplicons are plasmids bearing the gene of interest, the HSV origin of replication, and a packaging signal (Spaete and Frenkel, 1982). Following transfection into eukaryotic cells, amplicons are packaged as concatemers into HSV virions in the presence of a helper virus. Helper viruses were initially replication-defective viruses containing a deletion within an essential IE gene, such as ICP4 (Geller et al., 1990). Replication of the defective helper virus and packaging of the amplicon occur in a cell line capable of complementing the mutations in the deleted genes in trans. The main limitation of this system is that with each passage there is a chance of recombination between amplicon, helper viral genomes, and the complementing cell line, resulting in the potential production of replication-competent virus (During et al., 1994). Recently, it has been possible to package amplicons free of helper virus by providing a packaging-deficient helper virus genome via a bacterial artificial chromosome (BAC). The HSV BAC is deleted for ICP27, and the addition of DNA sequences renders it too large to be packaged into the capsid (Saeki et al., 2001).

Amplicons can be easily manipulated, contain multiple copies of the gene of interest, and have a large transgene capacity (up to 22 kb and potentially up to 150 kb). In addition, the choice of promoter is not critical for long-term expression, as amplicons do not enter latency but continue to express the gene until they are degraded. This has allowed high levels of reasonably long-term and cell-type specific expression to be obtained in the central nervous system (Kaplitt et al., 1994; Jin et al., 1996; Song et al., 1997; Sandler et al., 2002).

Replication-Defective Vectors

The alternative system, which is discussed in detail, involves the introduction of the gene of interest directly into the HSV-1 genome. This is achieved by insertion of the gene into a plasmid that contains the expression cassette flanked by specific HSV sequences. Following cotransfection into complementing cells, the cassette is inserted into the HSV genome by homologous recombination.

Deletion of either of the essential IE genes (ICP4 and ICP27) results in replication-defective viruses. These can be propagated directly to high titers in vitro in appropriate cell lines, which complement the deleted gene products in trans, without the need of a contaminating helper virus. Complementing cell lines for such deletions have been described, including E5, which complements ICP4 (DeLuca et al., 1985); B130/2, which complements ICP27 (Howard et al., 1998); and E26, which complements both ICP4 and ICP27 (Samaniego et al., 1995). In vivo, the temporal cascade of viral gene expression is incapable of proceeding past the IE phase, resulting in recombinants that can establish a persistent state very similar to latency. In addition, replication-defective vectors are unable to reactivate form latency and therefore persist for long periods of time in both neuronal and nonneuronal cells.

Minimizing Toxicity

Although deletion of ICP4 is sufficient to create a replication-defective vector, the remaining IE gene products, which are highly toxic to cells, are expressed abundantly (DeLuca et al., 1985) and thus, ICP4, ICP4/ICP22, or ICP4/ICP47 mutants are still toxic to neurons (Johnson et al., 1992). To prevent cytotoxicity, vectors containing multiple IE deletions have been engineered. HSV-1 recombinants deleted for all IE genes are entirely nontoxic to cells, but grow very poorly in the absence of ICP0 (Samaniego et al., 1997, 1998). The efficient propagation of such viruses is problematic, because it requires that all IE gene products are provided in trans by a single complementing cell line. This is difficult to produce due to the toxicity of the IE gene products. In addition, the elimination of all IE genes significantly reduces transgene expression (Samaniego et al., 1997). Retention of ICP0, which is a promiscuous transactivator of gene expression, allows efficient expression of transgenes and the virus to be propagated to high titers. Moreover, the $ICP4^-/ICP22^-/ICP27^-$ vector was found to be virtually nontoxic to both cultured cortical or dorsal root ganglia neurons and in the brain in vivo (Wu et al., 1996; Krisky et al., 1998).

Mutations in VP16, which can easily be complemented by addition of hexamethylbisacetamide (HMBA) to the growth medium, reduce or abolish transactivation of IE genes and present an alternative approach to inactivating all IE genes (Ace et al., 1989; Smiley and Duncan, 1997; Mossman and Smiley, 1999). At a high multiplicity of infection (MOI) value, however, the virus is still capable of replicating, and mutations in VP16 are therefore accompanied by deletion of IE genes such as ICP4 and/or ICP27. In that case, HMBA is not sufficient for virus growth, and complementing cell lines providing the equine herpesvirus 1 (EHV-1) homolog of VP16, together with ICP4 and ICP27, have been produced to eliminate the possibility of recombinational repair of the VP16 mutation (Thomas et al., 1999). A further block to replication in neurons is deletion of the nonessential gene ICP34.5, which is required for neurovirulence but allows the virus to replicate in several cell types in vitro (Coffin et al., 1996). Recombinant HSV-1 vectors with deletions in ICP27, ICP4, and ICP34.5 and an inactivating mutation in VP16 (in1814) are safe, nontoxic, and allow efficient gene delivery to neurons in culture and both the peripheral and central nervous system in vivo (Palmer et al., 2000; Lilley et al., 2001) (Figure 7.6).

Long-Term Expression During Latency

The ability of HSV-1 to establish a long-term latent infection in neurons has made it an attractive candidate as a vector for the delivery and expression of foreign genes into the nervous system. Obtaining prolonged expression of a transgene in latently infected neurons has, however, proven challenging, due to transcriptional silencing of most HSV promoters as well as exogenous promoters introduced into the latent viral genome (Fink et al., 1992; Lokensgard et al., 1994). For this reason, there is a great deal of interest in utilizing the latency promoters to drive expression of transgenes in neurons of the peripheral and central nervous system.

Insertion of a gene farther downstream of the LAP1 TATA box results in expression for longer periods (Ho and Mocarski, 1989) than when the gene is inserted immediately after the LAP1 TAT box (Dobson et al., 1989; Margolis et al., 1993). It therefore seemed that important elements in the sequences down-stream of LAP1 are required for the promoter to function during latency. LAP2, but not LAP1, is able to drive very low-level transgene expression during latency when inserted at an ectopic locus within the HSV genome, such as gC (Goins et al., 1994). When LAP1 linked to LAP2 was inserted into gC, expression was maintained during latency in the peripheral nervous system (PNS) (Lokensgard et al., 1997). Moreover, an approximately 800-bp fragment of LAP1 without the TATA box linked to the Moloney murine leukemia virus (MoMLV) long terminal repeat (LTR) and inserted into the gC locus was able to drive stable long-term expression of reporter genes in the PNS, although this was not possi-ble when a number of other promoters were linked to LAP1 (Lokensgard et al., 1994). Finally, insertion of an internal ribosome entry site (IRES) at a position 1.5 kb downstream of the 5′ end of the primary 2-kb LAT, which results in the maintenance of all cis-acting sequence elements for latent expression, allowed long-term expression of a reporter gene in the PNS (Lachmann and Efstathiou, 1997; Marshall et al., 2000). These findings suggest that although some of the elements necessary for expression during latency are present within LAP1, impor-tant sequences in LAP2 confer long-term expression on LAP1. The MoMLV LTR can substitute for LAP2 to achieve long-term expression in the PNS, further sug-gesting that the structure of LAP2 and its surrounding regions may be important for the LAT region to remain transcriptionally active during latency. Indeed, the dinucleotide content of the LAT region differs from that of the rest of the genome, which may reflect the chromatin structure of this region during latency (Coffin et al., 1995).

Based on this hypothesis, elements from the LAT region were utilized to confer long-term expression from heterologous promoters. A sequence 1.4-kb downstream of the LAP1 TATA box (referred to as LAT P2), linked to a strong heterologous promoter such as the cytomegalovirus (CMV) IE promoter, has been shown to drive high-level sustained expression of reporter genes during

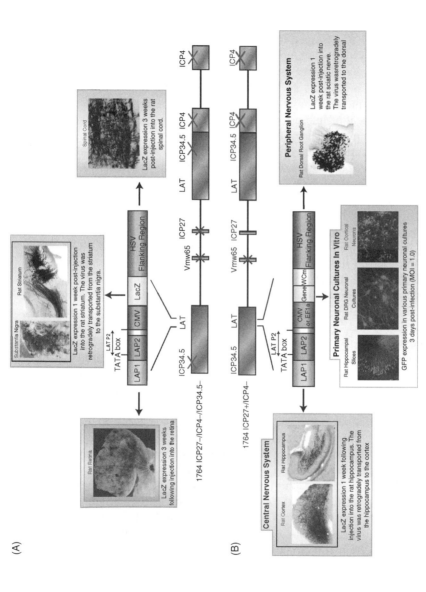

Figure 7.6 Widespread gene delivery to the nervous system using replication-defective HSV-1 vectors. (A) A multiply disabled (1764 ICP4-/ICP27-/ICP34.5-) HSV-1 vector expressing LacZ was injected into the rat retina, striatum, and spinal cord, resulting in high levels of expression into the central nervous system (Lilley et al., 2001). The LATP2 promoter system allows expression for at least 1 month postinjection, and taking advantage of the retrograde capability of HSV-1, the vector allows gene delivery to neurons distal from the site of injection. (B) A less disabled (1764 ICP27+/ICP4-) HSV-1 vector allows highly efficient gene delivery to neurons in culture and both the peripheral and central nervous system (unpublished data). Incorporation of the WCm element into the vector cassettes has resulted in improved expression levels.

latency (Palmer et al., 2000) (Figure 7.6). Importantly, genes could be expressed in the PNS from two promoters cloned in opposite orientations, with the LAT P2 sequence centrally located and inserted into the vhs locus (UL43).

Although, using these different approaches, long-term gene expression has been feasible in the PNS, obtaining long-term expression in the central nervous system (CNS) has been more challenging. This may be due to the different kinetics of gene expression from LAP, resulting in a gradual reduction in the number of transgene-expressing neurons. Nonetheless, when the CMV promoter was inserted after LAT P2, replication-defective vectors with ICP27, ICP4, and ICP35.4 deleted and an inactivating mutation in VP16 (in1814) have allowed widespread gene delivery to the CNS for extended periods of time (Lilley et al., 2001; Perez et al., 2004) (Figure 7.6A). These vectors were efficiently retrogradely transported, allowing high levels of gene expression not only at the injection site, but also at connected sites in the nervous system. Recent incorporation of the posttranscriptional regulatory element of the woodchuck hepatitis virus (WCm) into the vector cassettes has further improved expression levels (unpublished data) (Figure 7.6B).

APPLICATIONS HSV VECTORS

HSV-1 vectors are a valuable tool for the study of gene function in neuronal cells both in vitro and in vivo. Replication-defective vectors have been constructed expressing genes including amyloid precursor protein and presenilin 1 (Bursztajn et al., 1998), which are implicated in the pathogenesis of Alzheimer's disease, the glutamate receptor GluR6 (Telfeian et al., 2000) implicated in the development of temporal lobe epilepsy, the Brn3a transcription factor (Smith et al., 1998), the enzyme glutamatic acid decarboxylase (New et al., 1998), and numerous neurotrophins.

HSV-1 vectors have also been employed for therapeutic gene transfer in animal models of neurological disease. Replication-defective vectors have been used to deliver neurotrophins, such as neurotrophin-3 (NT3) and nerve growth factor (NGF), in animal models of peripheral neuropathy (Goss et al., 2002; Chattopadhyay et al., 2003, 2004). HSV-mediated delivery of proenkephalin in models of inflammatory pain (Goss et al., 2001), polyarthritis (Braz et al., 2001) and neuropathic pain (Hao et al., 2003a) has produced a long-term analgesic effect, which can be reestablished after reinoculation of the vector. Moreover, expression of glial-derived neurotrophic factor (GDNF) in dorsal root ganglia has been shown to provide an analgesic effect in a model of neuropathic pain (Hao et al., 2003b). In the CNS, replication-defective vectors expressing Bcl-2 and GDNF in the substantia nigra of the 6-hydroxydopamine model of Parkinson's disease prevented degeneration of dopaminergic neurons (Yamada et al., 1999; Natsume et al., 2001). HSV-mediated delivery of Bcl-2 and GDNF has also been shown to improve spinal motor neuron survival following root avulsion (Yamada et al., 2001; Natsume et al., 2002). Moreover, expression of the heat shock protein 27 (hsp27) protected neuronal cells against thermal and ischemic stress (Wagstaff et al., 1999). Finally, we are testing HSV vectors expressing NGF in animal models of Alzheimer's disease and vectors expressing other neurotrophins in various models of regeneration, such as spinal cord injury and optic nerve regeneration.

CONCLUSIONS

HSV has allowed efficient gene delivery to postmitotic, terminally differentiated neurons, which are traditionally very hard to transfect. In addition, the brain presents a complicated target, due to the heterogeneity of cell types, volumetric constraints, and the presence of the blood–brain barrier. HSV vectors have therefore become a valuable tool for the molecular analysis of brain function.

Major advances in the design of HSV vectors have led to vectors devoid of viral gene expression and toxicity. These nontoxic vector backbones have been combined with promoter systems capable of directing high levels of long-term transgene expression in neurons of both the peripheral and central nervous system. Taking advantage of the retrograde transport capability of HSV, such vectors have allowed widespread gene delivery to the nervous system.

Although this review has focused on gene delivery to neuronal cells, HSV is capable of infecting a wide variety of other cell types, including dendritic cells and hematopoetic stem cells, which are hard to transfect by other means (Coffin et al., 1998). This property has enabled HSV to be developed as a vaccine in infectious disease and cancer.

In recent years, considerable effort has been focused on developing means of delivering RNA interference (RNAi) to neurons for posttranslational gene silencing. HSV-1 vectors expressing short-hairpin RNA have been constructed by our laboratory and are currently being used to silence reporter genes in vitro and in vivo.

REFERENCES

Ace CI, McKee TA, Ryan JM, Cameron JM, Preston CM (1989). Construction and characterization of a herpes simplex virus type 1 mutant unable to transinduce immediate-early gene expression. *J Virol*. 63(5):2260–2269.

Braz J, Beaufour C, Coutaux A, et al. (2001). Therapeutic efficacy in experimental polyarthritis of viral-driven enkephalin overproduction in sensory neurons. *J Neurosci*. 21(20):7881–7888.

Bursztajn S, DeSouza R, McPhie DL, et al. (1998): Overexpression in neurons of human presenilin-1 or a presenilin-1 familial Alzheimer disease mutant does not enhance apoptosis. *J Neurosci*. 18(23):9790–9799.

Cai W, Schaffer PA (1992). Herpes simplex virus type 1 ICP0 regulates expression of immediate-early, early, and late genes in productively infected cells. *J Virol*. 66(5): 2904–2915.

Carter KL, Roizman B (1996). Alternatively spliced mRNAs predicted to yield frameshift proteins and stable intron 1 RNAs of the herpes simplex virus 1 regulatory gene alpha 0 accumulate in the cytoplasm of infected cells. *Proc Natl Acad Sci U S A*. 93(22):12535–12540.

Chattopadhyay M, Goss J, Lacomis D, et al. (2003). Protective effect of HSV-mediated gene transfer of nerve growth factor in pyridoxine neuropathy demonstrates functional activity of trkA receptors in large sensory neurons of adult animals. *Eur J Neurosci*. 17(4):732–740.

Chattopadhyay M, Goss J, Wolfe D, et al. (2004). Protective effect of herpes simplex virus–mediated neurotrophin gene transfer in cisplatin neuropathy. *Brain*. 127:929–939.

Chen X, Schmidt MC, Goins WF, Glorioso JC (1995). Two herpes simplex virus type 1 latency-active promoters differ in their contributions to latency-associated transcript expression during lytic and latent infections. *J Virol*. 69(12):7899–7908.

Chen SH, Kramer MF, Schaffer PA, Coen DM (1997). A viral function represses accumulation of transcripts from productive-cycle genes in mouse ganglia latently infected with herpes simplex virus. *J Virol*. 71(8):5878–5884.

Coffin RS, Howard MK, Latchman DS (1995). Altered dinucleotide content within the latently transcribed regions of the DNA of alpha herpes viruses: implications for latent RNA expression and DNA structure. *Virology*. 209(2):358–365.

Coffin RS, MacLean AR, Latchman DS, Brown SM (1996). Gene delivery to the central and peripheral nervous systems of mice using HSV1 ICP34.5 deletion mutant vectors. *Gene Ther*. 3(10):886–891.

Coffin RS, Thomas SK, Thomas NS, et al. (1998). Pure populations of transduced primary human cells can be produced using GFP expressing herpes virus vectors and flow cytometry. *Gene Ther*. 5(5):718–722.

DeLuca NA, Schaffer PA (1985). Activation of immediate-early, early, and late promoters by temperature-sensitive and wild-type forms of herpes simplex virus type 1 protein ICP4. *Mol Cell Biol*. 5(8):1997–1208.

DeLuca NA, McCarthy AM, Schaffer PA (1985). Isolation and characterization of deletion mutants of herpes simplex virus type 1 in the gene encoding immediate-early regulatory protein ICP4. *J Virol*. 56(2):558–570.

Dixon RA, Schaffer PA (1980). Fine-structure mapping and functional analysis of temperature-sensitive mutants in the gene encoding the herpes simplex virus type 1 immediate early protein VP175. *J Virol*. 36(1):189–203.

Dobson AT, Sederati F, Devi-Rao G, et al. (1989). Identification of the latency-associated transcript promoter by expression of rabbit beta-globin mRNA in mouse sensory nerve ganglia latently infected with a recombinant herpes simplex virus. *J Virol*. 63(9):3844–3851.

During MJ, Naegele JR, O'Malley KL, Geller AI (1994). Long-term behavioral recovery in parkinsonian rats by an HSV vector expressing tyrosine hydroxylase. *Science*. 266(5189):1399–1403.

Everett RD (1984). Trans activation of transcription by herpes virus products: requirement for two HSV-1 immediate-early polypeptides for maximum activity. *EMBO J*. 3(13):3135–3141.

Farrell MJ, Dobson AT, Feldman LT (1991). Herpes simplex virus latency-associated transcript is a stable intron. *Proc Natl Acad Sci U S A*. 88(3):790–794.

Fink DJ, Sternberg LR, Weber PC, Mata M, Goins WF, Glorioso JC (1992). In vivo expression of beta-galactosidase in hippocampal neurons by HSV-mediated gene transfer. *Hum Gene Ther*. 3(1):11–19.

Geller AI, Keyomarsi K, Bryan J, Pardee AB (1990). An efficient deletion mutant packaging system for defective herpes simplex virus vectors: potential applications to human gene therapy and neuronal physiology. *Proc Natl Acad Sci U S A*. 87(22):8950–8954.

Geraghty RJ, Krummenacher C, Cohen GH, Eisenberg RJ, Spear PG (1998). Entry of alphaherpesviruses mediated by poliovirus receptor-related protein 1 and poliovirus receptor. *Science*. 280(5369):1618–1620.

Goins WF, Sternberg LR, Croen KD, et al. (1994). A novel latency-active promoter is contained within the herpes simplex virus type 1 UL flanking repeats. *J Virol*. 68(4):2239–2252.

Gordon YJ, McKnight JL, Ostrove JM, Romanowski E, Araullo-Cruz T (1990). Host species and strain differences affect the ability of an HSV-1 ICP0 deletion mutant to establish latency and spontaneously reactivate in vivo. *Virology*. 178(2):469–477.

Goss JR, Mata M, Goins WF, Wu HH, Glorioso JC, Fink DJ (2001). Antinociceptive effect of a genomic herpes simplex virus–based vector expressing human proenkephalin in rat dorsal root ganglion. *Gene Ther*. 8(7):551–556.

Goss JR, Goins WF, Lacomis D, Mata M, Glorioso JC, Fink DJ (2002). Herpes simplex–mediated gene transfer of nerve growth factor protects against peripheral neuropathy in streptozotocin-induced diabetes in the mouse. *Diabetes*. 51(7):2227–2232.

Hao S, Mata M, Goins W, Glorioso JC, Fink DJ (2003a). Transgene-mediated enkephalin release enhances the effect of morphine and evades tolerance to produce a sustained antiallodynic effect in neuropathic pain. *Pain*. 102(1–2):135–142.

Hao S, Mata M, Wolfe D, Huang S, Glorioso JC, Fink DJ (2003b). HSV-mediated gene transfer of the glial cell–derived neurotrophic factor provides an antiallodynic effect on neuropathic pain. *Mol Ther*. 8(3):367–375.

Hardy WR, Sandri-Goldin RM (1994). Herpes simplex virus inhibits host cell splicing, and regulatory protein ICP27 is required for this effect. *J Virol*. 68(12):7790–7799.

Herold BC, Visalli RJ, Susmarski N, Brandt CR, Spear PG (1994). Glycoprotein C–independent binding of herpes simplex virus to cells requires cell surface heparan sulphate and glycoprotein B. *J Gen Virol*. 75:1211–1222.

Ho DY, Mocarski ES (1989). Herpes simplex virus latent RNA (LAT) is not required for latent infection in the mouse. *Proc Natl Acad Sci U S A*. 86(19):7596–7600.

Honess RW, Roizman B (1974). Regulation of herpesvirus macromolecular synthesis: I. Cascade regulation of the synthesis of three groups of viral proteins. *J Virol*. 14(1):8–19.

Howard MK, Kershaw T, Gibb B, et al. (1998). High efficiency gene transfer to the central nervous system of rodents and primates using herpes virus vectors lacking functional ICP27 and ICP34.5. *Gene Ther*. 5(8):1137–1147.

Jacob RJ, Morse LS, Roizman B (1979). Anatomy of herpes simplex virus DNA: XII. Accumulation of head-to-tail concatemers in nuclei of infected cells and their role in the generation of the four isomeric arrangements of viral DNA. *J Virol*. 29(2): 448–457.

Jin BK, Belloni M, Conti B, et al. (1996). Prolonged in vivo gene expression driven by a tyrosine hydroxylase promoter in a defective herpes simplex virus amplicon vector. *Hum Gene Ther*. 7(16):2015–2024.

Johnson PA, Yoshida K, Gage FH, Friedmann T (1992). Effects of gene transfer into cultured CNS neurons with a replication-defective herpes simplex virus type 1 vector. *Brain Res Mol Brain Res*. 12(1–3):95–102.

Kaplitt MG, Kwong AD, Kleopoulos SP, Mobbs CV, Rabkin SD, Pfaff DW (1994). Preproenkephalin promoter yields region-specific and long-term expression in adult brain after direct in vivo gene transfer via a defective herpes simplex viral vector. *Proc Natl Acad Sci U S A*. 91(19):8979–8983.

Krisky DM, Wolfe D, Goins WF, et al. (1998). Deletion of multiple immediate-early genes from herpes simplex virus reduces cytotoxicity and permits long-term gene expression in neurons. *Gene Ther*. 5(12):1593–1603.

Lachmann RH, Efstathiou S (1997). Utilization of the herpes simplex virus type 1 latency-associated regulatory region to drive stable reporter gene expression in the nervous system. *J Virol*. 71(4):3197–3207.

Lilley CE, Groutsi F, Han Z, et al. (2001). Multiple immediate-early gene-deficient herpes simplex virus vectors allowing efficient gene delivery to neurons in culture and widespread gene delivery to the central nervous system in vivo. *J Virol*. 75(9):4343–4356.

Lokensgard JR, Bloom DC, Dobson AT, Feldman LT (1994). Long-term promoter activity during herpes simplex virus latency. *J. Virol*. 68:7148–7158.

Lokensgard JR, Berthomme H, Feldman LT (1997). The latency-associated promoter of herpes simplex virus type 1 requires a region downstream of the transcription start site for long-term expression during latency. *J Virol*. 71(9):6714–6719.

Mabit H, Nakano MY, Prank U, et al. (2002). Intact microtubules support adenovirus and herpes simplex virus infections. *J Virol*. 76(19):9962–9971.

Mador N, Goldenberg D, Cohen O, Panet A, Steiner I (1998). Herpes simplex virus type 1 latency-associated transcripts suppress viral replication and reduce immediate-early gene mRNA levels in a neuronal cell line. *J Virol*. 72(6):5067–5075.

Marchand CF, Schwab ME (1986). Binding, uptake and retrograde axonal transport of herpes virus suis in sympathetic neurons. *Brain Res*. 383(1–2):262–270.

Margolis TP, Bloom DC, Dobson AT, Feldman LT, Stevens JG (1993). Decreased reporter gene expression during latent infection with HSV LAT promoter constructs. *Virology*. 197(2):585–592.

Marshall KR, Lachmann RH, Efstathiou S, Rinaldi A, Preston CM (2000). Long-term transgene expression in mice infected with a herpes simplex virus type 1 mutant severely impaired for immediate-early gene expression. *J Virol*. 74(2):956–964.

Mellerick DM, Fraser NW (1987). Physical state of the latent herpes simplex virus genome in a mouse model system: evidence suggesting an episomal state. *Virology*. 158(2):265–275.

Montgomery RI, Warner MS, Lum BJ, Spear PG (1996). Herpes simplex virus-1 entry into cells mediated by a novel member of the TNF/NGF receptor family. *Cell*. 87(3): 427–436.

Mossman KL, Smiley JR (1999). Truncation of the C-terminal acidic transcriptional activation domain of herpes simplex virus VP16 renders expression of the immediate-early genes almost entirely dependent on ICP0. *J Virol*. 73(12):9726–9733.

100 HERPES SIMPLEX VIRUS VECTORS

Natsume A, Mata M, Goss J, et al. (2001). Bcl-2 and GDNF delivered by HSV-mediated gene transfer act additively to protect dopaminergic neurons from 6-OHDA-induced degeneration. *Exp Neurol.* 169(2):231–238.

Natsume A, Mata M, Wolfe D, et al. (2002). Bcl-2 and GDNF delivered by HSV-mediated gene transfer after spinal root avulsion provide a synergistic effect. *J Neurotrauma.* 19(1):61–68.

New KC, Gale K, Martuza RL, Rabkin SD (1998). Novel synthesis and release of GABA in cerebellar granule cell cultures after infection with defective herpes simplex virus vectors expressing glutamic acid decarboxylase. *Brain Res Mol Brain Res.* 61(1–2):121–135.

O'Hare P, Hayward GS (1985). Evidence for a direct role for both the 175,000- and 110,000-molecular-weight immediate-early proteins of herpes simplex virus in the transactivation of delayed-early promoters. *J Virol.* 53(3):751–760.

Palmer JA, Branston RH, Lilley CE, et al. (2000). Development and optimization of herpes simplex virus vectors for multiple long-term gene delivery to the peripheral nervous system. *J Virol.* 74(12):5604–5618.

Perez MC, Hunt SP, Coffin RS, Palmer JA (2004). Comparative analysis of genomic HSV vectors for gene delivery to motor neurons following peripheral inoculation in vivo. *Gene Ther.* 11(13):1023–1032.

Perng GC, Slanina SM, Yukht A, et al. (1999). A herpes simplex virus type 1 latency-associated transcript mutant with increased virulence and reduced spontaneous reactivation. *J Virol.* 73(2):920–929.

Perng GC, Jones C, Ciacci-Zanella J, et al. (2000). Virus-induced neuronal apoptosis blocked by the herpes simplex virus latency-associated transcript. *Science.* 287:1500–1503.

Preston CM, Nicholl MJ (1997). Repression of gene expression upon infection of cells with herpes simplex virus type 1 mutants impaired for immediate-early protein synthesis. *J Virol.* 71:7807–7813.

Preston CM, Frame MC, Campbell ME (1988). A complex formed between cell components and an HSV structural polypeptide binds to a viral immediate early gene regulatory DNA sequence. *Cell.* 52(3):425–434.

Rice SA, Long MC, Lam V, Schaffer PA, Spencer CA (1995). Herpes simplex virus immediate-early protein ICP22 is required for viral modification of host RNA polymerase II and establishment of the normal viral transcription program. *J Virol.* 69(9): 5550–5559.

Sacks WR, Greene CC, Aschman DP, Schaffer PA (1985). Herpes simplex virus type 1 ICP27 is an essential regulatory protein. *J Virol.* 55(3):796–805.

Saeki Y, Fraefel C, Ichikawa T, Breakefield XO, Chiocca EA (2001). Improved helper virus-free packaging system for HSV amplicon vectors using an ICP27-deleted, over-sized HSV-1 DNA in a bacterial artificial chromosome. *Mol Ther.* 3(4):591–601.

Samaniego LA, Webb AL, DeLuca NA (1995). Functional interactions between herpes simplex virus immediate-early proteins during infection: gene expression as a consequence of ICP27 and different domains of ICP4. *J Virol.* 69(9):5705–5715.

Samaniego LA, Wu N, DeLuca NA (1997). The herpes simplex virus immediate-early protein ICP0 affects transcription from the viral genome and infected-cell survival in the absence of ICP4 and ICP27. *J Virol.* 71(6):4614–4625.

Samaniego LA, Neiderhiser L, DeLuca NA (1998). Persistence and expression of the herpes simplex virus genome in the absence of immediate-early proteins. *J Virol*. 72(4):3307–3320.

Sandler VM, Wang S, Angelo K, Lo HG, Breakefield XO, Clapham DE (2002). Modified herpes simplex virus delivery of enhanced GFP into the central nervous system. *J Neurosci Methods*. 121(2):211–219.

Sears AE, Halliburton IW, Meignier B, Silver S, Roizman B (1985). Herpes simplex virus 1 mutant deleted in the alpha 22 gene: growth and gene expression in permissive and restrictive cells and establishment of latency in mice. *J Virol*. 55(2):338–346.

Sekulovich RE, Leary K, Sandri-Goldin RM (1988). The herpes simplex virus type 1 alpha protein ICP27 can act as a *trans*-repressor or a *trans*-activator in combination with ICP4 and ICP0. *J Virol*. 62(12):4510–4512.

Shieh MT, WuDunn D, Montgomery RI, Esko JD, Spear PG (1992). Cell surface receptors for herpes simplex virus are heparan sulfate proteoglycans. *J Cell Biol*. 116(5): 1273–1281.

Smiley JR, Duncan J (1997). Truncation of the C-terminal acidic transcriptional activation domain of herpes simplex virus VP16 produces a phenotype similar to that of the in1814 linker insertion mutation. *J Virol*. 71(8):6191–6193.

Smith MD, Ensor EA, Coffin RS, Boxer LM, Latchman DS (1998). Bcl-2 transcription from the proximal P2 promoter is activated in neuronal cells by the Brn-3a POU family transcription factor. *J Biol Chem*. 273(27):16715–16722.

Song S, Wang Y, Bak SY, et al. (1997). An HSV-1 vector containing the rat tyrosine hydroxylase promoter enhances both long-term and cell type-specific expression in the midbrain. *J Neurochem*. 68(5):1792–1803.

Spaete RR, Frenkel N (1982). The herpes simplex virus amplicon: a new eukaryotic defective-virus cloning-amplifying vector. *Cell*. 30(1):295–304.

Stevens JG, Wagner EK, Devi-Rao GB, Cook ML, Feldman LT (1987). RNA complementary to a herpesvirus alpha gene mRNA is prominent in latently infected neurons. *Science*. 235(4792):1056–1059.

Tal-Singer R, Peng C, Ponce De Leon M, et al. (1995). Interaction of herpes simplex virus glycoprotein gC with mammalian cell surface molecules. *J Virol*. 69(7):4471–4483.

Telfeian AE, Federoff HJ, Leone P, During MJ, Williamson A (2000). Overexpression of GluR6 in rat hippocampus produces seizures and spontaneous nonsynaptic bursting in vitro. *Neurobiol Dis*. 7(4):362–374.

Thomas SK, Lilley CE, Latchman DS, Coffin RS (1999). Equine herpesvirus 1 gene 12 can substitute for vmw65 in the growth of herpes simplex virus (HSV) type 1, allowing the generation of optimized cell lines for the propagation of HSV vectors with multiple immediate-early gene defects. *J Virol*. 73(9):7399–7409.

Thompson RL, Sawtell NM (1997). The herpes simplex virus type 1 latency-associated transcript gene regulates the establishment of latency. *J Virol*. 71(7):5432–5440.

Wagstaff MJ, Collaco-Moraes Y, Smith J, de Belleroche JS, Coffin RS, Latchman DS (1999). Protection of neuronal cells from apoptosis by Hsp27 delivered with a herpes simplex virus–based vector. *J Biol Chem*. 274(8):5061–5069.

Wechsler SL, Nesburn AB, Watson R, Slanina SM, Ghiasi H (1988). Fine mapping of the latency-related gene of herpes simplex virus type 1: alternative splicing produces distinct latency-related RNAs containing open reading frames. *J Virol*. 62(11):4051–4058.

Wilcox CL, Johnson EM (1988). Characterization of nerve growth factor–dependent herpes simplex virus latency in neurons in vitro. *J Virol*. 62:393–399.

Wu N, Watkins SC, Schaffer PA, DeLuca NA (1996). Prolonged gene expression and cell survival after infection by a herpes simplex virus mutant defective in the immediate-early genes encoding ICP4, ICP27, and ICP22. *J Virol*. 70(9):6358–6369.

Yamada M, Oligino T, Mata M, Goss JR, Glorioso JC, Fink DJ (1999). Herpes simplex virus vector-mediated expression of Bcl-2 prevents 6-hydroxydopamine-induced degeneration of neurons in the substantia nigra in vivo. *Proc Natl Acad Sci U S A*. 96(7):4078–4083.

Yamada M, Natsume A, Mata M, et al. (2001). Herpes simplex virus vector-mediated expression of Bcl-2 protects spinal motor neurons from degeneration following root avulsion. *Exp Neurol*. 168(2):225–230.

York IA, Roop C, Andrews DW, Riddell SR, Graham FL, Johnson DC (1994). A cytosolic herpes simplex virus protein inhibits antigen presentation to CD8+ T lymphocytes. *Cell*. 77(4):525–535.

Zwaagstra JC, Ghiasi H, Nesburn AB, Wechsler SL (1991). Identification of a major regulatory sequence in the latency associated transcript (LAT) promoter of herpes simplex virus type 1 (HSV-1). *Virology*. 182(1):287–297.

8 Nonviral Gene Delivery Systems

TAKESHI SUDA and DEXI LIU

Department of Pharmaceutical Sciences, University of Pittsburgh
School of Pharmacy, Pittsburgh, Pennsylvania

Naked DNA cannot pass through undamaged cell membranes, due to its large molecular weight and lack of transporter on the cell surface. Delivery of DNA into the cell nucleus where the transcription machinery locates is the main objective of nonviral gene delivery. Factors taken into consideration for developing methods of gene delivery include the high sensitivity of genetic material to nucleases in tissues and the bloodstream, their limited access to individual cells in the tissue due to anatomical structures, and lack of permeability across the cell membrane. Although sometimes mutually inclusive, the nonviral approaches designed to overcome these biochemical and structural barriers can generally be divided into two categories: energy-based physical methods and carrier-based chemical methods. The physical methods employ a physical force, such as pressure, a shock wave, an electric pulse, ultrasound, or a laser beam, to create transient membrane pores on cells to allow DNA to defuse into or be placed directly inside a cell. With a few exceptions, physical methods normally require a device to generate proper force. The chemical methods, on the other hand, often use cationic compounds, either synthetic or naturally occurring, as a gene carrier. Chemical methods usually rely on a structure of preformed DNA–carrier complexes and endocytosis of target cells to bring DNA or RNA into cells. With many cationic lipids and polymers developed in recent years, one can reliably achieve a high level of gene delivery in cultured cells, although the in vivo success of the chemical methods has been limited to selected organs, such as the lung via intravenous or airway administration and solid tumor by intratumor injection. Compared to viral approaches, the unique features of nonviral methods are their simplicity, lack of immunogenicity, and flexibility. All types of nucleic acids, including circular plasmids, linear DNA (double or single stranded, long or short), and various RNAs can be delivered. Table 8.1 summarizes the unique

Concepts in Genetic Medicine, Edited by Boro Dropulic and Barrie Carter
Copyright © 2008 John Wiley & Sons, Inc.

TABLE 8.1 Characteristics of Nonviral Gene Delivery Systems[a]

Nonviral Method	Advantages	Disadvantages	Human Clinical Trial[b]	Limitation Toward Human Gene Therapy
Needle injection	Simple Good for DNA vaccine studies	Transfection limited to injection site Low efficiency	Yes (intramuscular gene delivery and DNA vaccine)	Low efficiency
Gene gun	Good in vitro and in vivo activity	Limited to topical use Causing tissue damage	Yes (topical application for DNA vaccine)	Production of homogeneous particles, tissue damage
Electroporation	Highly efficient in vitro and in vivo	Limited to small area in tissue Causing tissue damage	Yes (intratumor gene delivery)	Affecting only a small number of cells
Hydrodynamic delivery	Simple and highly effective for intravascular gene delivery	Transient tissue damage Hard to use in large animals	No	Large injection volume
Sonophoresis	Less invasive	Tissue damage Low efficiency	No	Low efficiency
Jet injection	Fairly efficient for topical application	Limited to topical use Low efficiency	No	Low efficiency
Laser	Less invasive	Limited to topical use Low efficiency	No	Low efficiency
Cationic lipids	Highly effective in vitro Targeting possible	Low activity and toxic in vivo	Yes (airway, oral, peritoneal, and pleural gene delivery)	Low in vivo activity and toxicity
Polycations	Highly effective in vitro Targeting possible	Low activity and toxic in vivo	No	Low in vivo activity and toxicity
Natural substance	Low toxicity Targeting possible	Low activity	No	Low activity

[a]The features listed are noninclusive and represent the characteristics of the current nonviral methods reviewed in this chapter.
[b]Clinical trial information registered with NIH is available at http://www.gemcris.od.nih.gov/.

features of the nonviral methods developed so far. The principles underlying each of these methods and their applications are described in the following sections.

PHYSICAL METHODS FOR GENE DELIVERY

Physical methods for gene delivery have the advantage of transferring genetic material directly into the cytoplasm or nucleus of cells, bypassing the need for cell surface binding, cell cycle status, and cellular function for internalization. In addition, high copy numbers of transgenes, large or small in size, can be delivered into the target cells. Several physical methods have been developed and a few have been used in clinical trials.

Needle Injection

Once considered unlikely, direct injection of DNA solution into a tissue to achieve gene transfer was reported in 1990 by Wolff et al. Using plasmid containing a reporter gene, Wolff and colleagues demonstrated a significant level of reporter gene expression in the muscle after a single intramuscular injection of plasmid DNA solution. The reporter gene expression appeared to be centralized near the needle track and the injection site. A similar procedure has also been performed for gene transfer to liver (Hickman et al., 1994), heart (Jiao et al., 1992), and skin (Hengge et al., 1995). Currently, the most common application of this procedure is intramuscular injection of DNA for vaccine development. A detailed procedure to achieve the optimal level of gene product has been established (Sasaki et al., 2003). Although the overall level of transgene expression achieved was low, preclinical examination in mice showed enhanced antitumor immunity by intramuscular injection of DNA vaccine expressing carcinoembryonic antigen and IL-12 (Song et al., 2000). Another promising result is significant improvement of the exercise capability of patients with severe ischemic heart diseases in a phase I/II clinical trial, in which naked DNA-encoding VEGF-2 was injected directly into the myocardium of the left ventricle through a catheter (Losordo et al., 2002).

A modified needle injection procedure was developed in the last few years. In 1999, we (F. Liu et al., 1999) and G. Zhang et al. 1999 reported that a rapid injection of a large volume of DNA solution via the tail vein of a mouse led to highly efficient gene delivery to hepatocytes. In this procedure, now known as *hydrodynamic delivery*, rapid injection of a large volume of DNA solution results in a transient cardiac congestion and retrograde flow of the injected DNA solution into the liver. The intravascular pressure in liver sinusoid enlarges liver fenestrae and generates pores on plasma membrane of hepatocytes. Consequently, DNA molecules diffuse into cells and are trapped inside when the membrane pores close (G. Zhang et al., 2004). Although the liver is the most transfected organ by this method, successful gene delivery has also been achieved in other organs, including the lung (Emerson et al., 2003), muscle (Hagstrom et al., 2004), heart (Mann et al., 1999), vascular endothelium (Mann et al., 1999), kidneys (Hamar et al., 2004), and even brain (Barnett et al., 2004). With modifications, hydrodynamic gene delivery has been applied successfully to several other vertebrates, including rat (Maruyama et al., 2002), fish (Romoren et al., 2004), rabbit (Eastman et al., 2002), dog (G. Zhang et al., 1997), ovine (Emerson et al., 2003), monkey (G. Zhang et al., 2001) and even human tissues (Mann et al., 1999). To date, the hydrodynamics-based procedure is the most effective nonviral method for in vivo gene delivery in rodents.

High efficiency and simplicity of the hydrodynamic delivery has raised interest in the gene therapy community to apply this method to humans. The current efforts have been placed on reducing the injection volume. In fact, recent work by Hagstrom et al. 2004 showed that highly efficient gene transfer into muscle tissue in dogs and primates can be achieved by a procedure involving injection of plasmid DNA or siRNA into a distal vein of a limb that is transiently isolated by a tourniquet or blood pressure cuff. Similarly, Eastman and colleagues had devised several methods for gene delivery to the isolated rabbit liver using minimally invasive catheter-based technique (Eastman et al., 2002). Employing balloon catheters or local injection, these studies indicate that successful gene transfer could be achieved with the volume and rates of injection within an acceptable range for rapid bolus delivery in humans. The remaining challenge is to optimize the experimental conditions, establish a clinical procedure, and demonstrate that hydrodynamic delivery is indeed applicable to and effective in humans.

Gene Gun Transfer

Gene gun transfer, also known as particle bombardment or ballistic DNA transfer, was originally developed for gene delivery to plants (Klein et al., 1987). Gene transfer by this method is achieved by propelling DNA-coated fine particles (~1 to 3 μm) directly against target tissue or cells using a helium-pressured device. The force created by the compressed shock wave of helium gas is able to accelerate DNA-coated gold or tungsten particles to a high speed with sufficient momentum to penetrate substantial physical barriers, such as plant cell walls, cell membrane, and the stratum corneum of mammalian epidermis (Yang et al., 1990). In animals, the gene gun approach has been demonstrated effective in a variety of tissues and organs, including skin (Yang et al., 1990), liver (Kuriyama et al., 2000), muscle (Lauritzen et al., 2002), spleen (Cheng et al., 1993), pancreas (Cheng et al., 1993), and other organs (Muramatsu et al., 1997; Matsuno et al., 2003). Ex vivo applications have included transfection of brain (Jiao et al., 1993), mammary (Thompson et al., 1993), leukocyte (Martiniuk et al., 2002), and a variety of tumor tissues (Tanigawa et al., 2000; Wang et al., 2001; S. Zhang et al., 2002). In vitro, several cell types have been transfected in suspension or as adherent cells (Heiser, 2004). Preclinical tests in animals for DNA vaccine studies (Trimble et al., 2003; Barfoed et al., 2004) have been reported. Direct transfer of particles into Langerhans antigen-presenting cells in the epidermis

(Condon et al., 1996), and generation of a Th2 response (Feltquate et al., 1997; Prayaga et al., 1997) in contrast to a Th1 response (Lima et al., 2003) have also been examined. The major limitations of the current gene gun technology are dose limitation (approximately 1 μg in each shot), difficulty to prepare uniform microparticles, and limited access to target cells deep in the tissue. Despite these limitations, as of July 2007, ballistic delivery has been approved in five clinical trials (http://www.wiley.co.uk/genetherapy/clinical/).

Electroporation

Electroporation, the transfer of DNA into living cells using electric fields, was first reported by Neumann and colleagues in 1982. When an electrical pulse is applied to cells placed between two electrodes, membrane pores are generated with a few milliseconds. These pores are transient and reseal within a few seconds. During this brief window of time, it is possible to introduce a wide variety of macromolecules into cells. Because of its simplicity and efficiency, this strategy of gene delivery spreads rapidly and has become a regular means for in vitro gene transfer in bacterial, yeast, plant, and animal cells, and for in vivo gene transfer. Vigorous studies revealed that three processes are involved in efficient electroporation; DNA distribution, membrane permeabilization and DNA electrophoresis (Andre and Mir, 2004). After injection of DNA to the site where electroporation will be applied, high-voltage pulses followed by low-voltage pulses lead to efficient gene delivery. A high-voltage pulse permeabilizes a cell membrane and the following low-voltage pulse pushes DNA into cells through permeabilized cell membranes by an electrophoretic mechanism. Electroporation has been broadly applicable to multiple cell types and is highly efficient, reproducible, and appropriate for both transient and stable transfections.

Preclinical in vivo electrotransfer has been conducted in mice for gene delivery into skeletal muscles (Aihara and Miyazaki, 1998), skin (Medi et al., 2005), cornea (Sakamoto et al., 1999), brain (Tanaka et al., 2000), lumbar intrathecal space (Lee et al., 2003), penile corpora cavernosa (Magee et al., 2002), testis (Yomogida et al., 2002), spleen (Tupin et al., 2003), kidney (Thanaketpaisarn et al., 2005), and various tumor tissues (Jaroszeski et al., 2004), such as colon adenocarcinoma (Tamura et al., 2001), melanoma (Rols et al., 1998), and hepatocellular carcinoma (Yamashita et al., 2001). Successful gene transfer was also reported (Mir et al., 2005) in rat, rabbit (Zampaglione et al., 2005), pig (Babiuk et al., 2002), sheep (Scheerlinck et al., 2004), goat (Tollefsen et al., 2003), dog (Draghia-Akli et al., 2003), cattle (Tollefsen et al., 2003), and monkey (Zampaglione et al., 2005). Furthermore, electroporation using needle-free meander and caliper electrodes has been demonstrated (L. Zhang et al., 2002). As of 2007, 4 clinical trials had been registered with NIH (http://www.gemcris.od.nih.gov). To date, electroporation is one of the most feasible nonviral gene delivery systems in clinical use.

Sonophoresis

In 1954, the successful treatment of digital polyarthritis was reported using a combination of hydrocortisone and ultrasound (Fellinger and Schmidt, 1954). Now this technique, sonophoresis, has emerged as a potential tool for facilitating delivery of nucleic acids into various cells in vitro and in vivo. The mechanism of ultrasonic gene delivery seems to be based on cavitation-induced permeabilization of the cell membrane (Mitragotri et al., 1995). Ultrasonic contrast agents are included in the procedure to enhance ultrasonic cavitation efficiency (Lawrie et al., 2000). Focused ultrasound has been shown to enhance in vivo gene transfer into rabbit carotid arteries in the presence of gas-filled albumin microspheres (Huber et al., 2003). In another study, in vivo gene therapy of tumors by systemic administration of DNA–cationic lipid complexes followed by localized application of ultrasound in mice was reported (Anwer et al., 2000). Unfortunately, the overall gene transfer efficiency of sonophoresis is relatively low and the technology has not been tested in humans.

Other Physical Methods

Jet stream and laser are additional mechanisms employed for gene delivery. The jet injection uses mechanical compression to force DNA solution through a small orifice, producing high-pressure stream that can penetrate a number of different tissues. Walther et al. 2001 reported a new and versatile hand-held jet injector for gene transfer into tumors. Efficient induction of immunity was also reported by jet injection of mixture of DNA and proteins (Imoto and Konishi, 2005). Although it is simple and well tolerated, this system shares a limitation similar to that of the gene gun approach. The effectiveness in delivery genes into cells deep into the tissue is less than desirable.

Focused laser provides another energy source to facilitate gene transfer into cells. The mechanism of laser-based gene transfer is not clear but probably involves disruption of cell membrane. Successful gene transfer using this technique was first demonstrated in 2003 (Zeira et al., 2003) using tibial muscle as the target tissue. It was shown that gene delivery into mouse muscle can be accomplished by focusing cells with a femtosecond infrared light in the presence of plasmid DNA. It remains to be seen, however, if laser-based gene transfer can be scaled up significantly in studies of larger muscles or other tissues.

CHEMICAL METHODS FOR GENE DELIVERY

The major advantages of chemical methods or synthetic vectors are their simplicity, ease of production, active targeting capability at the cellular level, relative safe comparing to the viral method, and high gene loading capacity. Many excellent review articles on this subject have been published in recent years (Hirko et al., 2003; D. Liu et al., 2003; Miller, 2003; Demeneix et al., 2004; Neu et al., 2005) summarizing recent progress in synthetic vectors for gene delivery. Following is a brief summary of some of the most advanced synthetic vectors.

Lipid-Based Gene Carriers

The efficient transfection of eukaryotic cells using cationic lipids was first described by Felgner et al. 1987. Since this instrumental discovery, many cationic lipids have been synthesized and demonstrated to be effective in gene delivery. These cationic lipids share the common structure of a positively charged head group and a hydrophobic tail connected by a linker. The most commonly used head group contains one or multiple amines (primary, secondary, tertiary, and quaternary amines), while the hydrophobic tail is composed of two alkyl chains (Ferrari et al., 2002) or a cholesterol residue (Gao and Huang, 1991; Vigneron et al., 1996). Various structures have been used as the linker (D. Liu et al., 2003). The head group and the hydrophobic moiety are connected through various linkage bonds (Byk et al., 1998).

Most cationic lipids that are active in gene delivery form liposomes. Due to the polymeric nature of charges on both cationic liposomes and DNA, cationic liposomes and DNA form complexes (lipoplexes) spontaneously under physiological pH and ionic strength. Gene delivery efficiency of lipoplexes is influenced primarily by lipid structure, charge ratio, the environment where gene delivery is carried out, and the type of cells employed. The intensive studies in the last two decades, although remaining inconclusive, seem to suggest that the most active cationic lipids for gene delivery in vitro include those containing one to four amines as charged head groups and a hydrophobic tail of being either cholesterol residue or two hydrocarbon chains with unsaturated 18 carbons (C18:1) or 14 carbons (C14:0) (Ren et al., 2000). In some cases, inclusion of a neutral lipid such as dioleoylphosphatidylethanolamine (DOPE) or cholesterol into cationic liposomes enhances gene transfer activity (Y. Liu et al., 1997; Zuidam and Barenholz, 1998). Delivery efficiency of lipoplexes varies significantly from one type of cells to another. Evidence suggests that intracellular DNA transport involves progression through both endosomes and lysosomes. In addition, cytoplasmic release of DNA from early endosomal compartment takes place as shown by electron microscopy (Lappalainen et al., 1997). Development of strategies to facilitate endosomal release, dissociation of DNA from the complexes in cytosol and transfer of DNA into nucleus is the major goal for lipid-based gene delivery.

Systemic tail vein injection of lipoplexes into mice resulted in a significant gene expression in the lung (F. Liu et al., 1997; Smyth-Templeton et al., 1997; Song et al., 1997; Eliyahu et al., 2002). For maximal gene expression, a higher charge ratio ($+/-$) compared to that of in vitro gene delivery appears necessary for systemic gene delivery (F. Liu et al., 1997; Song et al., 1997). Unfortunately, lipoplexes with a higher charge ratio ($+/-$) readily aggregate in blood, leading to various toxicities (Sakurai et al., 2001). Lipoplexes are also shown to activate the complement system (Plank et al., 1996) and to induce acute immune response (Whitmore et al., 1999). Inclusion of polyethylene glycol (PEG) derivative into the lipoplexes to shield the excess amount of positive charges has been used successfully to reduce lipoplex aggregation in the blood (Yu et al., 2004). The steric stabilization effect of PEG is dependent on its chain length and its density on the surface of lipoplex particles.

Lipoplexes have been used in clinical trials and represent 7.8% ($n = 102$) of total gene therapy trials (http://www.wiley.co.uk/genetherapy/clinical/). The target diseases are primarily cancer and cystic fibrosis. Phase I/II clinical study against recurrent glioblastoma has been conducted by local injection of lipoplexs using a suicide gene therapy approach (Reszka et al., 2005). The therapy was well tolerated without major side effects, and a greater than 50% reduction of tumor volume was observed in two out of eight cases. For cystic fibrosis, eight clinical trials of liposome-mediated gene therapy have been published to date (Lee et al., 2005). Although patients have demonstrated evidence of vector-specific CFTR expression and some functional changes toward normality, this has been variable, and current levels of gene transfer efficiency are probably too low to result in clinical benefits. Thus, except for local administration, the efficacy of lipoplexes is not sufficient for clinical use.

Polymer-Based Gene Carriers

Synthetic and naturally occurring polymers have been used for gene delivery. Poly-L-lysine (Wolfert et al., 1999), polyallylamine derivatives (Boussif et al., 1999), polyethylenimine (PEI) (Boussif et al., 1995; Lungwitz et al., 2005), polyamidoamine dendrimer (Tang et al., 1996), cationic dextran (Hwang et al., 2001), and cationic proteins such as protamine (Park et al., 2003) and histone (Balicki and Beutler, 1997) are among the most studied. Although all cationic polymers are capable of condensing DNA into small particles and enhancing cellular uptake via endocytosis through charge–charge interaction with anionic polysaccharides on the cell surface, their transfection activity and toxicity differ dramatically.

PEI is probably the most studied polycation for gene delivery. PEI is made from acid-catalyzed polymerization of aziridine through a ring-opening mechanism and has been used primarily in the paper industry and in water treatment. Jean-Paul Behr's group introduced PEI as an efficient and economical nonviral gene transfer reagent (Boussif et al., 1995). PEI with a variety of sizes in branched (B-PEI) or linear (L-PEI) configuration is readily available. PEI is the most densely charged polymer, with one of every third atoms being nitrogen that can be protonated. Branched PEI has a ratio of primary/secondary/tertiary amine groups close to $1 : 1 : 1$, according to the most recently revised estimation (von Harpe et al., 2000). Most of the amine groups in linear PEI are secondary amines, except for two terminal groups. Both linear and branched forms of PEI have excellent transfection activities in vitro. Dendrimers are unique polymers with a symmetric and sphere configuration and a narrow size distribution (Kukowska-Latallo et al., 1996). Szoka's group first reported that dendrimers could transfect cells (Haensler and Szoka, 1993). Similar results were reported by Baker's group in collaboration with Tomalia's group except that dendrimers with large MW are more active and the presence of DEAE–dextran is essential (Kukowska-Latallo et al., 1996). Szoka's group also reported that fractured dendrimers by partial hydrolysis improved the transfection efficiency over that of perfectly symmetric dendrimers (Tang et al., 1996). Besides many primary amines located on the surface, both PEI and dendrimer have abundant secondary and/or tertiary amine groups in the interior, which are essential to their transfection activity. Portions of the internal amine groups are believed to have lowered pK_a values and remain uncharged at the physiological pH value. They contribute to the transfection activity by absorbing protons inside endosomes, therefore blocking the endosome–lysosome transition, a cellular process that is dependent on the accumulation of vesicular protons. DNA/PEI complexes (polyplexes) are therefore kept away from the harsh environment in lysosomes. Moreover, PEI-induced accumulation of protons and its counterion Cl^- within the endosomes can create substantial osmotic pressure, which triggers the influx of water molecules and causes the vesicles to swell and burst (Sonawane et al., 2003), although other mechanisms may also involve the transfection process mediated by DNA/PEI complexes (Pollard et al., 1998). PEI is able to facilitate nucleic entry of the DNA/polymer complexes (Godbey et al., 1999), whereas DNA/cationic lipid complexes are not able to do so (Zabner et al., 1995). DNA/L-PEI complexes appear to be more active than DNA/B-PEI complexes in intravascular routes (Wightman et al., 2001), whereas DNA/dendrimer complexes are less active in vivo.

A limitation for PEI as a transfection reagent is its toxicity. In fact, PEI and poly L lysine are two of the most cytotoxic agents among several polycations studied so far. Excessive charges in DNA/PEI complexes can trigger membrane damage that leads to cell death (Moghimi et al., 2005). Lack of degradation of PEI may contribute further to the overall toxicity (Lecocq et al., 2000; Forrest et al., 2003). Other drawbacks, such as inducing aggregation of blood cells and platelets and activation of the complement system, have also been implicated in organs such as liver and lung (Ogris et al., 1999; Chollet et al., 2002). One discouraging observation is that the transfection activity of PEI always seems to associate with its toxicity to a certain degree (Thomas and Klibanov, 2002). This may relate to the fact that in order to rupture the endosome membrane and to transfect cells effectively, a threshold level of DNA/PEI complexes that accumulate in these vesicles has to be reached, which could cause cell damage.

Naturally Occurring Substances as Gene Carriers

Naturally occurring cationic compounds, including poly-L-lysine (Wu and Wu, 1987), protamine (Park et al., 2003), histone (Balicki and Beutler, 1997), and chitosine (Mansouri et al., 2004), are biodegradable and biocompatible. Thus, they are more desirable candidates for gene delivery. Poly-L-lysine is one of the first reagents used in gene delivery (Wu and Wu, 1987; Wolfert et al., 1999). Unfortunately, poly-L-lysine shows rather weak activity and modest to high toxicity, due primarily to its poor endosomolytic activity. Other proteins-based gene carriers, such as histone and protamin, suffer from very similar problems. Chitosan is another naturally occurring compound used as a gene carrier. Chitason is nontoxic polysaccharide capable of condensing DNA. With unlimited natural resources, chitosan could be an ideal gene carrier if its gene delivery efficiency could be improved (MacLaughlin et al., 1998; Kim et al., 2005). Enhancement of endosomal release by addition of a pH-sensitive endosomolytic peptide was reported to lead to a significant increase in reporter gene expression of all polycation-based transfection, with the exception of PEI.

Targeted Gene Delivery

The reduction of toxicity by PEGylation or other chemical modifications is in agreement with diminished binding of the complexes to cells. To restore gene transfer ability and acquire active targeting capability, several conjugations have been investigated, including integrin (Erbacher et al., 1999), transferrin (Kircheis et al., 2001), folate (Lu and Low, 2002), glycosylation (Kawakami et al., 2002), antibody (Tan et al., 2003), low-density lipoplotein (Yu et al., 2001), growth factors (Sosnowski et al., 1996; Ma et al., 2004), and others (Barrett et al., 2004; Schlachetzki et al., 2004). Integrins are heterodimeric membrane receptors containing the highly conserved arginine–glycine–aspartic acid (RGD) motif. RGD containing DNA complexes exhibited approximately 200-fold higher transgene expression in targeted cells (Muller et al., 2001). Transferrin has been incorporated into polyplexes with or without PEG spacers. It was demonstrated that transferrin-containing polyplexes show a significant increase in reporter gene expression (Vinogradov et al., 1999; Wightman et al., 1999). Transferrin has also been demonstrated to effectively shield the surface charges of polyplexes (Kircheis et al., 2001). Promising results on hepatocyte targeting in vivo has been achieved by intravenous injection of DNA complexes containing galactose decorated poly-L-ornithine and fusogenic peptides (Nishikawa et al., 2000). Epidermal growth factor has also been covalently coupled to PEI and led to a 300-fold increase in transfection efficiency (Blessing et al., 2001). Significant targeting was also reported using folate (Xu et al., 2001) and low-density lipoprotein (Affleck et al., 2001). Although antibody has been used for targeted gene delivery, the transfection efficiency of antibody-containing DNA complexes remains low (Mohr et al., 2004), probably due to their huge size and interference in interaction between DNA and cationic carriers.

CONCLUSIONS AND FUTURE PERSPECTIVES

Concerted efforts to develop a nonviral method for gene delivery to date have resulted in many useful tools for studies involving delivery into cells of DNA, RNA, proteins, or other types of molecules. The principle of nonviral gene delivery has now been proved through preclinical and clinical studies. The field of nonviral gene delivery has advanced significantly in recent years in basic research and application, and the level of gene expression resulting from a few nonviral gene delivery systems (e.g., gene expression in liver by hydrodynamic delivery and electroporation in skin and muscle), are approaching those for viral vectors. However, as a whole, the majority of nonviral methods are still much less efficient than viral methods in vivo. In addition, inflammation responses due to treatment-related tissue damage and toxic effects of carriers compounded with the innate immune response to unmethylated CpG content in DNA have been documented. Technically, there are a number of hurdles to overcome before a safe and efficient method of gene delivery can be developed for human use. Significant improvement needs to be achieved in (1) the efficiency of gene transfer by gene gun, electroporation, sonophoresis, and laser beam–based gene delivery; (2) the procedure with reduced injection volume for hydrodynamic delivery; (3) the safety profile of lipoplexes and polyplexes; (4) our understanding of the mechanisms regulating intracellular trafficking of transgene; (5) the targeting ability of synthetic vectors for their function in avoiding clearance by the reticuloendothelial system, in passing through the endothelium, and in entering parenchyma cells; and (6) our understanding of the difference in transfection between in vitro and in vivo. Although these are challenging tasks, it is likely that as our understanding of the gene delivery process improves, more efficacious synthetic vectors or physical methods will emerge.

Acknowledgments

This work was supported in part by the National Institutes of Health through grants RO1 HL075542 and RO1 EB002946.

REFERENCES

Affleck DG, Yu L, Bull DA, Bailey SH, Kim SW (2001). Augmentation of myocardial transfection using TerplexDNA: a novel gene delivery system. *Gene Ther*. 8:349–353.

Aihara H, Miyazaki J (1998). Gene transfer into muscle by electroporation in vivo. *Nat Biotechnol*. 16:867–870.

Andre F, Mir LM (2004). DNA electrotransfer: its principles and an updated review of its therapeutic applications. *Gene Ther*. 11 (Suppl 1):S33–S42.

Anwer K, Kao G, Proctor B, et al. (2000). Ultrasound enhancement of cationic lipid-mediated gene transfer to primary tumors following systemic administration. *Gene Ther*. 7:1833–1839.

Babiuk S, Baca-Estrada ME, Foldvari M, et al. (2002). Electroporation improves the efficacy of DNA vaccines in large animals. *Vaccine*. 20:3399–3408.

Balicki D, Beutler E (1997). Histone H2A significantly enhances in vitro DNA transfection. *Mol Med*. 3:782–787.

Barfoed AM, Kristensen B, Dannemann-Jensen T, et al. (2004). Influence of routes and administration parameters on antibody response of pigs following DNA vaccination. *Vaccine*. 22:1395–1405.

Barnett FH, Scharer-Schuksz M, Wood M, Yu X, Wagner TE, Friedlander M (2004). Intra-arterial delivery of endostatin gene to brain tumors prolongs survival and alters tumor vessel ultrastructure. *Gene Ther*. 11:1283–1289.

Barrett LB, Berry M, Ying W-B, et al. (2004). CTb targeted non-viral cDNA delivery enhances transgene expression in neurons. *J Gene Med*. 6:429–438.

Blessing T, Kursa M, Holzhauser R, Kircheis R, Wagner E (2001). Different strategies for formation of pegylated EGF-conjugated PEI/DNA complexes for targeted gene delivery. *Bioconjug Chem*. 12:529–537.

Boussif O, Lezoualc'h F, Zanta MA, et al. (1995). A versatile vector for gene and oligonucleotide transfer into cells in culture and in vivo: polyethylenimine. *Proc Natl Acad Sci U S A*. 92:7297–7301.

Boussif O, Delair T, Brua C, Veron L, Pavirani A, Kolbe HV (1999). Synthesis of polyallylamine derivatives and their use as gene transfer vectors in vitro. *Bioconjug Chem*. 10:877–883.

Byk G, Dubertret C, Escriou V, et al. (1998). Synthesis, activity, and structure–activity relationship studies of novel cationic lipids for DNA transfer. *J Med Chem*. 41:229–235.

Cheng L, Ziegelhoffer PR, Yang NS (1993). In vivo promoter activity and transgene expression in mammalian somatic tissues evaluated by using particle bombardment. *Proc Natl Acad Sci U S A*. 90:4455–4459.

Chollet P, Favrot MC, Hurbin A, Coll J-L (2002). Side-effects of a systemic injection of linear polyethylenimine–DNA complexes. *J Gene Med*. 4:84–91.

Condon C, Watkins SC, Celluzzi CM, Thompson K, Falo LD Jr (1996). DNA-based immunization by in vivo transfection of dendritic cells. *Nat Med*. 2:1122–1128.

Demeneix B, Hassani Z, Behr JP (2004). Towards multifunctional synthetic vectors. *Cur Gene Ther*. 4:445–455.

Draghia-Akli R, Cummings KK, Khan AS, Brown PA, Carpenter RH (2003). Effects of plasmid-mediated growth hormone releasing hormone supplementation in young, healthy beagle dogs. *J Anim Sci*. 81:2301–2310.

Eastman SJ, Baskin KM, Hodges BL, et al. (2002). Development of catheter-based procedures for transducing the isolated rabbit liver with plasmid DNA. *Hum Gene Ther*. 13:2065–2077.

Eliyahu H, Servel N, Domb AJ, Barenholz Y (2002). Lipoplex-induced hemagglutination: potential involvement in intravenous gene delivery. *Gene Ther*. 9:850–858.

Emerson M, Renwick L, Tate S, et al. (2003). Transfection efficiency and toxicity following delivery of naked plasmid DNA and cationic lipid–DNA complexes to ovine lung segments. *Mol Ther*. 8:646–653.

Erbacher P, Remy JS, Behr JP (1999). Gene transfer with synthetic virus-like particles via the integrin-mediated endocytosis pathway. *Gene Ther*. 6:138–145.

Felgner PL, Gadek TR, Holm M, et al. (1987) Lipofection: a highly efficient, lipid-mediated DNA-transfection procedure. *Proc Natl Acad Sci U S A*. 84:7413–7417.

Fellinger K, Schmidt J (1954). *Klinik and Therapies des chromischen Gelenkreumatismus*. Vienna, Austria: Maudrich; 549–552.

Feltquate DM, Heaney S, Webster RG, Robinson HL (1997). Different T helper cell types and antibody isotypes generated by saline and gene gun DNA immunization. *J Immunol*. 158:2278–2284.

Ferrari ME, Rusalov D, Enas J, Wheeler CJ (2002). Synergy between cationic lipid and co-lipid determines the macroscopic structure and transfection activity of lipoplexes. *Nucleic Acids Res*. 30:1808–1816.

Forrest ML, Koerber JT, Pack DW (2003). A degradable polyethylenimine derivative with low toxicity for highly efficient gene delivery. *Bioconjug Chem*. 14:934–940.

Gao X, Huang L (1991). A novel cationic liposome reagent for efficient transfection of mammalian cells. *Biochem Biophys Res Commun*. 179:280–285.

Godbey WT, Wu KK, Mikos AG (1999). Tracking the intracellular path of poly(ethylenimine)/DNA complexes for gene delivery. *Proc Natl Acad Sci U S A*. 96:5177–5181.

Haensler J, Szoka FC Jr (1993). Polyamidoamine cascade polymers mediate efficient transfection of cells in culture. *Bioconjug Chem*. 4:372–379.

Hagstrom JE, Hegge J, Zhang G, et al. (2004): A facile nonviral method for delivering genes and siRNAs to skeletal muscle of mammalian limbs. *Mol Ther*. 10:386–398.

Hamar P, Song E, Kokeny G, Chen A, Ouyang N, Lieberman J (2004). Small interfering RNA targeting Fas protects mice against renal ischemia-reperfusion injury. *Proc Natl Acad Sci U S A*. 101:14883–14888.

Heiser WC (2004). Delivery of DNA to cells in culture using particle bombardment. *Methods Mol Biol*. 245:175–184.

Hengge UR, Chan EF, Foster RA, Walker PS, Vogel JC (1995). Cytokine gene expression in epidermis with biological effects following injection of naked DNA. *Nat Genet*. 10:161–166.

Hickman MA, Malone RW, Lehmann-Bruinsma K, et al. (1994). Gene expression following direct injection of DNA into liver. *Hum Gene Ther*. 5:1477–1483.

Hirko A, Tang F, Hughes JA (2003). Cationic lipid vectors for plasmid DNA delivery. *Cur Med Chem*. 10:1185–1193.

Huber PE, Mann MJ, Melo LG, et al. (2003). Focused ultrasound (HIFU) induces localized enhancement of reporter gene expression in rabbit carotid artery. *Gene Ther*. 10:1600–1607.

Hwang SJ, Bellocq NC, Davis ME (2001). Effects of structure of β-cyclodextrin-containing polycations on gene delivery. *Bioconjug Chem*. 12:280–290.

Imoto J-I, Konishi E (2005). Needle-free jet injection of a mixture of Japanese encephalitis DNA and protein vaccines: a strategy to effectively enhance immunogenicity of the DNA vaccine in a murine model. *Viral Immunol*. 18:205–212.

Jaroszeski MJ, Heller LC, Gilbert R, Heller R (2004). Electrically mediated plasmid DNA delivery to solid tumors in vivo. *Methods Mol Biol*. 245:237–244.

Jiao S, Williams P, Berg RK, et al. (1992). Direct gene transfer into nonhuman primate myofibers in vivo. *Hum Gene Ther*. 3:21–33.

Jiao S, Cheng L, Wolff JA, Yang NS (1993). Particle bombardment–mediated gene transfer and expression in rat brain tissues. *Biotechnology (NY)*. 11:497–502.

Kawakami S, Yamashita F, Nishida K, Nakamura J, Hashida M (2002). Glycosylated cationic liposomes for cell-selective gene delivery. *Crit Rev Ther Drug Carrier Syst*. 19:171–190.

Kim TH, Kim SI, Akaike T, Cho CS (2005). Synergistic effect of poly(ethylenimine) on the transfection efficiency of galactosylated chitosan/DNA complexes. *J Control Release*. 105:354–366.

Kircheis R, Wightman L, Schreiber A, et al. (2001). Polyethylenimine/DNA complexes shielded by transferrin target gene expression to tumors after systemic application. *Gene Ther*. 8:28–40.

Klein RM, Wolf ED, Wu R, Sanford JC (1987). High-velocity microprojectiles for delivering nucleic acids into living cells. *Nature*. 327:70–73.

Kukowska-Latallo JF, Bielinska AU, Johnson J, Spindler R, Tomalia DA, Baker JR Jr (1996). Efficient transfer of genetic material into mammalian cells using Starburst polyamidoamine dendrimers. *Proc Natl Acad Sci U S A*. 93:4897–4902.

Kuriyama S, Mitoro A, Tsujinoue H, et al. (2000). Particle-mediated gene transfer into murine livers using a newly developed gene gun. *Gene Ther*. 7:1132–1136.

Lappalainen K, Miettinen R, Kellokoski J, Jaaskelainen I, Syrjanen S (1997). Intracellular distribution of oligonucleotides delivered by cationic liposomes: light and electron microscopic study. *J Histochem Cytochem*. 45:265–274.

Lauritzen HPMM, Reynet C, Schjerling P, et al. (2002). Gene gun bombardment-mediated expression and translocation of EGFP-tagged GLUT4 in skeletal muscle fibres in vivo. *Pflugers Arch*. 444:710–721.

Lawrie A, Brisken AF, Francis SE, Cumberland DC, Crossman DC, Newman CM (2000). Microbubble-enhanced ultrasound for vascular gene delivery. *Gene Ther*. 7: 2023–2027.

Lecocq M, Wattiaux-De Coninck S, Laurent N, Wattiaux R, Jadot M (2000). Uptake and intracellular fate of polyethylenimine in vivo. *Biochem Biophys Res Commun*. 278:414–418.

Lee TH, Yang LC, Chou AK, et al. (2003). In vivo electroporation of proopiomelanocortin induces analgesia in a formalin-injection pain model in rats. *Pain*. 104:159–167.

Lee TWR, Matthews DA, Blair GE (2005). Novel molecular approaches to cystic fibrosis gene therapy. *Biochem J*. 387:1–15.

Lima KM, dos Santos SA, Santos RR, Brandao IT, Rodrigues JM Jr, Silva CL (2003). Efficacy of DNA-hsp65 vaccination for tuberculosis varies with method of DNA introduction in vivo. *Vaccine* 22:49–56.

Liu D, Ren T and Gao X (2003). Cationic transfection lipids. *Cur Med Chem*. 10: 1307–1315.

Liu F, Qi H, Huang L, Liu D (1997). Factors controlling the efficiency of cationic lipid-mediated transfection in vivo via intravenous administration. *Gene Ther*. 4: 517–523.

Liu F, Song Y, Liu D (1999). Hydrodynamics-based transfection in animals by systemic administration of plasmid DNA. *Gene Ther*. 6:1258–1266.

Liu Y, Mounkes LC, Liggitt HD, et al. (1997). Factors influencing the efficiency of cationic liposome-mediated intravenous gene delivery. *Nat Biotechnol*. 15:167–173.

Losordo DW, Vale PR, Hendel RC, et al. (2002). Phase 1/2 placebo-controlled, double-blind, dose-escalating trial of myocardial vascular endothelial growth factor 2 gene transfer by catheter delivery in patients with chronic myocardial ischemia. *Circulation*. 105:2012–2018.

Lu Y, Low PS (2002). Folate-mediated delivery of macromolecular anticancer therapeutic agents. *Adv Drug Deliv Rev*. 54:675–693.

Lungwitz U, Breunig M, Blunk T, Gopferich A (2005). Polyethylenimine-based non-viral gene delivery systems. *Eur J Pharm Biopharm*. 60:247–266.

Ma N, Wu SS, Ma YX, et al. (2004). Nerve growth factor receptor-mediated gene transfer. *Mol Ther*. 9:270–281.

MacLaughlin FC, Mumper RJ, Wang J, et al. (1998). Chitosan and depolymerized chitosan oligomers as condensing carriers for in vivo plasmid delivery. *J Control Release*. 56:259–272.

Magee TR, Ferrini M, Garban HJ, et al. (2002) Gene therapy of erectile dysfunction in the rat with penile neuronal nitric oxide synthase. *Biol Reprod*. 67:20–28.

Mann MJ, Gibbons GH, Hutchinson H, et al. (1999). Pressure-mediated oligonucleotide transfection of rat and human cardiovascular tissues. *Proc Natl Acad Sci U S A*. 96:6411–6416.

Mansouri S, Lavigne P, Corsi K, Benderdour M, Beaumont E, Fernandes JC (2004). Chitosan-DNA nanoparticles as non-viral vectors in gene therapy: strategies to improve transfection efficacy. *Eur J Pharm Biopharm*. 57:1–8.

Martiniuk F, Chen A, Mack A, et al. (2002). Helios gene gun particle delivery for therapy of acid maltase deficiency. *DNA Cell Biol*. 21:717–725.

Maruyama H, Higuchi N, Nishikawa Y, et al. (2002). High-level expression of naked DNA delivered to rat liver via tail vein injection. *J Gene Med*. 4:333–341.

Matsuno Y, Iwata H, Umeda Y, et al. (2003). Nonviral gene gun mediated transfer into the beating heart. *ASAIO J*. 49:641–644.

Medi BM, Hoselton S, Marepalli RB, Singh J (2005). Skin targeted DNA vaccine delivery using electroporation in rabbits. I: efficacy. *Int J Pharm*. 294:53–63.

Miller AD (2003). The problem with cationic liposome/micelle-based non-viral vector systems for gene therapy. *Cur Med Chem*. 10:1195–1211.

Mir LM, Moller PH, Andre F, Gehl J (2005). Electric pulse-mediated gene delivery to various animal tissues. *Adv Genet*. 54:83–114.

Mitragotri S, Edwards DA, Blankschtein D, Langer R (1995). A mechanistic study of ultrasonically-enhanced transdermal drug delivery. *J Pharm Sci*. 84:697–706.

Moghimi SM, Symonds P, Murray JC, Hunter AC, Debska G, Szewczyk A (2005). A two-stage poly(ethylenimine)-mediated cytotoxicity: implications for gene transfer/therapy. *Mol Ther*. 11:990–995.

Mohr L, Yeung A, Aloman C, Wittrup D, Wands JR (2004). Antibody-directed therapy for human hepatocellular carcinoma. *Gastroenterology*. 127:S225–S231.

Muller K, Nahde T, Fahr A, Muller R, Brusselbach S (2001). Highly efficient transduction of endothelial cells by targeted artificial virus-like particles. *Cancer Gene Ther*. 8:107–117.

Muramatsu T, Shibata O, Ryoki S, Ohmori Y, Okumura J (1997). Foreign gene expression in the mouse testis by localized in vivo gene transfer. *Biochem Biophys Res Commun*. 233:45–49.

Neu M, Fischer D, Kissel T (2005). Recent advances in rational gene transfer vector design based on poly(ethylene imine) and its derivatives. *J Gene Med*. 7:992–1009.

Neumann E, Schaefer-Ridder M, Wang Y, Hofschneider PH (1982). Gene transfer into mouse lyoma cells by electroporation in high electric fields. *EMBO J*. 1:841–845.

Nishikawa M, Yamauchi M, Morimoto K, Ishida E, Takakura Y, Hashida M (2000). Hepatocyte-targeted in vivo gene expression by intravenous injection of plasmid DNA complexed with synthetic multi-functional gene delivery system. *Gene Ther*. 7: 548–555.

Ogris M, Brunner S, Schuller S, Kircheis R, Wagner E (1999). PEGylated DNA/transferrin-PEI complexes: reduced interaction with blood components, extended circulation in blood and potential for systemic gene delivery. *Gene Ther*. 6:595–605.

Park YJ, Liang JF, Ko KS, Kim SW, Yang VC (2003). Low molecular weight protamine as an efficient and nontoxic gene carrier: in vitro study. *J Gene Med*. 5:700–711.

Plank C, Mechtler K, Szoka FC Jr, Wagner E (1996). Activation of the complement system by synthetic DNA complexes: a potential barrier for intravenous gene delivery. *Hum Gene Ther*. 7:1437–1446.

Pollard H, Remy JS, Loussouarn G, Demolombe S, Behr JP, Escande D (1998). Poly ethylenimine but not cationic lipids promotes transgene delivery to the nucleus in mammalian cells. *J Biol Chem*. 273:7507–7511.

Prayaga SK, Ford MJ, Haynes JR (1997). Manipulation of HIV-1 gp120-specific immune responses elicited via gene gun-based DNA immunization. *Vaccine*. 15:1349–1352.

Ren T, Song YK, Zhang G, Liu D (2000). Structural basis for DOTMA for its high intravenous transfection activity in mouse. *Gene Ther*. 7:764–768.

Reszka RC, Jacobs A, Voges J (2005). Liposome-mediated suicide gene therapy in humans. *Methods Enzymol*. 391:200–208.

Rols MP, Delteil C, Golzio M, Dumond P, Cros S, Teissie J (1998). In vivo electrically mediated protein and gene transfer in murine melanoma. *Nat Biotechnol*. 16:168–171.

Romoren K, Thu BJ, Evensen O (2004). Expression of luciferase in selected organs following delivery of naked and formulated DNA to rainbow trout (*Oncorhynchus mykiss*) by different routes of administration. *Fish Shellfish Immunol*. 16:251–264.

Sakamoto T, Oshima Y, Nakagawa K, Ishibashi T, Inomata H, Sueishi K (1999). Target gene transfer of tissue plasminogen activator to cornea by electric pulse inhibits intracameral fibrin formation and corneal cloudiness. *Hum Gene Ther*. 10:2551–2557.

Sakurai F, Nishioka T, Saito H, et al. (2001). Interaction between DNA–cationic liposome complexes and erythrocytes is an important factor in systemic gene transfer via the intravenous route in mice: the role of the neutral helper lipid. *Gene Ther*. 8:677–686.

Sasaki S, Takeshita F, Xin KQ, Ishii N, Okuda K (2003). Adjuvant formulations and delivery systems for DNA vaccines. *Methods*. 31:243–254.

Scheerlinck J-PY, Karlis J, Tjelle TE, Presidente PJA, Mathiesen I, Newton SE (2004). In vivo electroporation improves immune responses to DNA vaccination in sheep. *Vaccine*. 22:1820–1825.

Schlachetzki F, Zhang Y, Boado RJ, Pardridge WM (2004). Gene therapy of the brain: the trans-vascular approach. *Neurology*. 62:1275–1281.

Smyth-Templeton NS, Lasic DD, Frederik PM, Strey HH, Roberts DD, and Palvlakis GN (1997). Improved DNA:liposome complexes for increased systemic delivery and gene expression. *Nature Biotechnol*. 15:647–652.

Sonawane ND, Szoka FC Jr, Verkman AS (2003). Chloride accumulation and swelling in endosomes enhances DNA transfer by polyamine–DNA polyplexes. *J Biol Chem*. 278:44826–44831.

Song YK, Liu F, Chu S, Liu D (1997). Characterization of cationic liposome-mediated gene transfer in vivo by intravenous administration. *Hum Gene Ther*. 8:1585–1594.

Song K, Chang Y, Prud'homme GJ (2000). Regulation of T-helper-1 versus T-helper-2 activity and enhancement of tumor immunity by combined DNA-based vaccination and nonviral cytokine gene transfer. *Gene Ther*. 7:481–492.

Sosnowski BA, Gonzalez AM, Chandler LA, Buechler YJ, Pierce GF, Baird A (1996). Targeting DNA to cells with basic fibroblast growth factor (FGF2). *J Biol Chem*. 271:33647–33653.

Tamura T, Nishi T, Goto T, et al. (2001). Intratumoral delivery of interleukin 12 expression plasmids with in vivo electroporation is effective for colon and renal cancer. *Hum Gene Ther*. 12:1265–1276.

Tan PH, Manunta M, Ardjomand N, et al. (2003). Antibody targeted gene transfer to endothelium. *J Gene Med*. 5:311–323.

Tanaka S, Uehara T, Nomura Y (2000). Up-regulation of protein–disulfide isomerase in response to hypoxia/brain ischemia and its protective effect against apoptotic cell death. *J Biol Chem*. 275:10388–10393.

Tang MX, Redemann CT, Szoka FC Jr (1996). In vitro gene delivery by degraded polyamidoamine dendrimers. *Bioconjug Chem*. 7:703–714.

Tanigawa K, Yu H, Sun R, Nickoloff BJ, Chang AE (2000). Gene gun application in the generation of effector T cells for adoptive immunotherapy. *Cancer Immunol Immunother*. 48:635–643.

Thanaketpaisarn O, Nishikawa M, Yamashita F, Hashida M (2005). Tissue-specific characteristics of in vivo electric gene: transfer by tissue and intravenous injection of plasmid DNA. *Pharm Res*. 22:883–891.

Thomas M, Klibanov AM (2002). Enhancing polyethylenimine's delivery of plasmid DNA into mammalian cells. *Proc Natl Acad Sci U S A*. 99:14640–14645.

Thompson TA, Gould MN, Burkholder JK, Yang NS (1993). Transient promoter activity in primary rat mammary epithelial cells evaluated using particle bombardment gene transfer. *In Vitro Cell Dev Biol*. 29A:165–170.

Tollefsen S, Vordermeier M, Olsen I, et al. (2003). DNA injection in combination with electroporation: a novel method for vaccination of farmed ruminants. *Scand J Immunol*. 57:229–238.

Trimble C, Lin C-T, Hung C-F, et al. (2003). Comparison of the CD8+ T cell responses and antitumor effects generated by DNA vaccine administered through gene gun, biojector, and syringe. *Vaccine*. 21:4036–4042.

Tupin E, Poirier B, Bureau MF, Khallou-Laschet J, Vranckx R, Caligiuri G, Gaston A-T, Duong Van Huyen J-P, Scherman D, Bariety J, Michel J-B, Nicoletti A (2003). Non-viral gene transfer of murine spleen cells achieved by in vivo electroporation. *Gene Ther*. 10:569–579.

Vigneron JP, Oudrhiri N, Fauquet M, et al. (1996). Guanidinium–cholesterol cationic lipids: efficient vectors for the transfection of eukaryotic cells. *Proc Natl Acad Sci U S A*. 93:9682–9686.

Vinogradov S, Batrakova E, Li S, Kabanov A (1999). Polyion complex micelles with protein-modified corona for receptor-mediated delivery of oligonucleotides into cells. *Bioconjug Chem*. 10:851–860.

von Harpe A, Petersen H, Li Y, Kissel T (2000). Characterization of commercially available and synthesized polyethylenimines for gene delivery. *J Control Release*. 69:309–322.

Walther W, Stein U, Fichtner I, Malcherek L, Lemm M, Schlag PM (2001). Nonviral in vivo gene delivery into tumors using a novel low volume jet-injection technology. *Gene Ther*. 8:173–180.

Wang J, Murakami T, Hakamata Y, et al. (2001). Gene gun-mediated oral mucosal transfer of interleukin 12 cDNA coupled with an irradiated melanoma vaccine in a hamster model: successful treatment of oral melanoma and distant skin lesion. *Cancer Gene Ther*. 8:705–712.

Whitmore M, Li S, Huang L (1999). LPD lipopolyplex initiates a potent cytokine response and inhibits tumor growth. *Gene Ther*. 6:1867–1875.

Wightman L, Patzelt E, Wagner E, Kircheis R (1999). Development of transferrin-polycation/DNA based vectors for gene delivery to melanoma cells. *J Drug Target*. 7:293–303.

Wightman L, Kircheis R, Rossler V, et al. (2001). Different behavior of branched and linear polyethylenimine for gene delivery in vitro and in vivo. *J Gene Med*. 3:362–372.

Wolfert MA, Dash PR, Nazarova O, et al. (1999). Polyelectrolyte vectors for gene delivery: influence of cationic polymer on biophysical properties of complexes formed with DNA. *Bioconjug Chem*. 10:993–1004.

Wolff JA, Malone RW, Williams P, et al. (1990). Direct gene transfer into mouse muscle in vivo. *Science*. 247:1465–1468.

Wu GY and Wu CH (1987). Receptor-mediated in vitro gene transformation by a soluble DNA carrier system. *J Biol Chem*. 262:4429–4432.

Xu L, Pirollo KF, Chang EH (2001). Tumor-targeted p53-gene therapy enhances the efficacy of conventional chemo/radiotherapy. *J Control Release*. 74:115–128.

Yamashita YI, Shimada M, Hasegawa H, et al. (2001). Electroporation-mediated interleukin-12 gene therapy for hepatocellular carcinoma in the mice model. *Cancer Res*. 61:1005–1012.

Yang NS, Burkholder J, Roberts B, Martinell B, McCabe D (1990). In vivo and in vitro gene transfer to mammalian somatic cells by particle bombardment. *Proc Natl Acad Sci U S A*. 87:9568–9572.

Yomogida K, Yagura Y, Nishimune Y (2002). Electroporated transgene-rescued spermato-genesis in infertile mutant mice with a Sertoli cell defect. *Biol Reprod*. 67:712–717.

Yu L, Suh H, Koh JJ, Kim SW (2001). Systemic administration of TerplexDNA system: pharmacokinetics and gene expression. *Pharm Res*. 18:1277–1283.

Yu W, Pirollo KF, Rait A, et al. (2004). A sterically stabilized immunolipoplex for systemic administration of a therapeutic gene. *Gene Ther*. 11:1434–1440.

Zabner J, Fasbender AJ, Moninger T, Poellinger KA, Welsh MJ (1995). Cellular and molecular barriers to gene transfer by a cationic lipid. *J Biol Chem*. 270:18997–19007.

Zampaglione I, Arcuri M, Cappelletti M, et al. (2005). In vivo DNA gene electro-transfer: a systematic analysis of different electrical parameters. *J Gene Med*. Jul:1.

Zeira E, Manevitch A, Khatchatouriants A, et al. (2003). Femtosecond infrared laser-an efficient and safe in vivo gene delivery system for prolonged expression. *Mol Ther*. 8:342–350.

Zhang G, Vargo D, Budker V, Armstrong N, Knechtle S, Wolff JA (1997). Expression of naked plasmid DNA injected into the afferent and efferent vessels of rodent and dog livers. *Hum Gene Ther*. 8:1763–1772.

Zhang G, Budker V, Wolff JA (1999). High levels of foreign gene expression in hepato-cytes after tail vein injections of naked plasmid DNA. *Hum Gene Ther*. 10:1735–1737.

Zhang G, Budker V, Williams P, Subbotin V, Wolff JA (2001). Efficient expression of naked DNA delivered intraarterially to limb muscles of nonhuman primates. *Hum Gene Ther*. 12:427–438.

Zhang G, Gao X, Song YK, et al. (2004). Hydroporation as the mechanism of hydrody-namic delivery. *Gene Ther*. 11:675–682.

Zhang L, Nolan E, Kreitschitz S, Rabussay DP (2002). Enhanced delivery of naked DNA to the skin by non-invasive in vivo electroporation. *Biochim Biophys Acta*. 1572:1–9.

Zhang S, Gu J, Yang N-S, et al. (2002). Relative promoter strengths in four human prostate cancer cell lines evaluated by particle bombardment–mediated gene transfer. *Prostate*. 51:286–292.

Zuidam NJ, Barenholz Y (1998). Electrostatic and structural properties of complexes involving plasmid DNA and cationic lipids commonly used for gene delivery. *Biochim Biophys Acta*. 1368:115–128.

9 Therapeutic Gene Transfer to Skeletal Muscle

PAUL GREGOREVIC and JEFFREY S. CHAMBERLAIN
Department of Neurology, Division of Neurogenetics, The University
of Washington School of Medicine, Seattle, Washington

Development of safe, efficient methods for the delivery of therapeutic genes to skeletal muscles is highly desirable for the treatment of a range of serious clinical conditions. Progress in the field of gene therapy has seen the development of a number of gene transfer technologies that may be adapted for the treatment of muscle-based conditions. Among the various systems, recombinant viral vectors derived from adeno-associated viruses (rAAVs) presently offer considerable potential for systemic delivery of gene constructs. In this chapter we briefly review some of the challenges to developing strategies for therapeutic gene transfer to muscle, and discuss the potential for rAAV vectors as a therapeutic gene delivery system.

Many conditions associated with muscle disease may be amenable to treatment by gene replacement or supplementation. Principal among these are severe forms of muscular dystrophy and myopathy that arise from single gene mutations that disrupt production of critical proteins. Gene transfer may also prove useful for the treatment of other conditions associated with muscle dysfunction, such as muscle wasting attributed to advanced aging, forms of cancer, chronic obstructive pulmonary diseases, and disuse mediated by inactivity due to preexisting illness. Also, it has been proposed that skeletal muscle may serve as an endocrine organ for the production of secretable products following transduction with an appropriate gene expression construct. Any intervention intending to achieve a therapeutic effect as a consequence of gene transfer to muscle must address a number of challenges associated with the efficiency and safety of vector delivery and the duration of transgene expression. As rAAV vectors have shown considerable promise as tools for gene transfer to skeletal muscle, they might ultimately prove valuable for the treatment of muscle-related disease.

VECTOR REQUIREMENTS AND PRODUCTION

Skeletal muscle may comprise as much as 40% of a person's mass. In an adult this may translate to more than 30 kg of skeletal muscle tissue, comprising more than 10^{12} myonuclei actively maintaining myofiber structure and function.[1] Treatment of severe muscle disorders such as Duchenne muscular dystrophy may require the transduction of individual myonuclei along the length of individual muscle fibers. Furthermore, because transduction efficiency is influenced by factors such as the route of administration and vector uptake by nonmuscle tissues (discussed later), successful treatment of a patient's entire musculature may require administration of considerably more vector than is needed to transduce just the estimated myonuclear population.[2] Such vector requirements may present a significant challenge regarding production logistics and cost.

Recombinant AAV vectors are typically generated by substituting the majority of the ~4.8-kb wild-type genome with an expression cassette of interest, and providing the viral genes associated with replication and capsid formation on an adenovirus-derived helper plasmid. Vector production entails transient transfection of HEK293 cells with a two-plasmid system and subsequent vector harvest. This system can generate vector at a yield approaching 10^5 vector genomes (vg) per cell.[3] An alternative vector production system under development using recombinant baculoviruses to provide the genes required for production in insect cells in culture has been reported to attain yields approaching 10^4 vg/cell.[4] This is an exciting prospect, as technical improvements to raise efficiency and the potential for scaling suspension culture may offer a promising means of reducing labor and cost requirements associated with large-scale vector production. Enrichment of vectors to a highly pure state will also prove essential for safe administration to patients. Purification of rAAV vectors via a combination of chromatography and density gradient centrifugation can generate titers on the order of 10^{14} vg/mL.

VECTOR SELECTIVITY FOR SKELETAL MUSCLE
AND EFFICIENCY OF MUSCLE TRANSDUCTION

The selectivity (or tropism) of a vector for the target tissue is critical to the practicality of a potential intervention, especially when administered via the bloodstream. Appropriate selectivity ensures that practical numbers of the therapeutic gene will be taken up by the cells of interest without undue uptake by other tissue types. The latter point is a critical factor, as it influences the dose requirement to transduce the target tissue effectively. Furthermore, vector uptake by nontarget cells may pose a risk to intervention tolerance, should it be associated with cellular toxicity or immune-cell presentation. Recombinant AAV vectors comprising alternative naturally occurring capsid isoforms (dubbed *serotypes*) exhibit differing propensity to transduce cell types in vivo, and a number of investigators have demonstrated that modification of the capsid gene can alter the tropism (or selectivity for transduction of a given tissue) of the vectors generated.[5,6]

Notably, serotype-6 rAAV vectors are particularly effective at transducing striated musculature, with comparatively little transduction of nonmuscle tissue via intravascular administration.[2,3] By comparison, vector systems based on plasmid DNA, adenoviruses, and retroviruses either fail to achieve an equivalent degree of muscle transduction per vector dose and/or elicit increased expression in nonmuscle tissues. While expression constructs can be designed to incorporate muscle-specific promoters to constrain the pattern of transgene expression, restricting vector tropism should also be considered an important factor when designing an intervention that may be distributed throughout the body of a patient. With the identification of over 100 AAV capsid variants to date, it remains to be seen whether novel serotypes will prove even better suited than more commonly used examples to muscle-based gene transfer. Alternatively, strategic modification of the capsid protein structure may endow a vector with modified tropism and limit gene transfer to nontarget cell types.

DELIVERY OF VECTORS TO THE MUSCLE MEMBRANE

Intramuscular administration of vectors is constrained by the distance of dissemination from the point of administration. Furthermore, vector dispersal in diseased muscles can be hampered as a consequence of the increased presence of intramuscular connective tissue, fat, and fibrous deposition. Given the challenges of achieving widespread transduction of even a single human muscle via direct injection, as many as hundreds of thousands of intramuscular injections would be required to attain saturable transduction of a patient's entire musculature. An efficient strategy for gene transfer will therefore probably require intravascular vector administration and subsequent extravasation. Historically, attempts to realize bodywide vector dissemination and transduction of skeletal musculature in animals have proven unsuccessful, owing to significant uptake of vector by nontarget tissues and/or limited extravastion across the microvascular endothelium.

We have observed that rAAV6 vectors are amenable to low-pressure introduction into the circulatory system of mice to achieve simultaneous transduction of the axial and appendicular musculature.[2] Intravascular infusion of rAAV serotypes that possess tropism for skeletal muscle can also transduce muscles in larger rodents and dogs.[7,8] Targeting cardiac, respiratory, and limb muscles of an adult mammal in a single administration represents an exciting strategy for minimally invasive systemic gene transfer to muscle. However, interventions intended for humans may also require pre-coadministration of agents capable of transiently increasing microvascular permeability, to maximize muscle transduction and minimize nonmuscle uptake. In this regard, agents such as recombinant vascular endothelial growth factor and compounds with related properties may prove useful, as their administration can elicit acute changes in microvascular permeability and facilitate extravasation of rAAV-sized particles.[2] Further research is required to completely define the role of such agents in the potential to achieve vasculature-mediated systemic vector dissemination.

VECTOR TOLERANCE: CELLULAR TOXICITY AND IMMUNOGENICITY

Clinically viable gene transfer must avoid potentially harmful side effects for patients. Such events may include:

- Cellular toxicity associated with uptake of viral proteins following transduction
- Immunologically mediated degradation of transduced tissue initiated following uptake and presentation of virus-derived proteins

Regarding cellular toxicity, AAV is presently considered nonpathogenic in humans, as it has not been linked conclusively with any known disease state. Furthermore, rAAV vectors typically do not contain any of the wildtype genome other than the ~140-bp flanking terminal repeat sequences, and therefore do not express viral proteins upon transduction. rAAV vectors appear capable of being administered in considerable doses via intravascular route to at least mice and dogs without evidence of significant organ toxicity.[2,7] In comparison, adenovirus- and retrovirus-derived vectors can elicit serious toxicity in nonmuscle organs following intravascular administration, even at doses far below that which might be required to attempt systemic gene transfer.

Regarding immunogenic clearance of transduced tissues, the probability of adverse event is influenced by a number of factors, including:

- Tropism specificity of the vector employed
- Expression pattern of the promoter incorporated in the construct design
- Previous exposure to wild-type AAV or rAAV serotypes

Initial assessments suggest that a significant proportion of the human population have been exposed to at least one serotype of AAV.[9,10] This exposure may limit the potential for particular vector serotypes to be administered to patient subsets without eliciting an immune response. Ongoing studies are currently considering the merits of employing transient immune suppression in conjunction with vector administration to facilitate transduction and cellular clearance of the capsid peptides without immunogenic reaction. Encouragingly, it would seem that not all serotypes equally prime the immune system against other variants.[11] Therefore, different serotyped vectors may be useful for different patients, subject to screening evaluation. Additionally, individual vector serotypes appear differentially amenable to repeat administration in animals, which suggests that hybrid capsid designs may elicit comparatively reduced immunological reactions, yet still maintain the tropism of desired serotypes.[11,12] Although the complex issues of immunology associated with recombinant viral vector administration may appear intimidating, concerted efforts to understand the interaction of vector capsids and the immune system will in time establish the true scope for administration of high doses of rAAV to humans.

PERSISTENCE OF EXPRESSION WITHOUT DISRUPTION
OF HOST GENOME INTEGRITY

The therapeutic potential of vectors must also consider the scope for achieving lasting transgene expression in muscle fibers in a manner that does not disrupt transcriptional events associated with cellular homeostasis. Retroviral vectors can achieve sustained transgene expression via integration into the recipient's genome. However, integration events in vivo remain largely uncontrolled, and the risk for insertional mutagenesis constitutes a significant shortcoming. Recombinant AAV vectors present an attractive option for sustained transgene expression, as the recombinant genomes form episomal DNA concatamers that persist in a nonintegrated fashion for years at a time (up to two years in mice and more than five years in dogs and primates) in mammalian musculature, subject to immune tolerance. Studies to date have not detected significant integration of AAV genomes in the nuclei of striated muscles. With appropriate methodological development, a single administration of rAAV vectors may elicit stable transduction of striated musculature beyond five years. Assuming that the safety of long-term gene expression is established in appropriate studies, maximizing transgene persistence would minimize the need for periodic readministration to sustain therapeutic effects and reduce the dependency of patients on continued medical interventions.

Cell turnover may deplete genomes introduced following transduction. In skeletal muscle, individual myofibers exist as terminally differentiated structures, which may persist for years. Myofiber turnover in the course of vigorous physical activity or injury may in time still deplete the population of transduced cells and therefore the therapeutic effect of the initial intervention. In such instances, periodic readministration of the intervention may be required to restore efficacy. However, in the absence of strategies designed to introduce the expression permanently construct into the muscle of the progenitor cell population, any gene transfer system will confront the same problem. Therefore, establishing the full potential for sustaining efficacious transduction in skeletal musculature via administration of rAAV vectors may not be as important as monitoring the degree of therapeutic effect upon disease state indices in anticipation of a potential need to readminister the intervention.

In summary, to develop a clinically viable strategy for attaining whole-body transduction of skeletal musculature in patients, many technical and logistic challenges must be confronted. Although rAAV vectors are not without their shortcomings, they presently represent the most promising strategy for efficient systemic gene transfer to muscle. In particular, intravascular administration of rAAV vectors has proven an attractive approach for achieving therapeutic levels of gene transfer bodywide in the musculature of adult mice. Further technical advances in rAAV vector biology will hopefully enhance the efficiency of gene transfer in this manner and reduce absolute vector requirements. Scaling promising rAAV-based interventions to mammalian models approximating the physical size and immunological profile of patients will also be necessary to ascertain the validity of these approaches for clinical applications.

REFERENCES

1. Ohira Y, Yoshinaga T, Ohara M, et al. Myonuclear domain and myosin phenotype in human soleus after bed rest with or without loading. *J Appl Physiol*. 1999;87:1776–1785.

2. Gregorevic P, Blankinship MJ, Allen JM, et al. Systemic delivery of genes to striated muscles using adeno-associated viral vectors. *Nat Med*. 2004;10:828–834.

3. Blankinship MJ, Gregorevic P, Allen JM, et al. Efficient transduction of skeletal muscle using vectors based on adeno-associated virus serotype 6. *Mol Ther*. 2004;10:671–678.

4. Urabe M, Ding C, Kotin RM. Insect cells as a factory to produce adeno-associated virus type 2 vectors. *Hum Gene Ther*. 2002;13:1935–1943.

5. Grimm D, Zhou S, Nakai H, et al. Preclinical in vivo evaluation of pseudotyped adeno-associated virus vectors for liver gene therapy. *Blood*. 2003;102:2412–2419.

6. Wu Z, Asokan A, Samulski RJ. Adeno-associated virus serotypes: vector toolkit for human gene therapy. *Mol Ther*. 2006;14:316–327.

7. Arruda VR, Stedman HH, Nichols TC, et al. Regional intravascular delivery of AAV-2-F.IX to skeletal muscle achieves long-term correction of hemophilia B in a large animal model. *Blood*. 2005;105:3458–3464.

8. Gregorevic P, Chamberlain JS. Functional enhancement of skeletal muscle by gene transfer. *Phys Med Rehabil Clin N Am*. 2005;16:875–887, vii–viii.

9. Halbert CL, Miller AD, McNamara S, et al. Prevalence of neutralizing antibodies against adeno-associated virus (AAV) types 2, 5, and 6 in cystic fibrosis and normal populations: implications for gene therapy using AAV vectors. *Hum Gene Ther*. 2006;17:440–447.

10. Gao G, Vandenberghe LH, Alvira MR, et al. Clades of adeno-associated viruses are widely disseminated in human tissues. *J Virol*. 2004;78:6381–6388.

11. Halbert CL, Rutledge EA, Allen JM, Russell DW, Miller AD. Repeat transduction in the mouse lung by using adeno-associated virus vectors with different serotypes. *J Virol*. 2000;74:1524–1532.

12. Riviere C, Danos O, Douar AM. Long-term expression and repeated administration of AAV type 1, 2 and 5 vectors in skeletal muscle of immunocompetent adult mice. *Gene Ther*. 2006;13:1300–1308.

10 Gene Therapy for Cardiovascular Disease

CHRISTINA A. PACAK, KERRY O. CRESAWN, and BARRY J. BYRNE

Department of Molecular Genetics and Microbiology, Gene Therapy Center, University of Florida, Gainesville, Florida

The cardiac gene delivery field offers a favorable alternative to options presently available for the treatment of many forms of cardiovasular disease (CVD).[1] Although drugs and surgical procedures are able to improve outcomes with varying degrees of success, gene therapy may one day enable physicians to provide long-lasting single-administration solutions to such problems.

When developing a gene delivery technique for the treatment of a specific disease, several considerations must be taken into account. The first consideration is to determine precisely what tissue is to be targeted for transgene delivery. Whether the disease is multi systemic, including a cardiac component, or one in which cardiac tissue alone is affected, researchers can choose a gene delivery system designed to provide transduction on a global scale, localized to one tissue or contained within a specific area of that tissue.

An example of a cardiac-specific problem that could potentially be ameliorated using a preemptive gene therapy approach was developed by Pachori et al. for recurring myocardial ischemia.[2] A closed chest model of chronic recurring myocardial ischemia and reperfusion was used to investigate the efficacy of overexpressing the antioxidant enzyme HO-1 using an AAV2 delivery vehicle. The approach protected myocytes successfully through a combination of protective-response activation and inhibition of cardiac remodeling.[2]

One example of an inherited disease with a cardiac component that is a good candidate for the development of a gene delivery treatment is Pompe disease, an autosomal recessive disorder characterized by the accumulation of glycogen in lysosomes due to a deficiency in the lysosomal enzyme acid α-glucosidase (Gaa). In this disease the function of skeletal muscle, diaphragm, and many other tissues is compromised, due to the accumulation of glycogen. Patients suffering from the most severe form (making less than 1% of normal levels of functional enzyme) die from cardio respiratory failure within the first one to two years of life.[3,4]

Pompe gene therapy studies have been performed using adenoviral (Ad) vectors, recombinant adeno-associated viral (rAAV) vectors, or plasmid-mediated gene delivery systems.[5] The first Ad-mediated gene delivery studies for Pompe disease were performed in patient fibroblasts, myoblasts, and myotubes.[6,7] These early studies demonstrated the ability to achieve overexpression of Gaa from Ad vectors up to 19- to 20-fold over untreated normal cells.[6,7] The studies also showed clearance of accumulated glycogen in treated cells, secretion of the 110-kDa precursor form into the culture media, localization of the Ad-delivered Gaa protein to the lysosomes, and M6P receptor-mediated uptake of Gaa secreted from transduced cells by Gaa-deficient cells.[6,7]

Once investigators established that viral vector–delivered Gaa is able to restore biochemical function and a natural histological phenotype in transduced cells and can cross-correct untransduced cells, researchers performed in vivo assessments of Ad-mediated Gaa delivery in animals. Both intracardiac and intramuscular delivery of Ad-human *Gaa* (h*Gaa*) were performed in newborn rats and resulted in 10- and sixfold (respectively) normal levels of Gaa in injected tissues.[7]

Recombinant adeno-associated virus (rAAV) is another gene delivery vehicle that has been studied extensively for use in treating Pompe disease. rAAV has emerged as an attractive option for cardiovascular gene therapy, due to its small size, safety, and its proven ability to persist in skeletal muscle for long periods of time.[8–13] The recent emergence of new serotypes of AAV and capsid manipulations of those serotypes have made it possible for researchers to alter natural tropisms to target specific organs.[14–20] Similar to Ad vectors, rAAV can infect both dividing and non-dividing cells; however, in contrast to Ad vectors, rAAV vectors have a packaging capacity of about 4.9 kb.

Several methods of rAAV-mediated correction of Pompe disease have been reported. The first group of studies established both that rAAV-mediated gene delivery of *Gaa* can overexpress Gaa in transduced cells in vitro with cross-correction of Gaa-deficient cells and that direct intramuscular or intramyocardial injections of rAAV-*Gaa* are able to restore Gaa to nearby normal levels in injected tissues.[21] Following intramuscular administration of rAAV serotype 2 (rAAV2) and rAAV serotype 1 (rAAV1) *Gaa*-carrying vectors, Fraites et al. observed 18-fold greater levels of expression with rAAV1 vectors than with rAAV2 vectors in the injected tissue, with rAAV1 vectors yielding levels of Gaa that were 450-fold over normal. The enzyme levels restored in the injected skeletal muscle resulted in glycogen clearance and muscle function improvement. Additionally, intramyocardial delivery with rAAV2 vectors resulted in 70% of normal Gaa levels in the heart.[21]

Due to the global presentation of Pompe disease, systemic transduction of multiple tissues or the transduction of a single depot organ able to provide cross-correction to other tissues will be necessary to create a successful therapy. One of the least invasive delivery route options for the administration of gene therapy is the intravenous (IV) route. To fully understand the ability of IV-delivered rAAV1-h*Gaa* vectors to provide disease correction, Mah et al.[22]

used the IV administration route to deliver rAAV1-h*Gaa* vectors to 1-day-old *Gaa*$^{-/-}$ mice and evaluated long-term correction one year after treatment. The immune system is not fully developed in mice until after birth. For this reason, the immune system of a neonate will accept a foreign protein (such as h*Gaa*) as a self-protein and fail to elicit an immune response. This method resulted in 81% of normal levels of Gaa activity in the heart at one year postinjection. The demonstrated ability of a single IV injection to achieve such high levels of sustained Gaa activity in the heart is promising and suggests that the far more invasive direct intracardiac injection route may not be necessary.

Currently, at least 12 distinct AAV serotypes have been isolated and studied.[23] Pseudotyping is the approach typically used to produce rAAV vectors of alternative serotypes. This involves packaging the transgene cassette containing AAV2 inverted terminal repeat (ITR) elements into the capsid of alternative serotypes.[24] Both in vitro and in vivo comparisons of these serotypes have revealed important information regarding which are optimal for targeting specific tissues.[15,25]

Recently, investigators have shown that the AAV9 capsid has a high natural affinity for cardiac tissue following a single intravenous administration of virus to newborn or adult mice via the superficial temporal vein or jugular vein (respectively) or to nonhuman primates (via a peripheral vein at birth),[18] suggesting that this capsid is particularly well suited for cardiac-specific gene delivery.

Overall, the rAAV-mediated gene delivery system does show great promise in the field of cardiac gene therapy, although one of its major limitations is its relatively small capacity for transgene size. This challenge has been overcome successfully by investigators studying Duchenne's muscular dystrophy (DMD) through creation of a mini-dystrophin gene that contains only those sequences that are essential for the translation of a functional dystrophin protein.[26] Over 90% of all patients with DMD develop cardiomyopathy, and many die of heart failure, making the development of a gene therapy treatment very desirable.[27] DMD is caused by a lack of dystrophin, a protein that is important for maintaining the integrity of muscle cell membranes. The onset of DMD occurs in early childhood and being X-linked recessive, affects boys primarily, although female carriers can suffer the effects of the cardiomyopathy. The disease is characterized by progressive muscle wasting: first in hips, pelvic area, thighs, and shoulders and subsequently in skeletal and cardiac tissues.[28]

Direct injections of rAAV carrying the mini-dystrophin gene into murine neonate chest cavities has demonstrated successful restoration of the dystrophin–glycoprotein complex in cardiac tissue up to 10 months postadministration.[26] Evans Blue dye (EBD) uptake is a hallmark for dystrophin-deficient myofibers and demonstrates the susceptibility of these fibers to mechanical stress. To create a mechanical challenge to the heart, β-isoproterenol was administered to the virus-infected *mdx* mouse. The rAAV-delivered microdystrophin expression improved the integrity of the sarcolemma and successfully prevented EBD uptake, demonstrating functional correction of the cardiomyopathy.[26]

Through use of the cardiomyopathic hamster model, researchers have been able to show that rAAV-mediated cardiac gene delivery of a pseudophosphorylated mutant of phospholamban was able to enhance myocardial uptake of calcium and suppress impairment of left ventricular (LV) systolic function for up to 30 weeks.[29] This demonstrated the potential use of rAAV as a vector for therapies involving progressive dilated cardiomyopathies and associated heart failure.[29] Other investigators have shown that cardiac allograft vasculopathy (CAV) can be treated using AAV- mediated delivery of angiopoietin-1 and-2.[30] Expression of these transgenes decreased inflammatory and apoptotic effects in rat allografts.[30]

By performing direct intramyocardial injections of naked vascular endothelial growth factor (VEGF) DNA into the streptozotocin-induced diabetic rat model, Yoon et al. were able to show an increase in capillary density, a decrease in endothelial cell and cardiomyocyte apoptosis, and significant improvements in cardiac function.[31] This demonstrated a successful gene therapy approach for the treatment of diabetic cardiomyopathy (DCM).

While transgene expression can be detected anywhere from 2 to 4 weeks following naked DNA injections, it then abruptly stops, due to what is believed to be an immune response to the high levels of naked DNA. Other studies have shown that when DNA was complexed to cationic liposomes, it was far better tolerated.[32] Investigators have also been able to show that delivery of antisense c-myb oligonucleotides can inhibit intimal arterial smooth muscle cell accumulation in a rat carotid injury model[33] demonstrating the ability of naked DNA gene therapy to be a useful delivery system for the provision of a short duration of transgene expression.

The lysosomal disease mucopolysaccharidosis VII (MPS) is caused by a deficiency in β-glucuronidase (GUSB) activity, which results in the defective catabolism of glycosaminoglycans (GAGs). In humans, the cardiac presentations of this disease include thickening of the mitral valve with regurgitation or stenosis, aortic valve thickening, hypertrophic cardiomyopathy, endocardial thickening, and dialated cardiomyopathy.[34] Using an MPS dog model, Sleeper et al. were able to show that using retroviral-mediated gene therapy at 2 to 3 days of age to deliver canine GUSB was a successful method to ameliorate the effects of the disease for up to 24 months.[35] There are several limitations to using the retroviral delivery system. Among these are the vector's inability to transduce nonproliferating target cells[36] and the potential for insertional mutagenesis and activation of oncogenes following host chromosome integration.[37]

Research into the development and optimization of gene transfer strategies for cardiovascular disease are ongoing. The volume of pre clinical data demonstrating safe and successful cardiac gene delivery and subsequent disease ablation warrants the current momentum in the cardiovascular field toward introducing these methods in near-future clinical trials.

REFERENCES

1. American Heart Association. 2004. www.americanheart.org.
2. Pachori AS, Melo LG, Zhang L, Solomon SD, Dzau VJ. Chronic recurrent myocardial ischemic injury is significantly attenuated by pre-emptive adeno-associated virus heme oxygenase-1 gene delivery. *J Am Coll Cardiol*. February 7, 2006;47(3):635–643.

3. Kishnani PS, Hwu WL, Mandel H, Nicolino M, Yong F, Corzo D. A retrospective, multinational, multicenter study on the natural history of infantile-onset Pompe disease. *J Pediatr*. May 2006;148(5):671–676.

4. Raben N, Plotz P, Byrne BJ. Acid alpha-glucosidase deficiency (glycogenosis type II, Pompe disease). *Curr Mol Med*. March 2002;2(2):145–166.

5. Martiniuk F, Chen A, Mack A, et al. Helios gene gun particle delivery for therapy of acid maltase deficiency. *DNA Cell Biol*. October 2002;21(10):717–725.

6. Nicolino MP, Puech JP, Kremer EJ, et al. Adenovirus-mediated transfer of the acid alpha-glucosidase gene into fibroblasts, myoblasts and myotubes from patients with glycogen storage disease type II leads to high level expression of enzyme and corrects glycogen accumulation. *Hum Mol Genet*. October 1998;7(11):1695–1702.

7. Pauly DF, Johns DC, Matelis LA, Lawrence JH, Byrne BJ, Kessler PD. Complete correction of acid alpha-glucosidase deficiency in Pompe disease fibroblasts in vitro, and lysosomally targeted expression in neonatal rat cardiac and skeletal muscle. *Gene Ther*. April 1998;5(4):473–480.

8. Carter BJ, Khoury G, Denhardt DT. Physical map and strand polarity of specific fragments of adenovirus-associated virus DNA produced by endonuclease R-EcoRI. *J Virol*. September 1975;16(3):559–568.

9. Clark KR, Sferra TJ, Johnson PR. Recombinant adeno-associated viral vectors mediate long-term transgene expression in muscle. *Hum Gene Ther*. April 10, 1997;8(6):659–669.

10. Kessler PD, Podsakoff GM, Chen X, et al. Gene delivery to skeletal muscle results in sustained expression and systemic delivery of a therapeutic protein. *Proc Natl Acad Sci U S A*. November 26, 1996;93(24):14082–14087.

11. Podsakoff G, Wong KK, Jr., Chatterjee S. Efficient gene transfer into nondividing cells by adeno-associated virus-based vectors. *J Virol*. September 1994;68(9):5656–5666.

12. Srivastava A, Lusby EW, Berns KI. Nucleotide sequence and organization of the adeno-associated virus 2 genome. *J Virol*. 1983;45:555–564.

13. Xiao X, Li J, Samulski RJ. Efficient long-term gene transfer into muscle tissue of immunocompetent mice by adeno-associated virus vector. *J Virol*. November 1996;70(11):8098–8108.

14. Chao H, Liu Y, Rabinowitz J, Li C, Samulski RJ, Walsh CE. Several log increase in therapeutic transgene delivery by distinct adeno-associated viral serotype vectors. *Mol Ther*. December 2000;2(6):619–623.

15. Du LL, Kido M, Lee DV, et al. Differential myocardial gene delivery by recombinant serotype-specific adeno-associated viral vectors. *Mol Ther*. September 2004;10(3):604–608.

16. Hauck B, Chen L, Xiao W. Generation and characterization of chimeric recombinant AAV vectors. *Mol Ther*. March 2003;7(3):419–425.

17. Nicklin SA, White SJ, Buning H, et al. Site-specific gene delivery to the vasculature in vivo using peptide-targeted adeno-associated virus (AAV) vectors. *Atherosclerosis*. July 2003;169(1):200.

18. Pacak CA, Mah CS, Thattaliyath BD, et al. Recombinant adeno-associated virus serotype 9 leads to preferential cardiac transduction in vivo. *Circ Res*. July 27, 2006.

19. Warrington KH, Jr, Gorbatyuk OS, Harrison JK, Opie SR, Zolotukhin S, Muzyczka N. Adeno-associated virus type 2 VP2 capsid protein is nonessential and can tolerate large peptide insertions at its N terminus. *J Virol*. June 2004;78(12):6595–6609.

20. Muller OJ, Leuchs B, Pleger ST, et al. Improved cardiac gene transfer by transcriptional and transductional targeting of adeno-associated viral vectors. *Cardiovasc Res.* April 1, 2006;70(1):70–78.

21. Fraites TJ, Jr, Schleissing MR, Shanely RA, et al. Correction of the enzymatic and functional deficits in a model of Pompe disease using adeno-associated virus vectors. *Mol Ther.* May 2002;5(5 Pt 1):571–578.

22. Mah C, Cresawn KO, Fraites TJ, Jr, et al. Sustained correction of glycogen storage disease type II using adeno-associated virus serotype 1 vectors. *Gene Ther.* September 2005;12(18):1405–1409.

23. Gao GP, Alvira MR, Wang L, Calcedo R, Johnston J, Wilson JM. Novel adeno-associated viruses from rhesus monkeys as vectors for human gene therapy. *Proc Natl Acad Sci U S A.* September 3, 2002;99(18):11854–11859.

24. Zolotukhin S, Potter M, Zolotukhin I, et al., Production and purification of serotype 1, 2, and 5 recombinant adeno-associated viral vectors. *Methods.* October 2002;28(2):158–167.

25. Su H, Huang Y, Takagawa J, et al. AAV serotype-1 mediates early onset of gene expression in mouse hearts and results in better therapeutic effect. *Gene Ther.* June 15, 2006.

26. Yue Y, Li Z, Harper SQ, Davisson RL, Chamberlain JS, Duan D. Microdystrophin gene therapy of cardiomyopathy restores dystrophin–glycoprotein complex and improves sarcolemma integrity in the *mdx* mouse heart. *Circulation.* September 30, 2003;108(13):1626–1632.

27. Melacini P, Vianello A, Villanova C, et al. Cardiac and respiratory involvement in advanced stage Duchenne muscular dystrophy. *Neuromuscul Disord.* October 1996;6(5):367–376.

28. Muscular Dystrophy Association. 2006. www.mdausa.org.

29. Hoshijima M, Ikeda Y, Iwanaga Y, et al. Chronic suppression of heart-failure progression by a pseudophosphorylated mutant of phospholamban via in vivo cardiac rAAV gene delivery. *Nat Med.* August 2002;8(8):864–871.

30. Nykanen AI, Pajusola K, Krebs R, et al. Common protective and diverse smooth muscle cell effects of AAV-mediated angiopoietin-1 and -2 expression in rat cardiac allograft vasculopathy. *Circ Res.* June 9, 2006;98(11):1373–1380.

31. Yoon YS, Uchida S, Masuo O, et al. Progressive attenuation of myocardial vascular endothelial growth factor expression is a seminal event in diabetic cardiomyopathy: restoration of microvascular homeostasis and recovery of cardiac function in diabetic cardiomyopathy after replenishment of local vascular endothelial growth factor. *Circulation.* April 26, 2005;111(16):2073–2085.

32. San H, Yang ZY, Pompili VJ, et al. Safety and short-term toxicity of a novel cationic lipid formulation for human gene therapy. *Hum Gene Ther.* December 1993;4(6):781–788.

33. Simons M, Edelman ER, DeKeyser JL, Langer R, Rosenberg RD. Antisense c-myb oligonucleotides inhibit intimal arterial smooth muscle cell accumulation in vivo. *Nature.* September 3, 1992;359(6390):67–70.

34. Dangel JH. Cardiovascular changes in children with mucopolysaccharide storage diseases and related disorders: clinical and echocardiographic findings in 64 patients. *Eur J Pediatr.* July 1998;157(7):534–538.

35. Sleeper MM, Fornasari B, Ellinwood NM, et al. Gene therapy ameliorates cardio-vascular disease in dogs with mucopolysaccharidosis VII. *Circulation*, August 17, 2004;110(7):815–820.

36. Psarras S, Karagianni N, Kellendonk C, et al. Gene transfer and genetic modification of embryonic stem cells by Cre- and Cre-PR-expressing MESV-based retroviral vectors. *J Gene Medi*. January 2004;6(1):32–42.

37. Haviernik P, Bunting KD. Safety concerns related to hematopoietic stem cell gene transfer using retroviral vectors. *Curr Gene Ther*. September 2004;4(3):263–276.

11 Intraarticular Vector Delivery for Inflammatory Joint Disease

HAIM BURSTEIN

Targeted Genetics Corporation, Seattle, Washington

Rheumatoid arthritis (RA), the most common inflammatory joint disease, is a chronic autoimmune disorder that affects approximately 1% of the population and causes significant morbidity, disability, and increased mortality. The etiology of RA is largely unknown, although current evidence suggests contributions from both environmental and genetic components (Harris, 1990). Chronic inflammation in the arthritic joint is characterized by recruitment of immune cells, including lymphocytes, macrophages, and plasma cells, leading to massive thickening of the synovium, accompanied by release of inflammatory mediators, ultimately leading to invasion and irreversible destruction of articular cartilage and bone. At the molecular level, chronic inflammatory arthritis is characterized by diminution of T-cell factors and an abundance of cytokines and growth factors such as interleukin-6 (IL-6), tumor necrosis factor (TNF)α, and IL-1β that are produced by macrophages and synovial fibroblasts and play a major role in the progression of joint destruction (Brennan and Feldmann, 1992). IL-1β, in particular, is a key cytokine that induces cartilage degradation, whereas TNFα is a major cytokine involved in joint inflammation (Arend and Dayer, 1995).

Conventional therapy manages the symptoms of arthritis using general anti-inflammatory agents, including both steroidal and nonsteroidal drugs, and disease-modifying drugs such as methotrexate. However, none of these pharmacologic agents has yet proven effective in halting the progression of disease. Significant progress in molecular technology facilitated the identification of cell subsets and disease molecules contributing to the inflammatory and destructive components of RA, prompting development of specifically targeted therapies. As a result, several biological agents that more effectively ameliorate arthritis symptoms and halt the progression of disease were identified. In particular, agents that modulate the proinflammatory activities of TNFα, and to a lesser degree IL-1β, have proven effective in preclinical studies as well as in human clinical trials, confirming the validity of these proinflammatory cytokines as therapeutic targets

Concepts in Genetic Medicine, Edited by Boro Dropulic and Barrie Carter
Copyright © 2008 John Wiley & Sons, Inc.

(Elliot et al., 1994; Moreland et al., 1997; Bresnihan et al., 1998; Jiang et al., 2000). Indeed, the U.S. Food and Drug Administration has approved the use of IL-1 receptor antagonist (IL-1Ra; anakinra), soluble TNFα receptor (etanercept), and two anti-TNFα monoclonal antibodies (infliximab and adalimumab) for the treatment of RA.

The use of biologics for arthritis therapy raises difficult challenges, including the need for costly daily or weekly repeat dosing. Effective levels of the therapeutic protein cannot be maintained for extended periods of time because their in vivo half-life is relatively short. In addition, repeated systemic administration of high doses of these biologics required to achieve local biological responses in affected joints may impose a significant risk of adverse effects, including increased susceptibility to bacterial infections (tuberculosis) and motor neural degeneration (multiple sclerosis). Reactivation of latent tuberculosis has been a particular problem, so that patients have to be screened before treatment is begun (Keane et al., 2001). Moreover, discontinuation of systemic protein therapy results in rapid relapse, and over 30% of patients are either refractory to systemic treatment or lose their initial responses (Olsen and stein, 2004). Direct intraarticular injection of protein therapeutics results in clinical benefit but has the disadvantages of rapid clearance by the lymphatics of materials reaching the joint space, of being prohibitively expensive, and of having only a short-lived effect. Thus, there continues to be a compelling need for the development of new therapeutic strategies.

Delivery of genes encoding therapeutic proteins, rather than administration of the proteins themselves, promises to obviate these problems. In particular, local gene therapy that involves the direct intraarticular administration of a gene transfer vector to obtain local transgene expression in the inflamed synovium may provide an attractive and potentially more effective alternative to protein-based drug delivery for the treatment of RA (Figure 11.1). This strategy offers the prospects of achieving high local concentrations of a therapeutic gene product in a sustained manner while minimizing exposure of nontarget organs. If persistent transgene expression could be achieved locally following gene transfer, it may circumvent the need for frequent repeat dosing. In addition, it may allow attainment of steady levels of the product, as opposed to the peaks and troughs associated with intermittent protein administration, thus improving the pharmacokinetics of these otherwise relatively short-lived proteins.

The feasibility and efficacy of transfering therapeutic genes encoding proteins with antiarthritic properties to the synovial tissue after intraarticular administration has been demonstrated in several experimental models of RA. The initial studies of gene delivery to the joint employed an ex vivo strategy in which synoviocytes, isolated from rabbit joint tissue, were transduced in culture with a retroviral vector encoding IL-1Ra cDNA. The genetically modified cells were then transplanted to the knee joint, colonized the synovial lining, and locally expressed the transgene. This procedure proved to be feasible and safe, first in animal models (Bandara et al., 1993; Otani et al., 1996) and then in a phase I clinical study in RA patients (Evans et al., 1996, 2005).

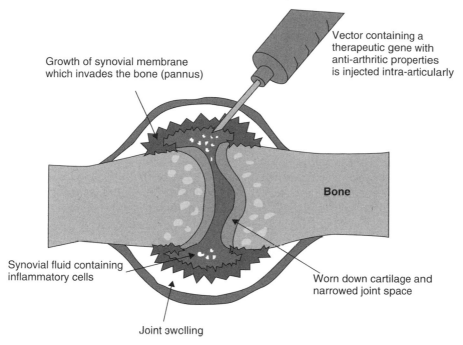

Growth of synovial membrane which invades the bone (pannus)

Vector containing a therapeutic gene with anti-arthritic properties is injected intra-articularly

Bone

Synovial fluid containing inflammatory cells

Worn down cartilage and narrowed joint space

Joint swelling

Figure 11.1 Direct intraarticular administration of a gene transfer vector containing a gene for a therapeutic protein with antiarthritic properties. For example, AAV2-TNFR:Fc, a vector containing a gene that encodes an anti-TNFα inhibitor protein is delivered to an arthitic joint where TNFα, a proinflammatory cytokine implicated in disease-related inflammation that causes tenderness, swelling, and tissue damage, is overexpressed. Joint cells transduced with the vector express and secrete soluble TNFR:Fc protein molecules into the joint space where they bind TNFα molecules and inhibit them from binding to their cognate receptors in the membrane of target joint cells. Thus blocked, TNFα is unable to cause joint inflammation

Although useful for establishing proof of concept, the ex vivo gene transfer method, which requires selection of synovial fibroblasts and their transplantaion into the arthritic joint, is invasive, labor intensive, time-consuming, and expensive, and thus not suitable for widespread clinical application. Thus, local gene therapy for RA would be better served by the development of safe and effective in vivo vectors that facilitate long-term transgene expression.

A variety of vectors, derived from several types of viruses, have been evaluated as gene transfer vehicles in preclinical animal models of RA, including retrovirus, lentivirus, adenovirus, adeno-associated virus (AAV), and herpes simplex virus (HSV) (Ghivizzani et al., 2001). In addition, several nonviral vectors, including liposomes and naked DNA, have been employed to deliver genes to the joint (Nita et al., 1996; Tomita et al., 1997). Although widely used for proof-of-concept studies to evaluate potential therapeutic genes with antiarthritic properties, adenoviral-mediated synovial gene transfer has generally resulted in short-term transgene expression and has been associated with antiviral inflammatory response (Sawchuk et al., 1996; Apparailly et al., 1998). Retroviral vectors have been employed to deliver reporter genes intraarticularly to the inflamed joints of rabbits (Ghivizzani et al., 1997) and rats (Nguyen et al., 1998) and have demonstrated the ability to stably transduce the dividing synovial cells in the inflamed joint and achieve levels of transgene expression similar to those achieved when using the ex vivo gene transfer method. Furthermore, intraarticular injection of a high-titer retrovirus encoding IL-4 to rats having adjuvant-induced arthritis was effective in reducing paw swelling and suppressing bone destruction (Boyle et al., 1999). Similarly, direct injection of recombinant lentiviral vectors, which are capable of transducing dividing and nondividing host cells, to the joints of rodents also appears to be efficient and durable in transducing the synovium of arthritic rat joints and effective in inhibiting the inflammatory effects of experimental arthritis (Gouze et al., 2002, 2003). However, from a safety consideration, a major disadvantage of using either retroviral or lentiviral vectors is the fact that they integrate their genome into that of the host cell in order to establish long-term transduction, which has the potential to activate cellular proto-oncogenes.

Among potential vector systems for intraarticular gene therapy of RA, AAV vectors appear particularly promising. They do not encode any viral proteins, are not inflammatory, and are able to infect both dividing and nondividing cells. Importantly, unlike its wild-type counterpart, AAV vector generally does not integrate but persists in the nucleus of the host cell as large circular concatamers. Thus, it represents a good candidate vector for a chronic inflammatory disease, such as RA, in which long-term expression of the therapeutic gene product will be required. Furthermore, the wild-type AAV is not pathogenic in humans, and AAV serotype 2 (AAV2)–based vectors, so far tested in a number of human clinical trials, demonstrate a favorable safety profile with clinical follow-up data out over eight years for patients treated in the first AAV clinical trials.

The feasibility and efficacy of direct in vivo AAV vector–mediated delivery of reporter and therapeutic genes to arthritic joints of mice and rats exhibiting experimental arthritis have been well demonstrated (Pan et al., 1999; Pan 2000; Goater et al., 2000; Watanabe et al., 2000; Zhang et al., 2000). A study in SCW-induced arthritis in rats which demonstrated the efficacy of AAV-TNFR:Fc has progressed to a phase I clinical trial in patients with RA (Chan et al., 2002). Progress has also been made to increase AAV vector transduction to the synovium. Pseudotyped AAV vectors of serotypes other than type 2 or the use of proteasome inhibitors has demonstrated a significant improvement in transduction of the synovium (Adiaansen et al., 2005; Apparailly et al., 2005; Jennings et al., 2005).

An impressive number of genes with antiarthritic properties have demonstrated efficacy in mouse, rat, and rabbit models of experimental arthritis. These include proinflammatory cytokine antagonists (TNFR:Fc, IL-1Ra) (Bandara et al., 1993; Ghivizzani et al., 1998; Pan et al., 2000; Chan et al., 2002), anti-inflammatory immunomodulators (IL-10, vIL-10, IL-4, IFNβ, CTLA-4) (Apparailly et al., 1998;

Boyle et al., 1999; Lechman et al., 1999; Triantaphyllopoulos et al., 1999; Whalen et al., 1999; Quattrocchi et al., 2000; Watanabe et al., 2000), apoptotic agents (Fas ligand and Fas-associated death domain) (Zhang et al., 1997; Kobayashi et al., 2000), inhibitors of synovial cell invasion and cartilage degradation (thymidine kinase) (Goossens et al., 1999), inhibitors of signaling pathways (IκBα, NFκB decoys, C-terminal Src kinase, cycline-dependent kinase inhibitors such as p16INK4a) (Miagkov et al., 1998; Takayanagi et al., 1999; Taniguchi et al., 1999; Tomita et al., 1997), and genes that promote cartilage regeneration (insulin-like growth factor 1) (Mi et al., 2000).

Particular interest has been generated by the observation that adenoviral gene transfer of anti-inflammatory genes such as soluble receptors for IL-1 or TNF, IL-4, and vIL-10 to a single arthritic joint of an animal with bilateral disease can also suppress disease in the uninjected contralateral joint (Ghivizzani et al., 1998; Lechman et al., 1999; Whalen et al., 1999; Kim et al., 2000). This contralateral effect has been observed following in vivo and ex vivo delivery of different candidate therapeutic genes in several animal models of arthritis (Miagkov et al., 1998; Boyle et al., 1999; Chan et al., 2002; Kim et al., 2001, 2002). Additional studies aimed at further understanding this effect have provided evidence that antigen-presenting cells such as macrophages and dendritic cells (DCs) as well as DC-derived exosomes may have an important role in conferring the anti-inflammatory protective effect in both the injected and noninjected contralateral joints (Lechman et al., 1999, 2001; Kim et al., 2000; Morita et al., 2001; Whalen et al., 2001; Lechman et al., 2003; Kim et al., 2005).

In summary, intraarticular gene transfer to the joint as a drug delivery system offers a promising strategy for treating inflammatory joint diseases. Viral DNA delivery systems with a variety of candidate therapeutic genes have been employed to demonstrate proof of concept in multiple animal models of RA. Of all the viral vectors evaluated so far, AAV is emerging as a vector of choice for future clinical studies, primarily because of its safety profile. Following a successful early phase I safety and feasibility study, based on ex vivo gene transfer to the joint, another phase I clinical trial involving direct intraarticular injection of AAV2-TNFR:Fc to arthritic joints of RA patients is in progress, and data should be available soon.

REFERENCES

Adiaansen J, Tas SW, Klarenbeek PL, et al. (2005). Enhanced gene transfer to arthritic joints using adeno-associated virus type 5: implications for intra-articular gene therapy. *Ann Rheum Dis* (ARD Online first).

Apparailly F, Verwaerde C, Jacquet C, Auriault C, Sany J, Jorgensen C (1998). Adenovirus-mediated transfer of viral IL-10 gene inhibits murine collagen-induced arthritis. *J Immunol*. 160:5213–5220.

Apparailly F, Khoury M, Vervoordeldonk MJB, et al. (2005). Adeno-associated virus pseudotype 5 vector improves gene transfer in arthritic joints. *Hum Gene Ther*. 16:426–434.

Arend WP, Dayer JM (1995). Inhibition of the production and effects of interleukin-1 and tumor necrosis factor alpha in rheumatoid arthritis. *Arthritis Rheum*. 38:151–160.

Bandara G, Mueller GM, Galea-Lauri J, et al. (1993). Intraarticular expression of biologically active interleukin 1-receptor-antagonist protein by ex vivo gene therapy. *Proc Natl Acad Sci U S A*. 90:10764–10768.

Boyle DL, Nguyen KHY, Zhuang S, et al. (1999). Intra-articular IL-4 gene therapy in arthritis: anti-inflammatory effect and enhanced Th2 activity. *Gene Ther*. 6: 1911–1918.

Brennan FM, Feldmann M (1992). Cytokines in autoimmunity. *Curr Opin Immunol*. 4:754–759.

Bresnihan B, Alvaro-Gracia JM, Cobby M, et al. (1998). Treatment of rheumatoid arthritis with recombinant human interleukin-1 receptor antagonist. *Arthritis Rheum*. 41: 2196–2204.

Chan JM, Villarreal G, Jin WW, Stepan T, Burstein H, Wahl SM (2002). Intraarticular gene transfer of TNFR:Fc suppresses experimental arthritis with reduced systemic distribution of the gene product. *Mol Ther*. 6:727–736.

Elliott MJ, Maini RN, Feldmann M, et al. (1994). Randomised double-blind comparison of chimeric monoclonal antibody to tumour necrosis factor alpha (cA2) versus placebo in rheumatoid arthritis. *Lancet*. 344:1105–1110.

Evans CH, Robbins PD, Ghivizzani SC, et al. (1996). Clinical trial to assess the safety, feasibility, and efficacy of transferring a potentially anti-arthritic cytokine gene to human joints with rheumatoid arthritis. *Hum Gene Ther*. 7:1261–1280.

Evans CH, Robbins PD, Ghivizzani SC, et al. (2005). Gene transfer to human joints: progress toward a gene therapy of arthritis. *Proc Natl Acad Sci U S A*. 102:8698–8703.

Ghivizzani SC, Lechman ER, Tio C, et al. (1997). Direct retrovirus-mediated gene transfer to the synovium of the rabbit knee: implications for arthritis gene therapy. *Gene Ther*. 4:977–982.

Ghivizzani SC, Lechman ER, Kang R, et al. (1998). Direct adenovirus-mediated gene transfer of interleukin 1 and tumor necrosis factor a soluble receptors to rabbit knees with experimental arthritis has local and distal anti-arthritic effects. *Proc Natl Acad Sci U S A*. 95:4613–4618.

Ghivizzani SC, Oligino TJ, Glorioso JC, Robbins PD and Evans CH (2001). Direct gene delivery strategies for the treatment of rheumatoid arthritis. *Drug Discov Today*. 6:259–267.

Goater J, Muller R, Kollias G, et al. (2000). Empirical advantages of adeno associated viral vectors in vivo gene therapy for arthritis. *J Rheumatol*. 27:983–989.

Goossens PH, Schouten GJ, Hart BA, et al. (1999). Feasibility of adenovirus-mediated nonsurgical synovectomy in collagen-induced arthritis-affected rhesus monkeys. *Hum Gene Ther*. 10:1139–1149.

Gouze E, Pawliuk R, Pilapil C, et al. (2002). In vivo gene delivery to synovium by lentiviral vectors. *Mol Ther*. 5:397–404.

Gouze E, Pawliuk R, Gouze JN, et al. (2003). Lentiviral-mediated gene delivery to synovium: potent intra-articular expression with amplification by inflammation. *Mol Ther*. 7:460–466.

Harris EJ (1990). Rheumatoid arthritis: pathophysiology and implications for therapy. *N Engl J Med*. 3322:1277–1289.

Jennings K, Miyamae T, Traister R, et al. (2005). Proteasome inhibition enhances AAV-mediated transgene expression in human synoviocytes in vitro and in vivo. *Mol Ther*. 11:600–607.

Jiang Y, Genant HK, Watt I, et al. (2000). A multicenter, double-blind, dose-ranging, randomized, placebo-controlled study of recombinant human interleukin-1 receptor antagonist in patients with rheumatoid arthritis: radiologic progression and correlation of Genant and Larsen scores. *Arthritis Rheum*. 43:1001–1009.

Keane J, Gershon S, Wise RP, et al. (2001). Tuberculosis associated with infliximab, a tumor necrosis factor neutralizing agent. *N Engl J Med*. 345:1098–1104.

Kim SH, Evans CH, Kim S, Oligino T, Ghivizzani SC, Robbins PD (2000). Gene therapy for established murine collagen-induced arthritis by local and systemic adenovirus-mediated delivery of interleukin-4. *Arthritis Res*. 2:293–302.

Kim SH, Kim S, Evans CH, Ghivizzani SC, Oligino T, Robbins PD (2001). Effective treatment of established murine collagen-induced arthritis by systemic administration of dendritic cells genetically modified to express IL-4. *J Immunol*. 166:3499–3505.

Kim SH, Lechman ER, Kim S, Nash J, Oligino TJ, Robbins PD (2002). Ex vivo gene delivery of IL-1Ra and soluble TNF receptor confers a distal synergistic therapeutic effect in antigen-induced arthritis. *Mol Ther*. 6:591–600.

Kim SH, Lechman ER, Bianco N, et al. (2005). Exosomes derived from IL-10-treated dendritic cells can suppress inflammation and collagen-induced arthritis. *J Immunol*. 174:6440–6448.

Kobayashi T, Okamoto K, Kobata T, et al. (2000). Novel gene therapy for rheumatoid arthritis by FADD gene transfer: induction of apoptosis of rheumatoid synoviocytes but not chondrocytes. *Gene Ther*. 7:527–533.

Lechman ER, Jaffurs D, Ghivizzani SC, et al. (1999). Direct adenoviral gene transfer of viral IL-10 to rabbit knee with experimental arthritis ameliorates disease in both injected and contralateral control knees. *J Immunol*. 163:2202–2208.

Lechman ER, Kim SH, Gambotto A, et al. (2001). Role for antigen presenting cells and exosomes in conferring a contralateral effect in models of antigen induced arthritis. *Mol Ther*. 3(Suppl):141–142.

Lechman ER, Keravala A, Nash J, Kim SH, Mi Z, Robbins PD (2003). The contralateral effect conferred by intra-articular adenovirus-mediated gene transfer of viral IL-10 is specific to the immunizing antigen. *Gene Ther*. 10:2029–2035.

Mi Z, Ghivizzani SC, Lechman ER, et al. (2000). Adenovirus-mediated gene transfer of insulin-like growth factor 1 stimulates proteoglycan synthesis in rabbit joints. *Arthritis Rheum*. 43:2563–2570.

Miagkov AV, Kovalenko DV, Brown CE, et al. (1998). NF-κB activation provides the potential link between inflammation and hyperplasia in the arthritic joint. *Proc Natl Acad Sci U S A*. 95:13859–13864.

Moreland LW, Baumgartner SW, Schiff MH, et al. (1997). Treatment of rheumatoid arthritis with a recombinant human tumor necrosis factor receptor (p75)-Fc fusion protein. *N Engl J Med*. 337:141–147.

Morita Y, Yang J, Gupta R, et al. (2001). Dendritic cells genetically engineered to express IL-4 inhibit murine collagen-induced arthritis. *J Clin Invest*. 107:1275–1284.

Nguyen KHY, Boyle DL, McCormack JE, Chada S, Jolly DJ, Firestein GS (1998). Direct synovial gene transfer with retroviral vectors in rat adjuvant arthritis. *J Rheumatol*. 25:1118–1125.

Nita I, Ghivizzani SC, Galea-Lauri J, et al. (1996). Direct gene delivery to synovium: an evaluation of potential vectors in vitro and in vivo. *Arthritis Rheum*. 39:820–828.

Olsen NJ, Stein CM (2004). New drugs for rheumatoid arthritis. *N Engl J Med*. 350: 2167–2179.

Otani K, Nita I, Macaulay W, Georgescu HI, Robbins PD, Evans CH (1996). Suppression of antigen-induced arthritis in rabbits by ex vivo gene therapy. *J Immunol*. 156:3558–3562.

Pan RY, Xiao X, Chen SL, et al. (1999). Disease-inducible transgene expression from a recombinant adeno-associated virus vector in a rat arthritis model. *J Virol*. 73: 3410–3417.

Pan RY, Chen SL, Xiao X, Liu DW, Peng HJ, Tsao YP (2000). Therapy and prevention of arthritis by recombinant adeno-associated virus vector with delivery of interleukin-1 receptor antagonist. *Arthritis Rheum*. 43:289–297.

Quattrocchi E, Dallman MJ, Feldmann M (2000). Adenovirus-mediated gene transfer of CTLA-4Ig fusion protein in the suppression of experimental autoimmune arthritis. *Arthritis Rheum*. 43:1688–1697.

Sawchuk SJ, Boivin GP, Duwel LE, et al. (1996) Anti-T cell receptor monoclonal antibody prolongs transgene expression following adenovirus-mediated in vivo gene transfer to mouse synovium. *Hum Gene Ther*. 7:499–506.

Takayanagi H, Juji T, Miyazaki T, et al. (1999). Suppression of arthritic bone destruction by adenovirus-mediated *csk* gene transfer to synoviocytes and osteoblasts. *J Clin Invest*. 104:137–146.

Taniguchi K, Kohsaka H, Inoue N, et al. (1999). Induction of the *p16INK4a* senescence gene as a new therapeutic strategy for the treatment of rheumatoid arthritis. *Nat Med*. 5:760–767.

Tomita T, Hashimoto H, Tomita N, et al. (1997). In vivo direct gene transfer into articular cartilage by intraarticular injection mediated by HVJ (Sendai virus) and liposomes. *Arthritis Rheum*. 40:901–906.

Triantaphyllopoulos KA, Williams RO, Tailor H, Chernajovsky Y (1999). Amelioration of collagen-induced arthritis and suppression of interferon-γ, interleukin-12, and tumor necrosis factor α production by interferon-β gene therapy. *Arthritis Rheum*. 42:90–99.

Watanabe S, Imagawa T, Boivin GP, Gao G, Wilson JM, Hirsch R (2000). Adeno-associated virus mediated long-term gene transfer and delivery of chondroprotective IL-4 to murine synovium. *Mol Ther*. 2:147–152.

Whalen JD, Lechman EL, Carlos CA, et al. (1999). Adenoviral transfer of viral IL-10 gene periarticularly to mouse paws suppresses development of collagen-induced arthritis in both injected and uninjected paws. *J Immunol*. 162:3625–3632.

Whalen JD, Thomson AW, Lu L, Robbins PD, Evans CH (2001). Viral IL-10 gene transfer inhibits DTH responses to soluble antigens: evidence for involvement of genetically modified dendritic cells and macrophages. *Mol Ther*. 4:543–550.

Zhang H, Yang Y, Horton JL, et al. (1997). Amelioration of collagen-induced arthritis by CD95 (*Apo-1/Fas*)-ligand gene transfer. *J Clin Invest*. 100:1951–1957.

Zhang HG, Xie J, Yang P, Wang Y, Xu L, Liu D, Hsu HS, Zhou T, Edwards CK 3rd, Mountz JD (2000). Adeno-associated virus production of soluble tumor necrosis factor receptor neutralizes tumor necrosis factor alpha and reduces arthritis. *Hum Gene Ther*. 11:2431–2442.

12 The Respiratory System as a Platform for Gene Delivery

BARRIE J. CARTER

Targeted Genetics Corporation, Seattle, Washington

There are several compelling reasons for pursuing gene delivery to the lung. The lung is directly and easily accessible via the airway. Gene delivery may be used to treat diseases that occur within the lung, including genetic diseases such as cystic fibrosis, lung cancers, and inflammatory conditions. The lung may be a useful route of delivery as a secretory platform for expression of proteins that are required elsewhere in the body. Remarkably high bioavailability of therapeutics may be attained by pulmonary delivery.

There are some obstacles that may hinder pulmonary delivery, especially for gene delivery systems. Overall, the mucociliary clearance system tends to prevent access of particles and infectious agents to airway cells. In some diseases, such as cystic fibrosis, the lung may be occluded further by processes such as bronchiectasis. For viral delivery systems, there may be relatively few receptors on the apical (lumenal) surface of the airway. For synthetic lipid-based delivery systems airway surfactants may destabilize the formulations. Also, there are multiple cell types in the airway, and most turn over within several months, so that in many cases, repeated delivery will be required.

Repeated delivery of vectors with immunogenic components such as viral capsids may be affected by host immune responses. However, the lung is one route of delivery that is somewhat less immunogenic because it is not generally exposed to serum immunoglobulin. Some virus delivery systems that induce a pro-inflammatory response, such as adenovirus, may also be less useful in the lung. Similarly, nonviral systems comprising lipid and DNA may be inflammatory due both to the undermethylation of the plasmid DNA component, which is generally produced in bacterial systems, and because many lipids can also induce inflammatory responses.

BARRIERS TO GENE DELIVERY IN THE LUNG

The architecture of the lung is a dichotomously branched airway passage that extends from the trachea to the alvelovar sacs through about 23 generations and can be considered as a fractal tree (Weibel, 1997). All of the tree is accessible to inhaled air and thus, in principle, is accessible to an inhaled drug or gene delivery system. Inhaled aerosols can be directed to different regions by manipulation of the droplet size and speed of administration of the aerosol. The entire lumenal surface of the airway comprises a continuous layer of epithelial cells (Robbins and Rennard, 1997). However, succesful cellular uptake of a gene vector following deposition is influenced by physical barriers to accessing these cells and biological barriers to cell entry and trafficking (Weiss, 2002; Davies et al., 2003; Johnson, 2004).

Nonspecific barriers to gene delivery in the lung include the cellular epithelial layer overlaid by the airway surface liquid and the glycocalyx, comprised of a complex matrix of carbohydrates, glycolipids, and glycoproteins. Also present are mucous, bacteria, and inflammatory cells, all of which may be greatly enhanced in some disease conditions. The epithelial cell layer in the airway is continuous, but it is comprised of many different cells types, including both ciliated and nonciliated cells, which also have different distributions in proximal and distal airways and in the alveoli (Robbins and Rennard, 1997). In the proximal airways there are many more ciliated cells, as well as serous and mucus cells in the submucosal glands, whereas nonciliated Clara cells are more predominant in the distal airways. In the alveoli there are alveolar type I cells for gas exchange and type II cells, which regenerate type I cells. These varying cell types present biological obstacles in that many have receptors for viruses (e.g., integrins as used by adenovirus or heparin sulfate used by adeno-associated virus serotype 2 (AAV2) and cationic liposomes), which are more frequent on the basolateral surface than on the apical surface.

Most airway cells are nondividing, which makes them poor targets for retrovirus vectors. Also, they are terminally differentiated and turn over with a half-life of perhaps several months, which requires repeated delivery of the vectors. In addition, even after entry to the cell, trafficking to the nucleus for some vectors such as AAV may be influenced by cytoplasmic components such as the proteosome pathway.

Various approaches have been suggested for surmounting these obstacles, including pharmacological manipulation of the barriers, or use of virus systems for which receptors exist on the apical surface. Adjunct agents to disrupt tight junctions may provide access to receptors on the basolateral surface, and surfactants, thixotropic solutions, or inert perfluorochemical liquids may give better distribution (Weiss, 2002). For AAV vectors, cytoplasmic tafficking after entry may be enhanced by reagents that interact with the proteosome pathway (Zhang et al., 2004). More biologically oriented approaches may include use of viral vectors for which receptors appear to exist on the apical surface, such as AAV5 (Auricchio et al., 2002; Sandalon et al., 2004) or the paramyxovirus Sendai virus (SeV), which expresses in the cytoplasm (Yonemitsu et al., 2000). Other alternatives may be to incorporate capsid components of viruses that have apical receptors, such as the envelope glycoprotein of filoviruses (Ebola) or the Jaagsiekte sheep retrovirus into lentivirus-based vectors (Sinn et al., 2003, 2005).

The fact that most target cells in the airway are nondividing has two implications. First, such cells are not transduced by retrovirus-based vectors but are readily transduced by adenovirus, AAV, and lentivirus vectors and second, the need to repeat delivery, at least at intervals of perhaps one to several months, imposes additional issues of host immune responses. Some delivery systems, particularly adenoviruses, induce significant innate immune responses after a single dose. Such host responses may represent significant safety limitations for applications to chronic diseases and may also induce both cellular and humoral immune responses that impair effective repeated delivery. However, adenovirus vectors may have useful applications for cancer, where the adjuvant effect of induction of innate and adaptive immune responses may be beneficial. Some vectors, including AAV, do not readily induce innate immune response or adaptive cellular immunity. For AAV, the main host response that might affect delivery is induction of neutralizing antibodies to the viral capsid, but in the context of pulmonary delivery this appears to be particularly blunted, presumably because serum IgG generally does not enter the lung. Certainly, repeated pulmonary delivery can be conducted effectively in several animal species, including rodents (Auricchio et al., 2002; Sandalon et al., 2004), rabbits (Beck et al., 1999), and nonhuman primates (Fischer et al., 2003), and repeated delivery by inhaled aerosol of an AAV2 vector in cystic fibrosis (CF) patients was very safe and well tolerated (Moss et al., 2004).

LUNG DISEASES

In the initial development of gene delivery technologies, genetic diseases appeared to be amenable targets because of the ease of direct delivery. CF, the most common recessive genetic disease, results from a mutation in the CFTR gene coding for a chloride ion channel that functions on the apical surface of airway epithelial. The CFTR defect leads to a complex pathophysiology, including bacterial colonization, neutrophil IL-8-dominated inflammation, and bronchiectasis. The major cause of early mortality in CF patients is loss of pulmonary function. There are no small molecule drugs to address the underlying cause of the disease, and protein therapy is not feasible. Considerable effort over the last 15 years (Davies et al., 2003; Griesenbach et al., 2004; Carter, 2005) has contributed very significantly to development of gene delivery technologies and to increased understanding of CF pathophysiology, but unfortunately has not yet led to clear proof of concept that gene delivery will be therapeutic for CF (Flotte and Laube, 2001). This reflects the complexity of the disease, the lack of good animal models, the biology of the lung, and the additional occlusion of the airways. Adenovirus vectors and cationic liposome delivery systems were tested in phase I trials in CF patients by direct instillation with a bronchoscope or by inhaled aerosol. However, expression was only short term, and inflammatory responses were induced both by the adenovirus vector capsid and the lipid–DNA complex. An AAV2 vector administered by inhaled aerosol, which did not induce inflammatory responses and showed an excellent safety profile, was advanced to phase II trials. Although one phase II trial suggested a possible beneficial effect (Moss et al., 2004), a robust effect was not observed in a more extensive test in a larger phase II trial. In view of the good safety of AAV vectors, a CF gene therapy eventually might be developed by using vectors with a different capsid (Auricchio et al., 2002, Sandalon et al., 2004) and perhaps by increasing transduction efficiency with agents that enhance trafficking of AAV to the cell nucleus (Zhang et al., 2004).

Hereditary emphysema is a lung disease resulting from a mutation in a protease alpha-1-antitrypsin (A1AT). A1AT normally is secreted from the liver and transported to the lung. In an early clinical trial, a single dose of a cationic liposome containing the cDNA for the A1AT gene was administered nasally and showed some decrease in IL-8 levels in nasal secretions (Davies et al., 2003). However, ongoing clinical trials are evaluating delivery by a nonpulmonary route (intramuscular injection) of AAV-A1AT vectors (Flotte et al., 2004).

Cancers occurring within the lung may be amenable to treatment with gene therapy by direct administration via the airway. Non-small cell lung cancer has been targeted with vectors expressing the p53 tumor suppressor gene injected directly into localized tumor masses in the lung via a flexible needle bronchoscopic injection or percutaneously under computed tomographic guidance. Early clinical trials used a retrovirus vector, but more recent trials with an adenovirus vector have shown encouraging synergies with chemotherapy or radiation (Davies et al., 2003; Moon et al., 2003). Also, an approach to treating malignant mesothelioma, a non-metastatic tumor localized to the pleural cavity, is being tested by direct percutaneous injection of an adenovirus vector expressing the suicide gene, herpes virus thymidine kinase, to activate the pro-drug ganciclovir (Mastrangeli et al., 1997), and some antitumor responses have been observed. Both types of approaches to lung tumors with adenovirus appear to be safe and repeatable.

Several concepts have been proposed for use of gene delivery for other lung disease, such as asthma, acute lung injury, or acute respiratory distress syndrome, but work in this area has not progressed very far (Demoly et al., 1997; Davies et al., 2003; Factor, 2003). For asthma it is possible that cytokine genes could be delivered to the lung with the goal of redressing the imbalance in Th1 and Th2 helper T-cell responses, but the multifactorial nature of the disease may render gene delivery impractical (Nyce and Metzger, 1997).

LUNG AS A DELIVERY DEPOT

Despite the barrier properties of the lung epithelium, it may represent a useful route for delivery of therapeutics (Agu et al., 2001). The large surface area (about 75 m^2) and very high capacity for solute exchange may offer an efficient route for delivery for therapeutic biologics such as proteins and peptides that may be required systemically. Such biologics are often difficult to formulate in tablets or capsules and are more often delivered by injection. Also, the high cost of production of proteins coupled with the high dosages required and their generally short half-life leads to a very high expense for many such drugs. Gene delivery to the lung is an alternative since many vectors can be aerosolized, are probably cheaper to produce, and may provide long-term expression. In particular, AAV vectors may have utility for such applications since they have already demonstrated an excellent safety profile when delivered by inhaled aerosol in trials in a significant number of CF patients.

Systemic delivery of therapeutic proteins after pulmonary delivery of AAV vectors has been studied. Vectors with an AAV5 capsid transduced pulmonary epithelial cells more efficiently than did AAV1 or AAV2 vectors. In rats, a single endobronchial delivery of an AAV vector expressing the rat analog of a therapeutic human soluble TNFα receptor (etanercept) resulted in prolonged secretion into serum of the soluble protein at levels of several hundred ng/mL for up to eight months, and readministration of a subsequent dose extended the expression for an additional eight months (Sandalon et al., 2004). Similarly, mice administered AAV5 vectors expressing either Epo or hemophilia factor IX secreted into serum over a period of up to five months at levels sufficient to raise the hematocrit level in normal mice or reduce blood clotting times in factor IX–deficient mice and again a second dose of vector administered at five months enabled continued secretion (Auricchio et al., 2002). Systemic expression of the cytokine IL-10, at 50 ng/mL in serum, was observed two days after direct instillation of a recombinant SeV/IL-10 vector to the lungs of mice (Griesenbach et al., 2002). This serum level of IL-10 represented about 5% bioavailability of that secreted into the lumen of the lung, as measured in broncho-alveolar lavage fluid. However, administration of SeV vectors to lung was associated with an inflammatory response and long-term expression has not been examined, so its utility as a delivery system may be limited.

In summary, it appears to be feasible to use the lung as a delivery depot by using a vector such as AAV that provides persistent expression in the absence of a deleterious host immune response. Thus, the lung may be a very effective mode of delivery for biologic therapeutics via gene delivery, with the possible attendant advantages of reduced cost of goods and greatly decreased frequency of administration.

REFERENCES

Agu RU, Ugwoke MI, Armand M, Kinget R, Verbeke N (2001). The lung as a route for systemic delivery of therapeutic proteins and peptides. *Respir Res*. 2:198–209.

Auricchio A, O'Connor E, Weiner D, et al. (2002). Noninvasive gene transfer to the lung for systemic delivery of therapeutic proteins. *J Clin Invest*. 110:499–504.

Beck SE, Jones LA, Chesnut K, et al. (1999). Repeated delivery of adeno-associated virus vectors to the rabbit airway. *J Virol*. 73:9446–9455.

Carter BJ (2005). Adeno-associated virus vectors in clinical trials. *Hum Gene Ther*. 16:541–550.

Davies JC, Geddes DM, Alton EFW (2003). Pulmonary gene therapy. In: Rolland A, Sullivan SM, eds. *Pharmaceutical Gene Delivery Systems*. New York: Marcel Dekker, 363–396.

Demoly P, Mathieu M, Curiel DT, Godard P, Bousquet J, Michel FB (1997). Gene therapy for asthma. *Gene Ther*. 4:507–516.

Factor P (2003). Gene therapy for asthma. *Mol Ther*. 7:148–152.

Fischer AC, Beck SE, Smith CL, et al. (2003). Succesful transgene expression with serial doses of aerosolized rAAV2 vectors in rhesus macaques. *Mol Ther*. 8:918–926.

Flotte TR (2005). Adeno-associated virus-mediated gene transfer for lung diseases. *Hum Gene Ther*. 16:643–648.

Flotte TR, Laube BL (2001). Gene therapy for cystic fibrosis. *Chest*. 120:124S–131S.

Flotte TR, Brantly ML, Spencer LT, Baker CT, Humphries M (2004). Phase I trial of intramuscular injection of recombinant adeno-associated virus alpha-1-anti-trypsin (rAAV2-CD-hAAT) gene vector to AAT-deficient adults. *Hum Gene Ther*. 14:93–128.

Griesenbach U, Cassady RL, Ferrari S, et al. (2002). The nasal epithelium as a factory for systemic protein delivery. *Mol Ther*. 5:98–103.

Griesenbach U, Geddes DM, Alton EWFW (2004). Gene therapy for cystic fibrosis: an example for lung gene therapy. *Gene Ther*. 11:S43–S50.

Johnson LG (2004). Overcoming barriers to efficient airway epithelial gene transfer. In: Templeton N, ed. *Gene and Cell Therapy*. New York: Marcel Dekker; 585–595.

Mastrangeli A, Harvey B-G, Crystal RG (1997). Gene therapy for lung disease. In: Crystal RG, et al., eds. *The Lung: Scientific Foundations*. 2nd ed. Philadelphia, PA: Lippincott-Raven; 2795–2811.

Moon C, Oh Y, Roth JA (2003). Current status of gene therapy for lung cancer and head and neck cancer. *Clin Cancer Res*. 9:5055–5067.

Moss RB, Rodman, Spencer LT, et al. (2004). Repeated adeno-associated virus serotype 2 aerosol- mediated cystic fibrosis transmembrane regulator gene transfer to the lungs of patients with cystic fibrosis: multi-center double-blind, placebo-controlled trial. *Chest*. 125:509–521.

Nyce JW, Metzger WJ (1997). DNA anti-sense therapy for asthma in an animal model. *Nature*. 385:721–725.

Robbins RA, Rennard SI (1997). Biology of airway epithelial cells. In: Crystal RG, et al., eds. *The Lung: Scientific Foundations*. 2nd ed. Philadelphia, PA; Lippincott-Raven; 445–453.

Sandalon Z, Bruckheimer EM, Lustig KH, Rogers LC, Peluso RW, Burstein H. (2004). Secretion of a TNFR:Fc fusion protein following pulmonary administration of pseudotyped adeno-associated virus vectors. *J Virol*. 78:12355–121365.

Sinn PL, Hickey MA, Staber PD, et al. (2003). Lentivirus vectors pseudotyped with filoviral envelope glycoproteins transduce airway epithelia from the apical surface independently of the folate receptor alpha. *J Virol*. 77:5902–5910.

Sinn PL, Penisten AK, Burnight ER, et al. (2005). Gene transfer to respiratory epithelia with lentivirus pseudotyped with Jaagsiekte sheep retrovirus envelope glycoprotein. *Hum Gene Ther*. 16:479–488.

Weibel ER (1997). Design of airways and blood vessels considered as branching trees. In: Crystal RG, et al., eds. *The Lung: Scientific Foundations*. 2nd ed. Philadelphia, PA: Lippincott-Raven; 1061–1071.

Weiss DJ (2002). Delivery of gene transfer vectors to lung: obstacles and the role of adjunct therapies techniques for airway administration. *Mol Ther*. 6:148–151.

Yonemitsu Y, Kitson C, Ferrari S, et al. (2000). Efficient gene transfer to airway epithelium using recombinant Sendai virus. *Nat Biotechnol*. 18:970–973.

Zhang LN, Karp P, Gerard CJ, et al. (2004). Dual therapeutic utility of proteasome modulating agents or pharmaco-gene therapy of the cystic fibrosis airway. *Mol Ther*. 10:990–1002.

13 The Brain as a Target for Gene Therapy

PEDRO R. LOWENSTEIN and MARIA G. CASTRO

Gene Therapeutics Research Institute of the Cedars-Sinai Medical
Center, and Department of Molecular and Medical Pharmacology,
University of California–Los Angeles, Los Angeles, California

Neurological diseases are limited by the particular conditions pertaining to the cellular composition, anatomy, immune reactivity, and particular diseases that affect brain structure and function. Concerning the cellular composition, the brain is composed of mostly nondividing neurons and dividing glial cells. Neurodegenerative disorders affect neuronal survival. Thus, gene therapies that affect neurons must contend with the challenge of a finite, long-lived, mainly nondividing population of cells of very complex morphology. This influences the tight safety limitations on gene therapy targeting the brain.

Concerning the brain anatomy, the brain is surrounded by various barriers. First, at the gross morphological level it is enclosed by the bony skull and fibrous meninges. At the cellular level it is separated from the general bloodstream by a selective blood–brain barrier. At the functional level, the brain possesses a peculiar immune reactivity whose understanding remains to be dissected completely. This peculiar immune status of the brain is usually mislabeled as the brain's immune privilege. However, the brain is not immune-privileged in the naive manner of this description. The main limitation is to prime an immune response from antigens expressed exclusively within the brain parenchyma. This is an advantage for gene therapists. However, any antigen that primes the immune system systemically will target and eliminate antigen-expressing cells in the brain. A clinical example of this is the progressive brain autoimmune disease multiple sclerosis.

Concerning the diseases that affect the brain, the most common ones are the neurodegenerations, followed by brain tumors, infections, autoimmune diseases, and genetic diseases of the brain. Currently, those being treated clinically with gene therapy are the brain tumors and the recessively inherited brain diseases as well as Alzheimer's and Parkinson's diseases. Gene therapies for neurodegenerations

Concepts in Genetic Medicine, Edited by Boro Dropulic and Barrie Carter
Copyright © 2008 John Wiley & Sons, Inc.

such as autoimmune diseases (e.g., multiple sclerosis) and dominant diseases (e.g., Huntington's disease) are currently at the experimental level.

NEURODEGENERATIVE DISEASES

Neurodegenerative disorders are progressive brain diseases, each targeting specific regions of the brain, such as Alzheimer's disease, Parkinson's disease, or the dominantly inherited Huntington's disease. Each disease targets a specific brain area. Thus, gene therapies are based on the particular neuroanatomical areas affected by the disease, as well as our knowledge of the pathophysiology and genetic contributing factors.

ALZHEIMER'S DISEASE

Alzheimer's disease (AD) is characterized by deposition of extracellular amyloid plaques, intracellular neurofibrillary tangles, synaptic loss, and neurodegeneration. Amyloid plaques are composed of insoluble amyloid-beta (Aβ) fibril fragments of the high-molecular-weight amyloid precursor protein (APP). In familial AD, mutations in presenilin and APP alter the proteolytic cleavage of APP by secretases, leading to an extracellular accumulation of amyloid plaques. Neurofibrially tangles are composed of insoluble hyperphosphorylated tau. Normally, phosphorylated tau stabilizes neuronal microtubles. Tangles are thought to lead to neuronal dysfunction, neuronal loss, and synaptic loss. These neurodegenerative changes lead to a disruption of the connectivity among various brain regions [1].

Nerve growth factor (NGF) promotes survival of basal forebrain cholinergic neurons, which degenerate in this disease [2]. This has led to the use of NGF to attempt to rescue degenerating basal forebrain cholinergic neurons [3–6]. Since cholinergic dysfunction could be a primary defect, or it could be secondary to neocortical degeneration, understanding the disease pathophysiology will be important in determining the potential therapeutic benefit of cholinergic drugs in AD.

Infusion of NGF into the ventricles of patients with AD had serious side effects, such as pain and weight loss [7]. As an alternative delivery, transplantation of primary rat fibroblasts producing human NGF were first investigated in fimbria fornix–lesioned rats [5]. After safety and feasibility had been confirmed in primates [8–10], a phase I trial was initiated [10]. In the fibroblast transplant experiments, patients with mild AD showed no adverse effects 22 months after transplantation of autologous fibroblasts obtained from skin biopsies, infected with an NGF-expressing Moloney murine leukemia virus (MoMLV)–derived retroviral vector The lack of toxicity of NGF in this trial has led to a further phase I trial in patients with mild AD based on injection of adeno-associated virus (AAV)–mediating NGF expression into the basal forebrain.

Alternative strategies for AD include transduction of apoE2 [11] to reduce the Aβ burden and the subsequent development of neuritic plaques in AD. Work on immunization approaches to reduce intraparenchymal levels of Aβ, which may include techniques allied to gene therapy, are also currently being tested. Vaccination with a plasmid that encodes Aβ42 [12] or by intranasal administration of replication-incompetent adenovirus (AdV) carrying both Aβ and GM-CSF genes [13] have been tested. Alternative immunization paradigms are being developed, as active immunization with Aβ1-42 was effective in mouse models but led to meningoencephalitis in some treated patients [14,15].

Neprilysin, an enzyme that degrades Aβ, has been used as an alternative gene therapy utilizing lentiviral vectors, and as such, has been tested in a number of different models [16,17]. Also, IGF-1 was effective in experimental models of neuronal degenerations in mouse models of amyotrophic lateral sclerosis [18]. Equally, simianRNA has now been shown to be an effective manner of reducing the overexpression of pathogenic proteins in the case of experimental models of Huntington's disease (e.g., huntingtin), dominant-inherited ataxias, and torsion dystonia [19–22].

PARKINSON'S DISEASE

Parkinson's disease (PD) is a progressive loss of dopaminergic neurons in the substantia nigra and other brain stem nuclei. Patients with PD have motor impairment with resting tremor, bradykinesia, and rigidity, but also balance problems and autonomic nervous dysfunction, and they show cognitive and psychiatric features. Genetic contributing factors include mutations in the α-*synuclein* (PARK1) and *parkin* (PARK2) genes [23,24]. *Parkin* functions as an *E3* ubiquitin-protein ligase, and a loss of function results in the failure of intracellular protein processing, with consecutive accumulation of various proteins to toxic levels [25]. Although sporadic and inherited PD have different causes, they probably intersect in common pathways [26,27]. The central cause of sporadic PD seems to be a mitochondrial complex I inhibition, and complex I deficiency may cause α-synuclein aggregation, contributing to the degeneration of dopaminergic neurons [26,27].

Gene therapy for PD was first developed in rat models using transduction of a single gene encoding tyrosine hydroxylase [28,29]. Limitations of this approach included the side effects of the helper-dependent HSV-1 amplicon vector used at that time, low expression, and expression of tyrosine hydroxylase (TH) as the only gene. Currently, gene therapy for Parkinson's includes (1) transduction of multiple genes essential for the synthesis of dopamine, to restore dopamine levels; (2) transduction of genes encoding growth factors, differentiation factors, transcription factors, and antiapoptotic proteins to prevent ongoing neurodegeneration of nigrostriatal dopamine neurons; and (3) improvements and further developments of vector and promoter systems to reduce toxicity, and immune responses, to increase longevity of expression, and to regulate transgene expression.

Coexpression of multiple enzymes are needed for regulated physiological release of dopamine and their functions are (1) TH, which converts tyrosine to L-dopa in the presence of tetrahydrobiopterin (BH4); (2) GTP cyclohydroxylase I (GCHI), which is the rate-limiting enzyme in the biosynthesis of BH4;

(3) aromatic aminodecarboxylase (AADC), which converts L-dopa to dopamine; and (4) vesicular monoamine transporter type 2 (VMAT-2), which concentrates dopamine into synaptic vesicles. Gene therapy combinations have been implemented in rat and primate models of PD using AAV, HSV-1 amplicon, or lentiviral vectors: TH and GHI [30,31]; TH, GCHI, and AADC [32–34]; TH, GCHI, AADC, and VMAT-2 [35].

Neuroprotective gene therapy has been utilized in Parkinson's disease. Expression of glial cell–derived neurotrophic factor (GDNF [36]) and brain cell–derived neurotrophic factor (BDNF [37]), as well as other neurotrophic factors related to GDNF, such as neurturin, protect nigrostriatal neurons from neurotoxic insults in rat and primate models of PD [38–42]. Long-term consequences of growth factor expression, such as down-regulation of TH [43,44] and questions regarding timing and regulation of therapy [45] need to be addressed; nevertheless, it may be difficult to mimic long-term human expression in nonhuman species.

Alternatively, Sonic Hedgehog, a secreted neurodifferentiation factor [46,47], has been utilized. Sonic Hedgehog could act on local precursor neurons to differentiate them in the direction of nigrostriatal dopamine cells. Other paradigms of gene therapy for PD, which are currently being tested in animal models, include the transduction of dopaminergic neurons with JNK-interacting protein-1 (JIP-1), apoptosis protease activating factor-1 (APAF-1 [48]) dominant negative inhibitor, neuronal apoptosis inhibitor protein (NAIP [49]), Hsp70 [50], and *Parkin* [51,52] and are reviewed elsewhere [53].

Because of potentially unknown side effects of the gene therapies, especially in the very long term, it will be important that novel gene therapies include safety procedures for regulating and inhibiting gene expression.

Another gene therapy paradigm concerns the transduction of excitatory glutamatergic neurons of the subthalamic nucleus (STN), with AAV expressing glutamic acid decarboxylase (GAD), the enzyme that synthesizes the inhibitory transmitter GABA [54]. Electrical inhibition of the STN through deep brain stimulation is clinically effective. This paradigm has already been implemented in a clinical trial [55]. This is the first clinical gene therapy trial in humans suffering from PD.

Other clinical gene therapy trials for PD are based on the transduction of AADC and neurturin [56] using AAV vectors. Neurturin is a growth factor, and AADC expression is expected to lower the need for high doses of L-dopa. Intriguingly, due to a large number of current considerations, these trials are going ahead without using regulatory systems.

BRAIN TUMORS: GLIOBLASTOMA MULTIFORME

Glioblastoma is the most common, rapidly progressive brain tumors, with an incidence of 3 to 6 in 100,000. Molecular lesions in glioma cells include deregulation of the cell cycle, alterations of apoptosis and cell differentiation, endothelial proliferation, neovascularization, and tumor cell migration and invasion. Initially, gene therapy for glioblastoma was attempted with transplantations of fibroblasts genetically engineered to secrete retrovirus vectors carrying thymidine kinase [57]. Clinical application of this approach in a large phase III clinical trial did not show a benefit for patients [58–60]. Therefore, current gene therapies aim at (1) a combination of therapeutic genes for synergistic action, (2) a combination of viral therapy with gene and immunotherapy (Figure 13.1), (3) improved vector delivery based on convection-enhanced delivery, and (4) imaging of vector application and therapy [61,62]. The various gene therapeutic strategies that have been studied to treat glioma models have been reviewed recently [63–65] and they include (1) replicating viruses based on replication-conditional HSV-1 and Adv vectors, (2) prodrug-activating enzymes, (3) cell cycle–regulating proteins (e.g., p53, p16, p21, PTEN, Rb, p300), (4) pro-apoptotic

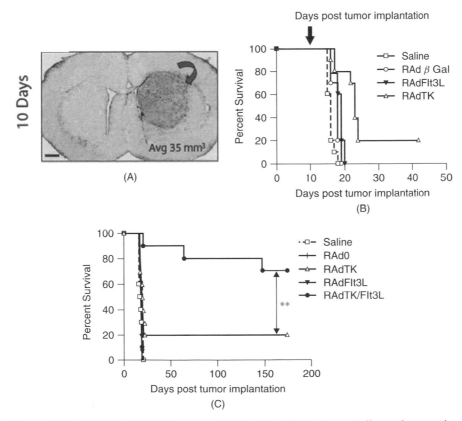

Figure 13.1   A stringent brain tumor model developed to test novel glioma therapeutics. Panel A illustrates a large CNS1 glioma tumor at the time of treatment. Panel B shows that treatment of a tumor of this size with either RAd-TK or RAd-Flt3L fails to rescue a significant percentage of animals. However, when animals are treated with both TK and Flt3L vectors (panel C), approximately 70% of animals survive. TK plus ganciclovir is given to kill dividing glioma cells and to provide tumor antigens to dendritic cells that are induced to infiltrate the tumor by Flt3 L.

genes (caspases, bax, Fas ligand) and angiogenesis inhibitors (endostatin, angio-station, etc.), and (5) immunomodulation.

Further, current clinical gene therapy protocols (http://www.gemcris.od.nih.gov) to investigate the safety and efficiency of (1) replication-competent oncolytic viruses (e.g., herpes simplex virus derived G207 [66] and 1716 [67–69] and adenovirus-derived Onyx-015 [70]; (2) prodrug therapy (e.g., thymidine kinase,); (3) cell-cycle regulation (e.g., p53); (4) antiangiogenesis; (5) immunomodula-tion (e.g., IL-4, TGFβ2 antisense, human interferon-beta (H5.010CMVhIFN-β) mediated by AdV or cationic liposomes [71,72], GM-CSF (IR851), IL-12, Flt3L [73,74]) and; (6) modification of dendritic cells [75,76], stem cells, and neural precursors targeting infiltrating brain GBMs [77–84].

SILENCING GENE EXPRESSION: AN APPROACH TO TREATING DOMINANTLY INHERITED DISEASES

The technologies developed by the gene therapy scientific community concern primarily the expression of genes in target tissues. However, the *reduction* of endogenous gene expression has been very challenging. This has left domi-nantly inherited diseases relatively untouched by gene therapy approaches. In dominantly inherited diseases the expression of a mutated protein causes the dis-ease: for example, in Huntington's disease, dominantly inherited ataxias, and dominantly inherited spinal cord degenerations such as the familial cases of amyotrophic lateral sclerosis. Recently, gene therapists have started to harness endogenous cellular mechanisms that regulate levels of endogenous mRNA (i.e., siRNA), to block expression of endogenous genes whose mutations causes disease [85–89]. These techniques have tested the role of individual genes in physiolog-ical processes, and more recently as an effective way to inhibit gene expression in a gene therapeutic context.

Gene therapists working with various different vectors have utilized siRNAs, and these have been tested for the treatment of brain [20,22,90], liver diseases [91–96], infectious diseases [97–104], and cancer [91,105–108]. Interestingly, because the treatment of inherited dominant diseases has so far been limited to palliative treatments, recent successes in experimental models of Huntington's disease [20,109] are likely to be translated clinically in a shorter time than exper-imental gene therapies for diseases that may already have effective, though not curative treatments available.

FUTURE CHALLENGES OF CLINICAL GENE THERAPY FOR NEUROLOGICAL DISEASES

The challenges for clinically effective gene therapy for brain diseases involve mainly limitations in establishing more clinical trials. Although clinical trials have proceeded for the treatment of brain tumors, inherited brain diseases, and cancer, very few of the many strategies developed have reached the clinical stage. In addition, many of these only reached the stage of phase I clinical trials. It is necessary to move novel strategies into larger phase III trials to truly indicate whether or not a novel treatment is working. At least one gene therapy with an adenovirus with a prodrug gene has been moved into a phase III trial in glioblastoma, by Ark Therapeutics in Europe. The problem is not to fail, but not to try. Sadly, some neurological gene therapy researchers, for reasons outside their control, are often limited by external limitations imposed on them by mistaken ethical, financial, scientific, and clinical concerns.

REFERENCES

1. De Lacoste MC, White CL III. The role of cortical connectivity in Alzheimer's disease pathogenesis: a review and model system. *Neurobiol Aging*. 1993;14:1–16.

2. Levi-Montalcini R. The nerve growth factor 35 years later. *Science*. 1987;237:1154–1162.

3. Hefti F. Nerve growth factor promotes survival of septal cholinergic neurons after fimbrial transections. *J Neurosci*. 1986;6:2155–2162.

4. Fischer WK, Wictorin A, Bjorklund LR, Williams SV, and Gage FH. Amelioration of cholinergic neuron atrophy and spatial memory impairment in aged rats by nerve growth factor. *Nature*. 1987;329:65–68.

5. Rosenberg MB, Friedmann T, Robertson RC, et al. Grafting genetically modified cells to the damaged brain: restorative effects of NGF expression. *Science*. 1988;242:1575–1578.

6. Tuszynski MH, U HS, Amaral DG, Gage FH. Nerve growth factor infusion in the primate brain reduces lesion-induced cholinergic neuronal degeneration. *J Neurosci*. 1990;10:3604–3614.

7. Eriksdotter Jonhagen M, Nordberg A, Amberla K, et al. Intracerebroventricular infusion of nerve growth factor in three patients with Alzheimer's disease. *Dement Geriatr Cogn Disord*. 1998;9:246–257.

8. Conner JM, Darracq MA, Roberts J, Tuszynski MH. Nontropic actions of neurotrophins: subcortical nerve growth factor gene delivery reverses age-related degeneration of primate cortical cholinergic innervation. *Proc Natl Acad Sci U S A*. 2001;98:1941–1946.

9. Smith DE, Roberts J, Gage FH, Tuszynski MH. Age-associated neuronal atrophy occurs in the primate brain and is reversible by growth factor gene therapy. *Proc Natl Acad Sci U S A*. 1999;96:10893–10898.

10. Tuszynski MH, Thal L, Pay M, et al. A phase 1 clinical trial of nerve growth factor gene therapy for Alzheimer disease. *Nat Med*. 2005;11:551–555.

11. Dodart JC, Marr RA, Koistinaho M, et al. Gene delivery of human apolipoprotein E alters brain Abeta burden in a mouse model of Alzheimer's disease. *Proc Natl Acad Sci U S A*. 2005;102:1211–1216.

12. Qu B, Rosenberg RN, Li L, Boyer PJ, Johnston SA. Gene vaccination to bias the immune response to amyloid-beta peptide as therapy for Alzheimer disease. *Arch Neurol*. 2004;61:1859–1864.

13. Kim HD, Kong FK, Cao Y, et al. Immunization of Alzheimer model mice with adenovirus vectors encoding amyloid beta-protein and GM-CSF reduces amyloid load in the brain. *Neurosci Lett*. 2004;370:218–223.

14. Hock C, Konietzko U, Papassotiropoulos A, et al. Generation of antibodies specific for beta-amyloid by vaccination of patients with Alzheimer disease. *Nat Med*. 2002;8:1270–1275.

15. Hock C, Konietzko U, Streffer JR, et al. Antibodies against beta-amyloid slow cognitive decline in Alzheimer's disease. *Neuron*. 2003;38:547–554.

16. Marr RA, Rockenstein E, Mukherjee A, et al. Neprilysin gene transfer reduces human amyloid pathology in transgenic mice. *J Neurosci*. 2003;23:1992–1996.

17. Marr RA, Guan H, Rockenstein E, et al. Neprilysin regulates amyloid beta peptide levels. *J Mol Neurosci*. 2004;22:5–11.

18. Kaspar BK, Llado J, Sherkat N, Rothstein JD, Gage FH. Retrograde viral delivery of IGF-1 prolongs survival in a mouse ALS model. *Science*. 2003;301:839–842.

19. Miller VM, Xia H, Marrs GL, et al. Allele-specific silencing of dominant disease genes. *Proc Natl Acad Sci U S A*. 2003;100:7195–7200.

20. Harper SQ, Staber PD, He X, et al. RNA interference improves motor and neuropathological abnormalities in a Huntington's disease mouse model. *Proc Natl Acad Sci U S A*. 2005;102:5820–5825.

21. Xia H, Mao Q, Paulson HL, Davidson BL. siRNA-mediated gene silencing in vitro and in vivo. *Nat Biotechnol*. 2002;20:1006–1010.

22. Xia H, Mao Q, Eliason SL, et al. RNAi suppresses polyglutamine-induced neurodegeneration in a model of spinocerebellar ataxia. *Nat Med*. 2004;10:816–820.

23. Kitada T, Asakawa S, Hattori N, et al. Mutations in the *parkin* gene cause autosomal recessive juvenile parkinsonism. *Nature*. 1998;392:605–608.

24. Polymeropoulos MH, Higgins JJ, Golbe LI, et al. Mapping of a gene for Parkinson's disease to chromosome 4q21-q23. *Science*. 1996;274:1197–1199.

25. Imai Y, Soda M, Inoue H, Hattori N, Mizuno Y, Takahashi R. An unfolded putative transmembrane polypeptide, which can lead to endoplasmic reticulum stress, is a substrate of parkin. *Cell*. 2001;105:891–902.

26. Dauer W, Przedborski S. Parkinson's disease: mechanisms and models. *Neuron*. 2003;39:889–909.

27. Dawson TM, Dawson VL. Molecular pathways of neurodegeneration in Parkinson's disease. *Science*. 2003;302:819–822.

28. Kaplitt MG, Leone P, Samulski RJ, et al. Long-term gene expression and phenotypic correction using adeno-associated virus vectors in the mammalian brain. *Nat Genet*. 1994;8:148–154.

29. During MJ, Naegele JR, O'Malley KL, Geller AI. Long-term behavioral recovery in parkinsonian rats by an HSV vector expressing tyrosine hydroxylase. *Science*. 1994;266:1399–1403.

30. Kirik D, Georgievska B, Burger C, et al. Reversal of motor impairments in parkinsonian rats by continuous intrastriatal delivery of L-dopa using rAAV-mediated gene transfer. *Proc Natl Acad Sci U S A*. 2002;99:4708–4713.

31. Mandel RJ, Rendahl KG, Spratt SK, Snyder RO, Cohen LK, Leff SE. Characterization of intrastriatal recombinant adeno-associated virus-mediated gene transfer of human tyrosine hydroxylase and human GTP-cyclohydrolase I in a rat model of Parkinson's disease. *J Neurosci*. 1998;18:4271–4284.

32. Muramatsu S, Fujimoto K, Ikeguchi K, et al. Behavioral recovery in a primate model of Parkinson's disease by triple transduction of striatal cells with adeno-associated viral vectors expressing dopamine-synthesizing enzymes. *Hum Gene Ther*. 2002;13:345–354.

33. Azzouz M, Martin-Rendon E, Barber RD, et al. Multicistronic lentiviral vector-mediated striatal gene transfer of aromatic L-amino acid decarboxylase, tyrosine hydroxylase, and GTP cyclohydrolase I induces sustained transgene expression, dopamine production, and functional improvement in a rat model of Parkinson's disease. *J Neurosci*. 2002;22:10302–10312.

34. Shen Y, Muramatsu SI, Ikeguchi K, et al. Triple transduction with adeno-associated virus vectors expressing tyrosine hydroxylase, aromatic-L-amino-acid decarboxylase, and GTP cyclohydrolase I for gene therapy of Parkinson's disease. *Hum Gene Ther*. 2000;11:1509–1519.

35. Sun M, Kong L, Wang X, et al. Coexpression of tyrosine hydroxylase, GTP cyclohydrolase I, aromatic amino acid decarboxylase, and vesicular monoamine transporter 2 from a helper virus-free herpes simplex virus type 1 vector supports high-level, long-term biochemical and behavioral correction of a rat model of Parkinson's disease. *Hum Gene Ther*. 2004;15:1177–1196.

36. Lin LF, Doherty DH, Lile JD, Bektesh S, Collins F. GDNF: a glial cell line-derived neurotrophic factor for midbrain dopaminergic neurons. *Science*. 1993;260:1130–1132.

37. Hyman C, Hofer M, Barde YA, et al. BDNF is a neurotrophic factor for dopaminergic neurons of the substantia nigra. *Nature*. 1991;350:230–232.

38. Kordower JH. In vivo gene delivery of glial cell line–derived neurotrophic factor for Parkinson's disease. *Ann Neurol*. 2003;53 (Suppl 3): S120–S132; discussion S132–S124.

39. Kordower JH, Emborg ME, Bloch J, et al. Neurodegeneration prevented by lentiviral vector delivery of GDNF in primate models of Parkinson's disease. *Science*. 2000;290:767–773.

40. Kirik D, Rosenblad C, Bjorklund A, Mandel RJ. Long-term rAAV-mediated gene transfer of GDNF in the rat Parkinson's model: intrastriatal but not intranigral transduction promotes functional regeneration in the lesioned nigrostriatal system. *J Neurosci*. 2000;20:4686–4700.

41. Choi-Lundberg DL, Lin Q, Chang YN, et al. Dopaminergic neurons protected from degeneration by GDNF gene therapy. *Science*. 1997;275:838–841.

42. Bjorklund A, Kirik D, Rosenblad C, Georgievska B, Lundberg C, Mandel RJ. Towards a neuroprotective gene therapy for Parkinson's disease: use of adenovirus, AAV and lentivirus vectors for gene transfer of GDNF to the nigrostriatal system in the rat Parkinson model. *Brain Res*. 2000;886:82–98.

43. Georgievska B, Kirik D, Bjorklund A. Overexpression of glial cell line–derived neurotrophic factor using a lentiviral vector induces time- and dose-dependent downregulation of tyrosine hydroxylase in the intact nigrostriatal dopamine system. *J Neurosci*. 2004;24:6437–6445.

44. Rosenblad C, Georgievska B, Kirik D. Long-term striatal overexpression of GDNF selectively downregulates tyrosine hydroxylase in the intact nigrostriatal dopamine system. *Eur J Neurosci*. 2003;17:260–270.

45. Georgievska B, Jakobsson J, Persson E, Ericson C, Kirik D, Lundberg C. Regulated delivery of glial cell line–derived neurotrophic factor into rat striatum, using a tetracycline-dependent lentiviral vector. *Hum Gene Ther*. 2004;15:934–944.

46. Hurtado-Lorenzo A, Millan E, Gonzalez-Nicolini V, Suwelack D, Castro MG, Lowenstein PR. Differentiation and transcription factor gene therapy in experimental Parkinson's disease: Sonic Hedgehog and Gli-1, but not Nurr-1, protect nigrostriatal cell bodies from 6-OHDA-induced neurodegeneration. *Mol Ther*. 2004;10:507–524.

47. Suwelack D, Hurtado-Lorenzo A, Millan E, et al. Neuronal expression of the transcription factor Gli1 using the Tubulin a-1 promoter is neuroprotective in an experimental model of Parkinson's disease. *Gene Ther*. 2004;11:1742–1752.

48. Mochizuki H, Hayakawa H, Migita M, et al. An AAV-derived Apaf-1 dominant negative inhibitor prevents MPTP toxicity as antiapoptotic gene therapy for Parkinson's disease. *Proc Natl Acad Sci U S A*. 2001;98:10918–10923.

49. Crocker SJ, Wigle N, Liston P, et al. NAIP protects the nigrostriatal dopamine pathway in an intrastriatal 6-OHDA rat model of Parkinson's disease. *Eur J Neurosci*. 2001;14:391–400.

50. Dong Z, Wolfer DP, Lipp HP, Bueler H. Hsp70 gene transfer by adeno-associated virus inhibits MPTP-induced nigrostriatal degeneration in the mouse model of Parkinson disease. *Mol Ther*. 2005;11:80–88.

51. Yamada M, Mizuno Y, Mochizuki H. Parkin gene therapy for alpha-synucleinopathy: a rat model of Parkinson's disease. *Hum Gene Ther*. 2005;16:262–270.

52. Lo Bianco C, Schneider BL, Bauer M, et al. Lentiviral vector delivery of *parkin* prevents dopaminergic degeneration in an alpha-synuclein rat model of Parkinson's disease. *Proc Natl Acad Sci U S A*. 2004;101:17510–17515.

53. Burton EA, Glorioso JC, Fink DJ. Gene therapy progress and prospects: Parkinson's disease. *Gene Ther*. 2003;10:1721–1727.

54. Luo J, Kaplitt MG, Fitzsimons HL, et al. Subthalamic GAD gene therapy in a Parkinson's disease rat model. *Science*. 2002;298:425–429.

55. During MJ, Kaplitt MG, Stern MB, Eidelberg D. Subthalamic GAD gene transfer in Parkinson disease patients who are candidates for deep brain stimulation. *Hum Gene Ther*. 2001;12:1589–1591.

56. Fjord-Larsen L, Johansen JL, Kusk P, et al. Efficient in vivo protection of nigral dopaminergic neurons by lentiviral gene transfer of a modified Neurturin construct. *Exp Neurol*. 2005;195:49–60.

57. Culver KW, Ram Z, Wallbridge S, Ishii H, Oldfield EH, Blaese RM. In vivo gene transfer with retroviral vector-producer cells for treatment of experimental brain tumors. *Science*. 1992;256:1550–1552.

58. Ram Z, Culver KW, Oshiro EM, et al. Therapy of malignant brain tumors by intratumoral implantation of retroviral vector-producing cells. *Nat Med*. 1997;3:1354–1361.

59. Rainov NG. A phase III clinical evaluation of herpes simplex virus type 1 thymidine kinase and ganciclovir gene therapy as an adjuvant to surgical resection and radiation in adults with previously untreated glioblastoma multiforme. *Hum Gene Ther*. 2000;11:2389–2401.

60. Klatzmann D, Valery CA, Bensimon G, et al. A phase I/II study of herpes simplex virus type 1 thymidine kinase "suicide" gene therapy for recurrent glioblastoma. Study Group on Gene Therapy for Glioblastoma. *Hum Gene Ther*. 1998;9:2595–2604.

61. Jacobs AH, Voges J, Kracht LW, et al. Imaging in gene therapy of patients with glioma. *J Neurooncol*. 2003;65:291–305.

62. Jacobs A, Voges J, Reszka R, et al. Positron-emission tomography of vector-mediated gene expression in gene therapy for gliomas. *Lancet*. 2001;358:727–729.

63. Lam PY, Breakefield XO. Potential of gene therapy for brain tumors. *Hum Mol Genet*. 2001;10:777–787.

64. Jacobs A, Breakefield XO, Fraefel C. HSV-1-based vectors for gene therapy of neurological diseases and brain tumors: I. HSV-1 structure, replication and pathogenesis. *Neoplasia*. 1999;1:387–401.

65. Castro MG, Cowen R, Williamson IK, et al. Current and future strategies for the treatment of malignant brain tumors. *Pharmacol Ther*. 2003;98:71–108.

66. Markert JM, Medlock MD, Rabkin SD, et al. Conditionally replicating herpes simplex virus mutant, G207 for the treatment of malignant glioma: results of a phase I trial. *Gene Ther*. 2000;7:867–874.

67. Papanastassiou V, Rampling R, Fraser M, et al. The potential for efficacy of the modified (ICP 34.5(-)) herpes simplex virus HSV1716 following intratumoural injection into human malignant glioma: a proof of principle study. *Gene Ther*. 2002;9:398–406.

68. Harrow S, Papanastassiou V, Harland J, et al. HSV1716 injection into the brain adjacent to tumour following surgical resection of high-grade glioma: safety data and long-term survival. *Gene Ther*. 2004;11:1648–1658.

69. Rampling R, Cruickshank G, Papanastassiou V, et al. Toxicity evaluation of replication-competent herpes simplex virus (ICP 34.5 null mutant 1716) in patients with recurrent malignant glioma. *Gene Ther*. 2000;7:859–866.

70. Chiocca EA, Abbed KM, Tatter S, et al. A phase I open-label, dose-escalation, multi-institutional trial of injection with an E1B-attenuated adenovirus, ONYX-015, into the peritumoral region of recurrent malignant gliomas, in the adjuvant setting. *Mol Ther*. 2004;10:958–966.

71. Eck SL, Alavi JB, Judy K, et al. Treatment of recurrent or progressive malignant glioma with a recombinant adenovirus expressing human interferon-beta (H5.010CMVhIFN-beta): a phase I trial. *Hum Gene Ther*. 2001;12:97–113.

72. Yoshida J, Mizuno M, Fujii M, et al. Human gene therapy for malignant gliomas (glioblastoma multiforme and anaplastic astrocytoma) by in vivo transduction with human interferon beta gene using cationic liposomes. *Hum Gene Ther*. 2004;15:77–86.

73. Ali S, King GD, Curtin JF, et al. Combined immunostimulation and conditional cytotoxic gene therapy provide long term survival in a large glioma model. *Cancer Res*. 2005;65:194–204.

74. Ali S, Curtin JF, Zirger JM, et al. Inflammatory and anti-glioma effects of an adenovirus expressing human soluble fms-like tyrosine kinase 3 ligand (hsFlt3L): treatment with hsflt3l inhibits intracranial glioma progression. *Mol Ther*. 2004;10:1071–1084.

75. Yu JS, Liu G, Ying H, Yong WH, Black KL, Wheeler CJ. Vaccination with tumor lysate-pulsed dendritic cells elicits antigen-specific, cytotoxic T-cells in patients with malignant glioma. *Cancer Res*. 2004;64:4973–4979.

76. Liau LM, Prins RM, Kiertscher SM, et al. Dendritic cell vaccination in glioblastoma patients induces systemic and intracranial T-cell responses modulated by the local central nervous system tumor microenvironment. *Clin Cancer Res*. 2005;11:5515–5525.

77. Shah K, Bureau E, Kim DE, et al. Glioma therapy and real-time imaging of neural precursor cell migration and tumor regression. *Ann Neurol*. 2005;57:34–41.

78. Brown AB, Yang W, Schmidt NO, et al. Intravascular delivery of neural stem cell lines to target intracranial and extracranial tumors of neural and non-neural origin. *Hum Gene Ther*. 2003;14:1777–1785.

79. Tang Y, Shah K, Messerli SM, Snyder E, Breakefield X, Weissleder R. In vivo tracking of neural progenitor cell migration to glioblastomas. *Hum Gene Ther*. 2003;14:1247–1254.

80. Aboody KS, Brown A, Rainov NG, et al. Neural stem cells display extensive tropism for pathology in adult brain: evidence from intracranial gliomas. *Proc Natl Acad Sci U S A*. 2000;97:12846–12851.

81. Herrlinger U, Woiciechowski C, Sena-Esteves M, et al. Neural precursor cells for delivery of replication-conditional HSV-1 vectors to intracerebral gliomas. *Mol Ther*. 2000;1:347–357.

82. Ehtesham M, Kabos P, Kabosova A, Neuman T, Black KL, Yu JS. The use of interleukin 12-secreting neural stem cells for the treatment of intracranial glioma. *Cancer Res*. 2002;62:5657–5663.

83. Ehtesham M, Kabos P, Gutierrez MA, et al. Induction of glioblastoma apoptosis using neural stem cell–mediated delivery of tumor necrosis factor-related apoptosis-inducing ligand. *Cancer Res*. 2002;62:7170–7174.

84. Ehtesham M, Yuan X, Kabos P, et al. Glioma tropic neural stem cells consist of astrocytic precursors and their migratory capacity is mediated by CXCR4. *Neoplasia*. 2002;6:287–293.

85. Bayne EH, Allshire RC. RNA-directed transcriptional gene silencing in mammals. *Trends Genet*. 2005;21:370–373.

86. Lecellier CH, Dunoyer P, Arar K, et al. A cellular microRNA mediates antiviral defense in human cells. *Science*. 2005;308:557–560.

87. Sontheimer EJ, Carthew RW. Silence from within: endogenous siRNAs and miRNAs. *Cell*. 2005;122:9–12.

88. Tomari Y, Zamore PD. Perspective: machines for RNAi. *Genes Dev*. 2005; 19:517–529.

89. Voinnet O. Induction and suppression of RNA silencing: insights from viral infections. *Nat Rev Genet*. 2005;6:206–220.

90. Davidson BL, Paulson HL. Molecular medicine for the brain: silencing of disease genes with RNA interference. *Lancet Neurol*. 2004;3:145–149.

91. Morrissey DV, Lockridge JA, Shaw L, et al. Potent and persistent in vivo anti-HBV activity of chemically modified siRNAs. *Nat Biotechnol*. 2005;23:1002–1007.

92. Li H, Fu X, Chen Y, et al. Use of adenovirus-delivered siRNA to target oncoprotein p28GANK in hepatocellular carcinoma. *Gastroenterology*. 2005;128:2029–2041.

93. Kronke J, Kittler R, Buchholz F, et al. Alternative approaches for efficient inhibition of hepatitis C virus RNA replication by small interfering RNAs. *J Virol*. 2004;78:3436–3446.

94. Radhakrishnan SK, Layden TJ, and Gartel AL. RNA interference as a new strategy against viral hepatitis. *Virology*. 2004;323:173–181.

95. McCaffrey AP, Meuse L, Pham TT, Conklin DS, Hannon GJ, Kay MA. RNA interference in adult mice. *Nature*. 2002;418:38–39.

96. McCaffrey AP, Nakai H, Pandey K, et al. Inhibition of hepatitis B virus in mice by RNA interference. *Nat Biotechnol*. 2003;21:639–644.

97. Bennink JR, and Palmore TN. The promise of siRNAs for the treatment of influenza. *Trends Mol Med*. 2004;10:571–574.

98. Bitko V, Musiyenko A, Shulyayeva O, Barik S. Inhibition of respiratory viruses by nasally administered siRNA. *Nat Med*. 2005;11:50–55.

99. Lee SK, Dykxhoorn DM, Kumar P, et al. Lentiviral delivery of short hairpin RNAs protects CD4 T cells from multiple clades and primary isolates of HIV. *Blood*. 2005;106:818–826.

100. Li BJ, Tang Q, Cheng D, et al. Using siRNA in prophylactic and therapeutic regimens against SARS coronavirus in Rhesus macaque. *Nat Med*. 2005;11:944–951.

101. Schubert S, Grunert HP, Zeichhardt H, Werk D, Erdmann VA, Kurreck J. Maintaining inhibition: siRNA double expression vectors against coxsackieviral RNAs. *J Mol Biol*. 2005;346:457–465.

102. Werk D, Schubert S, Lindig V, et al. Developing an effective RNA interference strategy against a plus-strand RNA virus: silencing of coxsackievirus B3 and its cognate coxsackievirus–adenovirus receptor. *Biol Chem*. 2005;386:857–863.

103. Zhang W, Singam R, Hellermann G, et al. Attenuation of dengue virus infection by adeno-associated virus–mediated siRNA delivery. *Genet Vaccines Ther*. 2004;2:8.

104. Zhang W, Yang H, Kong X, et al. Inhibition of respiratory syncytial virus infection with intranasal siRNA nanoparticles targeting the viral NS1 gene. *Nat Med*. 2005;11:56–62.

105. Hede K. Blocking cancer with RNA interference moves toward the clinic. *J Natl Cancer Inst*. 2005;97:626–628.

106. Liang Z, Yoon Y, Votaw J, Goodman MM, Williams L, Shim H. Silencing of CXCR4 blocks breast cancer metastasis. *Cancer Res*. 2005;65:967–971.

107. Sumimoto H, Yamagata S, Shimizu A, et al. Gene therapy for human small-cell lung carcinoma by inactivation of *Skp-2* with virally mediated RNA interference. *Gene Ther*. 2005;12:95–100.

108. Li S, Rosenberg JE, Donjacour AA, et al. Rapid inhibition of cancer cell growth induced by lentiviral delivery and expression of mutant-template telomerase RNA and anti-telomerase short-interfering RNA. *Cancer Res*. 2004;64:4833–4840.

109. Rodriguez-Lebron E, Denovan-Wright EM, Nash K, Lewin AS, Mandel RJ. Intrastriatal rAAV-mediated delivery of anti-huntingtin shRNAs induces partial reversal of disease progression in R6/1 Huntington's disease transgenic mice. *Mol Ther*. 2005;12:618–633.

14 Immune Responses to Viral Vectors Injected Systemically or into the CNS

PEDRO R. LOWENSTEIN and MARIA G. CASTRO
Gene Therapeutics Research Institute of the Cedars-Sinai Medical
Center, and Department of Molecular and Medical Pharmacology,
University of California–Los Angeles, Los Angeles, California

Despite major advances in both basic and clinical gene therapy, the hurdles imposed by the immune system have not yet been surmounted. A lack of understanding of how the immune system reacts to the vectors used in gene therapy, difficulties in measuring preexisting antivector immune responses in humans, and reliance of experimental studies in an unavoidably small number of animal species have challenged, and in a few cases stopped, the progress of very promising clinical trials. In this brief review we discuss the mechanisms of antivector immune responses and novel pathways and approaches to overcome one of the last hurdles to safe and effective clinical gene therapy.

INNATE IMMUNE RESPONSES

The innate immune response is the earliest line of defense generated by the host. Following injection of recombinant adenoviral vectors carrying therapeutic transgenes, the innate immune response is activated very rapidly (i.e., within minutes to hours). One of the initial aspects in the recognition of foreign infectious agents is performed by antigen-presenting cells (APCs). Examples of APCs include the dendritic cells and macrophages, which are located in many different tissues throughout the body. These cells demonstrate a high level of phagocytic activity, which allows for the capture of foreign antigens for further processing [1]. Although this recognition is nonspecific, the ability of the APCs to recognize foreign antigen is the first event in a sequence of events that leads to the eventual activation of effector T and B cells [2]. Importantly, dendritic cells are the

Concepts in Genetic Medicine, Edited by Boro Dropulic and Barrie Carter
Copyright © 2008 John Wiley & Sons, Inc.

main cells responsible for carrying antigenic epitopes from the infected tissues to lymph nodes, where these antigens will be presented to naive T lymphocytes to prime the adaptive immune response. Dendritic cells link nonspecific innate inflammatory responses to adaptive antigen-specific immune responses.

Other important components of the innate immune system include granulocytes, neutrophils, natural killer (NK) cells, and natural killer T (NKT) cells, in addition to macrophages and dendritic cells (DCs). All these cell types are rapidly recruited to the site of viral infection and participate in antiviral responses directly, by killing infected cells and producing antiviral cytokines, as well as indirectly, by the production of chemokines that act to recruit other immune cells into infected tissues. Later, these cytokines and chemokines can also be involved in activation of the adaptive immune response [3].

Interaction of viral vectors with receptors on cell surfaces lead to the stimulation of intracellular signaling pathways, including activation of NFκB [4], AT-2/c-Jun [5], interferon regulatory factors (IRFs) [6], and MAP kinases [7]. This increases the production of inflammatory cytokines, such as IFNα/β, IFNγ, IL-6, and IL-12 [8–10], and chemokines (e.g., CCL2, CCL5, CXCL10, and MIP-family chemokines) [11–15]. The production of antiviral cytokines and chemokines protects against viral infection but can also inhibit transcription of vector-encoded transgenes [16,17]. Systemic administration of first-generation adenoviral vectors results in inflammation that eliminates transgene expression from liver and lungs. This is mediated by macrophages, NK cells, and cytokines such as TNFα and IFNγ [18–21].

The immune response to the injection of adenoviral vectors into the central nervous system (CNS) differs greatly from the response seen following injection to peripheral organ systems. Several factors, including the presence of a blood–brain barrier (BBB), a lack of lymphatic capillaries, the absence of dendritic cells from the naive noninflamed brain, and a low level of major histocompatibility complex (MHC) expression, have caused the brain to be considered a relatively immune-privileged organ.

This localized inflammation is a nonspecific response characterized by influx of T cells, macrophages, and other cells of the innate immune system, and is found to be present for only a month after vector administration. Furthermore, this inflammatory response does not result in elimination of transgene expression [22–24]. As discussed previously, the inability to mount a response that eliminates transgene expression may be the result of the failure of the brain to produce an effective antigen-specific T-cell response against the injected adenoviral vector [22–24].

As a result, immune responses in the brain versus those seen in peripheral organs differ greatly (Figure 14.1). While injections of first-generation adenoviral vectors cause immune responses that result in complete elimination of both vector and transgene expression in two to three weeks [25] in the brain, transgene expression is sustained for much longer [22–24,26–30] (i.e., for up to 6 to 13 months). However, long-term expression in the CNS depends on the dose of vector injected. Injection of very high doses (i.e., above a threshold of 1×10^8

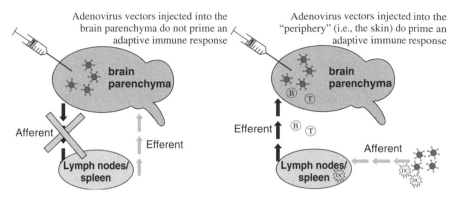

Figure 14.1 Brain immune system. The left side demonstrates that careful injection of viral vectors into the brain parenchyma does not stimulate an immune response, due to the lack of an afferent arm of the immune system that could carry antigens to the lymph nodes to initiate an adaptive immune response. In the absence of an effective afferent immune arm, there is no efferent immune arm capable of eliminating viral vectors from the brain. Nevertheless, injection of vectors will activate the innate immune system to release of cytokines and chemokines, but this response will be transient. The right side illustrates that if antigens are made available to the immune system (e.g., through the injection of viral vectors into the skin), active stimulation of the immune system will occur. Once priming has occurred, activated T cells will infiltrate the brain and eliminate transgene-expressing cells.

IU) causes a massive activation of the innate immune response in the brain that will completely eliminate transgene expression and cause a brain lesion, even in the absence of the priming of the systemic immune response [15,31,32].

Although the immune-privileged status of the CNS acts to limit the amount of immune cells that are able to gain access to the brain, brain endothelial cells, perivascular macrophages, microglia, and astrocytes can initiate an innate immune reaction in response to the delivery of viral vectors into the brain. Injection of first-generation adenovirus vectors (Ads) and novel HC-Ads into the brain results in stimulation of a rapid local inflammatory reaction. This early response is characterized by recruitment of macrophages and non-antigen-specific lymphocytes, and increased expression of MHC class I antigens and activation of local microglia and astrocytes are all found proximal to the site of infection [22]. This response can first be detected at vector doses above 1×10^6 to 1×10^7 IU. The existence of a threshold for adenoviral vector-mediated gene therapy has recently been established at 1×10^8 IU. Injections below this threshold result in cytokine and cellular-mediated inflammation that is acute, transient, and attenuated within 30 days and which does not clear transgene expression from the brain. Injection of vectors above this 1×10^8 IU threshold results in increased cytotoxicity, irreversible inflammation, elimination of transgene expression, and the loss of neurons and glia [15,31,33].

ADAPTIVE IMMUNE RESPONSES

The kinetics of the adaptive immune response is slower than the innate immune system. Its effector mechanisms increase over days rather than hours as do innate immune responses. Delivery of viral vectors to the liver or lung, or following systemic injection, triggers the innate immune inflammation, which is followed by the adaptive immune inflammation approximately 5 to 10 days later. Thus, both the innate and adaptive inflammatory processes become intimately linked in time and cannot be dissociated into individual components. In the brain, however, a vector delivered carefully to the brain parenchyma will cause innate immune inflammation but will fail to prime a systemic adaptive immune response (Figure 14.1). The causes of the lack of priming of the adaptive immune response from infectious antigens delivered to the brain parenchyma are to be found in the anatomy of the brain immune system, the lack of cells in the naive brain that can carry an infectious antigen to the lymph nodes to be presented to naive lymphocytes (i.e., dendritic cells), the lack of lymphatics, and the presence of numerous immune-suppressant molecules such as TGFβ.

In contrast to what is seen in other organs, however, transgene expression levels in the brain remains largely unaltered in the presence of these presumably antigen nonspecific T lymphocytes that enter the brain during early innate inflammatory responses [28]. This suggests that the mechanism underlying persistent transgene expression is due to an ineffective T-cell-mediated response in the brain, which results in a response that is unable to clear vector or transgene product from the naive brain [23,24,34,35]. This is thought to be due to the lack of a functional DC system present in the naive brain [35], although once brain inflammation occurs, various populations of DCs have been shown to be present within the brain parenchyma [35–48]. Despite low basal MHC class I and II expression in the brain, inflammation increases their expression, a necessary step to allow immune cell infiltration of the brain.

In peripheral organs such as the liver and lung, both CD8+ and CD4+ T cells, have a role in the anti-adenoviral vector response [49,50]. One of the predominant effector cells involved in the eventual clearance of virus from the host are the CD8+ cytotoxic T cells (CTLs) [49]. The immune response against adenoviral vectors recognizes antigenic epitopes present within the proteins that form the viral capsid (e.g., the fiber protein). Even though the adenoviral vectors are defective for replication within infected cells, due to the high multiplicity of infectin (MOI) values used to transduce cells, all transcriptional cassettes become activated. Thus, following infection with first-generation vector, these antigens are synthesized and presented by infected cells on MHC molecules.

Studies in a variety of immunodeficient mice have demonstrated the central role of adaptive immune response in eliminating transgene expression [49–56]. Yang et al. [51] first postulated direct killing of transduced hepatocytes by CTLs, potentially through apoptotic mechanisms. However, direct in situ demonstration of the killing of target cells by CD8+ in vivo has been elusive. Thus, recent work on the clearing of hepatitis B virus from the liver in a transgenic model (3) has provided strong evidence that CD8+ CTLs, through the secretion of IFNγ, inhibit viral genome replication with only limited toxicity to liver cells. Therefore, the precise cellular and immune mechanism for inhibition of transgene expression in the brain remains to be determined.

To overcome the limitations of vectors expressing wild-type viral proteins, a number of vectors not expressing any viral proteins have been produced. The most common of such vectors deleted of all wild-type viral genomic sequences are vectors derived from adenovirus (high-capacity helper-dependent adenoviral vectors), herpes simplex virus (HSV)-1 (amplicon vectors), adeno-associated virus (AAV) vectors, and lentiviral vectors.

The potential immunogenicity of completely deleted vectors hinges on whether gene expression from the viral vectors is necessary to initiate an adaptive immune response against adenovirus, or whether virions themselves would be sufficient. To this end, studies were undertaken that utilized adenoviral vectors that could not express genes from their genomes, due either to psoralen/ultraviolet (UV) inactivation, or because capsids were unable to package vector genomes. Even though all these vectors cause the same inflammation when injected into the brain [30], in mice systemic injection of psoralen/UV inactivated vectors did prime a systemic immune response detectable as CTLs [57], whereas in rats, injection of similar vectors did not prime a systemic immune response that could abolish transgene expression from the brain, suggesting that in rats, psoralen/UV-inactivated vectors did not prime a systemic immune response [31]. Thus, whether genome expression is needed to prime systemic antiadenoviral immune responses remains to be determined. Importantly, however, work by Samulski's group demonstrated by gene expression microarrays that the number of genes whose expression is altered following infection of target cells is reduced substantially compared to those containing vector genomes when infection proceeds with adenovirus virions devoid of genomes [58,59].

However, following infection with an HC-Adv vector (or any of the other completely deleted vectors), the potential antigenic epitopes will only be present within the vector capsid. As a consequence, these antigenic epitopes can be presented on MHC to the immune system only during early infection steps (i.e., while the vector is uncoating). Presentation of antigenic epitopes in this case will be transient, and can only occur until all virion proteins have been metabolized. Importantly, uncoating has been shown to be vector and serotype specific [60]. Consequently, vector-specific CTL recognition does not require de novo gene expression, and antigenic epitopes derived from virion proteins complexed with MHC class I molecules can serve as targets for CTL recognition and induction of antiviral CTL responses [22,57,61]. Thus, it is highly likely that systemic adaptive immune responses against completely deleted vectors, studied within the proper immunological context, will be shown to be the rule rather than the exception.

Once uncoating has been completed and all input virion proteins have been degraded, antigenic epitopes will no longer be produced from vectors not encoding for any wild-type viral proteins. Potential immune responses to antigenic epitopes present in the transgene, however, could continue. Thus, whereas the stimulation of immune responses against viral vectors can be inhibited almost completely, those potentially raised against the transgene will be more difficult to address. Nevertheless, similar problems have been faced by the treatment of any disease that necessitates the delivery of a protein [e.g., diabetes (insulin) or hemophilia (factor IX)]. This highlights one of the major challenges to the use of viral vectors, since immune responses against virions and transgenes have been detected when utilizing not only Adv but also AAV and lentiviral vectors [62,63].

Immune responses against transgenes will, of course, be more difficult to address; however, in the treatment of diabetes and hemophilia, a percentage of patients are known to develop blocking immune responses while continuing to respond to higher doses of therapeutic proteins. ^{51}Cr release assays have also shown that CTLs can be generated against the therapeutic transgene in mice [62,64], although various mechanisms are being developed to control one of the last frontiers in antivector immune responses [65,66]. Most recently, the genetic determinants of antiadenoviral immune responses have also been started to be elucidated, and it is promising that this work will identify the central factors that control antivector immunity [67–70].

Interestingly, the dynamics of the immune response against vectors completely deleted of wild-type genomic sequences suggests the use of transient immune-suppression during vector uncoating. Even if gene therapy has been somewhat reluctant in utilizing short term, transient immune-suppression regimes at the start of the therapies, their potential in making clinical trials safer is starting to be appreciated. This is now being discussed more openly in the clinical literature as a potential approach.

CONSEQUENCES FOR GENE THERAPY OF THE CNS

Because a large portion of the human population has been exposed to adenovirus, it is important to determine whether adenoviral vectors used as gene transfer systems are able to produce stable and long-term expression of transgene in the presence of a systemic immune challenge. Upon injection of first-generation adenoviral vector into brain parenchyma only, a local inflammatory response is elicited (Figure 14.1). This localized inflammation is a nonspecific response characterized by influx of T cells, macrophages, and other cells of the innate immune system, and is only found to be present for one month after vector administration. Furthermore, this inflammatory response does not result in elimination of transgene expression [22–24]. As discussed previously, the inability to mount a response that eliminates transgene expression may be the result of the failure of the brain to produce an effective antigen-specific T-cell response against the injected adenoviral vector [22–24].

Activation of antiviral T cells by previous exposure or peripheral immunization with adenovirus results in the infiltration of T lymphocytes into the brain parenchyma, activation of other immune effectors such as macrophages and microglia, and finally, the elimination of adenoviral-mediated transgene expression [23,71]. Further, recent experiments from our laboratory have demonstrated that the systemic immune response is dependent on both sets of CD4+ and CD8+ T cells, IFNγ, perforin, and TNFα and leads to the phagocytosis and cell death of at least a significant number of transduced cells (unpublished data). These experiments illustrate the challenge imposed on gene therapy by the immune system [62,63]. However, even if transgene expression is somewhat compromised, in the CNS HC-Ad vectors can achieve long-term transgene expression even in the presence of systemic antiadenoviral immune responses [30,71,72].

Viral vectors currently represent the best available vehicles for efficient gene transfer. Considerable gains in the field of gene therapy have been made in recent decades; however, the remaining immunogenic properties of these vectors is a major drawback to the use of adenoviral vectors in clinical procedures. Despite these potential problems, great advances have been made for the use of viral vectors as gene transfer vectors. The creation of newer vector gene transfer systems and the production of gene-deleted and "gutless" vectors that are less immunogenic will have a great impact on the clinical future of gene therapy.

The excitement about clinical trials in gene therapy has been tempered following the realization that the immune system can mount effective responses that have clinical consequences [73,74]. It is very encouranging that recent important advances in growing, producing [75–77], and testing novel vectors fully deleted of wild-type genomic sequences indicate exciting solutions to current immune challenges in ways that will overcome this last hurdle to clinically effective gene therapy [78–80]. Although it will also be important that future work using viral vectors expand our ability to target specific populations of cells and express therapeutic and regulated levels of transgene [81], it is also important to recognize the continued challenge imposed by the host immune system. Elucidation of all aspects of the immune response in the context of gene therapy and understanding of its mechanisms is paramount for the safe, clinically effective application of clinical gene therapy.

Acknowledgments

Gene therapy projects for neurological diseases are funded by the National Institutes of Health/National Institute of Neurological Disorders and Stroke grant 1RO1 NS44556.01; National Institute of Diabetes and Digestive and Kidney Diseases 1RO3 TW006273-01 to M.G.C.; National Institutes of Health/National Institute of Neurological Disorders and Stroke grants 1RO1 NS 42893.01, U54 NS045309-01, and 1R21 NS04729-01; the Bram and Elaine Goldsmith Chair in Gene Therapeutics to P.R.L.; the Medallions Group Chair in Gene Therapy to M.G.C.; and the Linda Tallen and David Paul Kane Annual Fellowship to M.G.C. and P.R.L. We also thank the generous funding that our institute receives from the board of governors at Cedars Sinai Medical Center. We thank the support and academic leadership of S. Melmed, and R. Katzman and D. Meyer for their superb administrative and organizational support.

REFERENCES

1. Banchereau J, Steinman RM. Dendritic cells and the control of immunity. *Nature*. 1998;392:245–252.

2. Jooss K, Chirmule N. Immunity to adenovirus and adeno-associated viral vectors: implications for gene therapy. *Gene Ther*. 2003;10:955–963.

3. Guidotti LG, Chisari FV. Noncytolytic control of viral infections by the innate and adaptive immune response. *Annu Rev Immunol*. 2001;19:65–91.

4. Alexopoulou L, Holt AC, Medzhitov R, and Flavell RA. Recognition of double-stranded RNA and activation of NF-kappaB by Toll-like receptor 3. *Nature*. 2001; 413:732–738.

5. Paludan SR, Ellermann-Eriksen S, Kruys V, Mogensen SC. Expression of TNF-alpha by herpes simplex virus–infected macrophages is regulated by a dual mechanism: transcriptional regulation by NF-kappa B and activating transcription factor 2/Jun and translational regulation through the AU-rich region of the 3' untranslated region. *J Immunol*. 2001;167:2202–2208.

6. Sato M, Suemori H, Hata N, et al. Distinct and essential roles of transcription factors IRF-3 and IRF-7 in response to viruses for IFN-alpha/beta gene induction. *Immunity*. 2000;13:539–548.

7. Dong C, Davis RJ, Flavell RA. MAP kinases in the immune response. *Annu Rev Immunol*. 2002;20:55–72.

8. Higginbotham JN, Seth P, Blaese RM, Ramsey WJ. The release of inflammatory cytokines from human peripheral blood mononuclear cells in vitro following exposure to adenovirus variants and capsid. *Hum Gene Ther*. 2002;13:129–141.

9. Malmgaard L, Salazar-Mather TP, Lewis CA, Biron CA. Promotion of alpha/beta interferon induction during in vivo viral infection through alpha/beta interferon receptor/STAT1 system-dependent and -independent pathways. *J Virol*. 2002;76: 4520–4525.

10. Schnell MA, Zhang Y, Tazelaar J, et al. Activation of innate immunity in nonhuman primates following intraportal administration of adenoviral vectors. *Mol Ther*. 2001;3:708–722.

11. Muruve DA, Barnes MJ, Stillman IE, Libermann TA. Adenoviral gene therapy leads to rapid induction of multiple chemokines and acute neutrophil-dependent hepatic injury in vivo. *Hum Gene Ther*. 1999;10:965–976.

12. Bowen GP, Borgland SL, Lam M, Libermann TA, Wong NC, Muruve DA. Adenovirus vector-induced inflammation: capsid-dependent induction of the C-C chemokine RANTES requires NF-kappa B. *Hum Gene Ther*. 2002;13:367–379.

13. Tibbles LA, Spurrell JC, Bowen GP, et al. Activation of p38 and ERK signaling during adenovirus vector cell entry lead to expression of the C-X-C chemokine IP-10. *J Virol*. 2002;76:1559–1568.

14. Borgland SL, Bowen GP, Wong NC, Libermann TA, Muruve DA. Adenovirus vector-induced expression of the C-X-C chemokine IP-10 is mediated through capsid-dependent activation of NF-kappaB. *J Virol*. 2000;74:3941–3947.

15. Zirger JM, Barcia C, Liu C, et al. Rapid upregulation of interferon-regulated and chemokine mRNAs upon injection of 108 international units, but not lower doses, of adenoviral vectors into the brain. *J Virol*. 2006;80:5655–5659.

16. Sung RS, Qin L, Bromberg JS. TNFalpha and IFNgamma induced by innate anti-adenoviral immune responses inhibit adenovirus-mediated transgene expression. *Mol Ther.* 2001;3:757–767.

17. Qin L, Ding Y, Pahud DR, Chang E, Imperiale MJ, Bromberg JS. Promoter attenuation in gene therapy: interferon-gamma and tumor necrosis factor-alpha inhibit transgene expression. *Hum Gene Ther.* 1997;8:2019–2029.

18. Peng Y, Trevejo J, Zhou J, et al. Inhibition of tumor necrosis factor alpha by an adenovirus-encoded soluble fusion protein extends transgene expression in the liver and lung. *J Virol.* 1999;73:5098–5109.

19. Worgall S, Singh R, Leopold PL, et al. Selective expansion of alveolar macrophages in vivo by adenovirus-mediated transfer of the murine granulocyte–macrophage colony-stimulating factor cDNA. *Blood.* 1999;93:655–666.

20. Worgall S, Wolff G, Falck-Pedersen E, Crystal RG. Innate immune mechanisms dominate elimination of adenoviral vectors following in vivo administration. *Hum Gene Ther.* 1997;8:37–44.

21. Lieber A, He CY, Meuse L, Himeda C, Wilson C, Kay MA. Inhibition of NF-kappaB activation in combination with bcl-2 expression allows for persistence of first-generation adenovirus vectors in the mouse liver. *J Virol.* 1998;72:9267–9277.

22. Byrnes AP, Rusby JE, Wood MJ, Charlton HM. Adenovirus gene transfer causes inflammation in the brain. *Neuroscience.* 1995;66:1015–1024.

23. Byrnes AP, Wood MJ, Charlton HM. Role of T cells in inflammation caused by adenovirus vectors in the brain. *Gene Ther.* 1996;3:644–651.

24. Kajiwara K, Byrnes AP, Charlton HM, Wood MJ, Wood KJ. Immune responses to adenoviral vectors during gene transfer in the brain. *Hum Gene Ther.* 1997;8:253–265.

25. Elkon KB, Liu CC, Gall JG, et al. Tumor necrosis factor alpha plays a central role in immune-mediated clearance of adenoviral vectors. *Proc Natl Acad Sci U S A.* 1997;94:9814–9819.

26. Byrnes AP, MacLaren RE, Charlton HM. Immunological instability of persistent adenovirus vectors in the brain: peripheral exposure to vector leads to renewed inflammation, reduced gene expression, and demyelination. *J Neurosci.* 1996;16:3045–3055.

27. Kajiwara K, Byrnes AP, Ohmoto Y, Charlton HM, Wood MJ, Wood KJ. Humoral immune responses to adenovirus vectors in the brain. *J Neuroimmunol.* 2000;103:8–15.

28. Wood MJ, Charlton HM, Wood KJ, Kajiwara K, Byrnes AP. Immune responses to adenovirus vectors in the nervous system. *Trends Neurosci.* 1996;19:497–501.

29. Zermansky AJ, Bolognani F, Stone D, et al. Towards global and long-term neurological gene therapy: unexpected transgene dependent, high-level, and widespread distribution of HSV-1 thymidine kinase throughout the CNS. *Mol Ther.* 2001;4:490–498.

30. Thomas CE, Abordo-Adesida E, Maleniak TC, Stone D, Gerdes G, Lowenstein PR. Gene transfer into rat brain using adenoviral vectors. In: Gerfen JN, McKay R, Rogawski MA, Sibley DR, Skolnick P, eds. *Current Protocols in Neuroscience.* New York: Wiley; 2000;4.23.21–24.23.40.

31. Thomas CE, Birkett D, Anozie I, Castro MG, Lowenstein PR. Acute direct adenoviral vector cytotoxicity and chronic, but not acute, inflammatory responses correlate with decreased vector-mediated transgene expression in the brain. *Mol Ther.* 2001;3:36–46.

32. Zirger J, Barcia C, Liu CS, et al. Immune system regulation of transgene expression in the brain 2: differential increase in mRNAs encoding for interferon-regulated, chemokine and T-cell genes during either innate acute or chronic systemic adaptive immune responses to first generation adenoviral vectors. *Mol Ther.* 2004;9(Suppl 1): 390–391.

33. Lowenstein PR, ed. Immune responses to viral vectors for gene therapy. *Gene Ther.* 2003;10:933–998.

34. Wood MJA, Byrnes AP, McMenamin M, et al. Immune responses to viruses: practical implications for the use of viruses as vectors for experimental and clinical gene therapy. In: Lowenstein LW, eds. *Protocols for Gene Transfer in Neuroscience.* New York: Wiley; 1996.

35. Lowenstein PR. Immunology of viral-vector-mediated gene transfer into the brain: an evolutionary and developmental perspective. *Trends Immunol.* 2002;23:23–30.

36. Fischer HG, Bonifas U, Reichmann G. Phenotype and functions of brain dendritic cells emerging during chronic infection of mice with *Toxoplasma gondii*. *J Immunol.* 2000;164:4826–4834.

37. Fischer HG, Bielinsky AK. Antigen presentation function of brain-derived dendriform cells depends on astrocyte help. *Int Immunol.* 1999;11:1265–1274.

38. Santambrogio L, Belyanskaya SL, Fischer FR, et al. Developmental plasticity of CNS microglia. *Proc Natl Acad Sci U S A.* 2001;98:6295–6300.

39. Fischer HG, Reichmann G. Brain dendritic cells and macrophages/microglia in central nervous system inflammation. *J Immunol.* 2001;166:2717–2726.

40. Matyszak MK, Perry VH. The potential role of dendritic cells in immune-mediated inflammatory diseases in the central nervous system. *Neuroscience.* 1996;74: 599–608.

41. Carson MJ, Reilly CR, Sutcliffe JG, Lo D. Disproportionate recruitment of CD8+ T cells into the central nervous system by professional antigen-presenting cells. *Am J Pathol.* 1999;154:481–494.

42. McMenamin PG. Distribution and phenotype of dendritic cells and resident tissue macrophages in the dura mater, leptomeninges, and choroid plexus of the rat brain as demonstrated in wholemount preparations. *J Comp Neurol.* 1999;405:553–562.

43. Stevenson PG, Austyn JM, Hawke S. Uncoupling of virus-induced inflammation and anti-viral immunity in the brain parenchyma. *J Gen Virol.* 2002;83:1735–1743.

44. Hart DN, Fabre JW. Demonstration and characterization of Ia-positive dendritic cells in the interstitial connective tissues of rat heart and other tissues, but not brain. *J Exp Med.* 1981;154:347–361.

45. Lowe J, MacLennan KA, Powe DG, Pound JD, Palmer JB. Microglial cells in human brain have phenotypic characteristics related to possible function as dendritic antigen presenting cells. *J Pathol.* 1989;159:143–149.

46. McMahon EJ, Bailey SL, Castenada CV, Waldner H, Miller SD. Epitope spreading initiates in the CNS in two mouse models of multiple sclerosis. *Nat Med.* 2005;11:335–339.

47. Greter M, Heppner FL, Lemos MP, et al. Dendritic cells permit immune invasion of the CNS in an animal model of multiple sclerosis. *Nat Med.* 2005;11:328–334.

48. Ponomarev ED, Shriver LP, Maresz K, Dittel BN. Microglial cell activation and proliferation precedes the onset of CNS autoimmunity. *J Neurosci Res.* 2005;81:374–389.

49. Yang Y, Nunes FA, Berencsi K, Furth EE, Gonczol E, Wilson JM. Cellular immunity to viral antigens limits E1-deleted adenoviruses for gene therapy. *Proc Natl Acad Sci U S A*. 1994;91:4407–4411.

50. Yang Y, Li Q, Ertl HC, Wilson JM. Cellular and humoral immune responses to viral antigens create barriers to lung-directed gene therapy with recombinant adenoviruses. *J Virol*. 1995;69:2004–2015.

51. Yang Y, Ertl HC, Wilson JM. MHC class I-restricted cytotoxic T lymphocytes to viral antigens destroy hepatocytes in mice infected with E1-deleted recombinant adenoviruses. *Immunity*. 1994;1:433–442.

52. Barr D, Tubb J, Ferguson D, et al. Strain related variations in adenovirally mediated transgene expression from mouse hepatocytes in vivo: comparisons between immunocompetent and immunodeficient inbred strains. *Gene Ther*. 1995;2:151–155.

53. Dai Y, Schwarz EM, Gu D, Zhang WW, Sarvetnick N, Verma IM. Cellular and humoral immune responses to adenoviral vectors containing factor IX gene: tolerization of factor IX and vector antigens allows for long-term expression. *Proc Natl Acad Sci U S A*. 1995;92:1401–1405.

54. Yang Y, Wilson JM. Clearance of adenovirus-infected hepatocytes by MHC class I-restricted CD4+ CTLs in vivo. *J Immunol*. 1995;155:2564–2570.

55. Yang Y, Trinchieri G, Wilson JM. Recombinant IL-12 prevents formation of blocking IgA antibodies to recombinant adenovirus and allows repeated gene therapy to mouse lung. *Nat Med*. 1995;1:890–893.

56. Zsengeller ZK, Wert SE, Hull WM, et al. Persistence of replication-deficient adenovirus-mediated gene transfer in lungs of immune-deficient (*nu/nu*) mice. *Hum Gene Ther*. 1995;6:457–467.

57. Kafri T, Morgan D, Krahl T, Sarvetnick N, Sherman L, Verma I. Cellular immune response to adenoviral vector infected cells does not require de novo viral gene expression: implications for gene therapy. *Proc Natl Acad Sci U S A*. 1998;95:11377–11382.

58. Stilwell JL, Samulski RJ. Role of viral vectors and virion shells in cellular gene expression. *Mol Ther*. 2004;9:337–346.

59. Stilwell JL, McCarty DM, Negishi A, Superfine R, Samulski RJ. Development and characterization of novel empty adenovirus capsids and their impact on cellular gene expression. *J Virol*. 2003;77:12881–12885.

60. Thomas CE, Storm TA, Huang Z, Kay MA. Rapid uncoating of vector genomes is the key to efficient liver transduction with pseudotyped adeno-associated virus vectors. *J Virol*. 2004;78:3110–3122.

61. Molinier-Frenkel V, Gahery-Segard H, Mehtali M, et al. Immune response to recombinant adenovirus in humans: capsid components from viral input are targets for vector-specific cytotoxic T lymphocytes. *J Virol*. 2000;74:7678–7682.

62. Abordo-Adesida E, Follenzi A, Barcia C, et al. Stability of lentiviral vector-mediated transgene expression in the brain in the presence of systemic antivector immune responses. *Hum Gene Ther*. 2005;16:741–751.

63. Peden CS, Burger C, Muzyczka N, Mandel RJ. Circulating anti-wild-type adeno-associated virus type 2 (AAV2) antibodies inhibit recombinant AAV2 (rAAV2)-mediated, but not rAAV5-mediated, gene transfer in the brain. *J Virol*. 2004;78:6344–6359.

64. Yang Y, Jooss KU, Su Q, Ertl HC, Wilson JM. Immune responses to viral antigens versus transgene product in the elimination of recombinant adenovirus-infected hepatocytes in vivo. *Gene Ther.* 1996;3:137–144.

65. Dobrzynski E, Fitzgerald JC, Cao O, Mingozzi F, Wang L, Herzog RW. Prevention of cytotoxic T lymphocyte responses to factor IX-expressing hepatocytes by gene transfer-induced regulatory T cells. *Proc Natl Acad Sci U S A.* 2006;103:4592–4597.

66. Bagley J, Iacomini J. Gene therapy progress and prospects: gene therapy in organ transplantation. *Gene Ther.* 2003;10:605–611.

67. Chen J, Hsu HC, Zajac AJ, et al. In vivo analysis of adenovirus-specific cytotoxic T lymphocyte response in mice deficient in CD28, Fas ligand, and perforin. *Hum Gene Ther.* 2006;6:669–682.

68. Chen J, Zajac AJ, McPherson SA, et al. Primary adenovirus-specific cytotoxic T lymphocyte response occurs after viral clearance and liver enzyme elevation. *Gene Ther.* 2005;12:1079–1088.

69. Zhang HG, Hsu HC, Yang PA, et al. Identification of multiple genetic loci that regulate adenovirus gene therapy. *Gene Ther.* 2004;11:4–14.

70. Zhang HG, High KA, Wu Q, et al. Genetic analysis of the antibody response to AAV2 and factor IX. *Mol Ther.* 2005;11:866–874.

71. Thomas CE, Schiedner G, Kochanek S, Castro MG, Lowenstein PR. Peripheral infection with adenovirus causes unexpected long-term brain inflammation in animals injected intracranially with first-generation, but not with high-capacity, adenovirus vectors: toward realistic long-term neurological gene therapy for chronic diseases. *Proc Natl Acad Sci U S A.* 2000;97:7482–7487.

72. Thomas CE, Schiedner G, Kochanek S, Castro MG, Lowenstein PR. Preexisting antiadenoviral immunity is not a barrier to efficient and stable transduction of the brain, mediated by novel high-capacity adenovirus vectors. *Hum Gene Ther.* 2001;12:839–846.

73. Raper SE, Chirmule N, Lee FS, et al. Fatal systemic inflammatory response syndrome in a ornithine transcarbamylase deficient patient following adenoviral gene transfer. *Mol Genet Metab.* 2003;80:148–158.

74. Manno CS, Pierce GF, Arruda VR, et al. Successful transduction of liver in hemophilia by AAV–factor IX and limitations imposed by the host immune response. *Nat Med.* 2006;12:342–347.

75. Kiang A, Hartman ZC, Liao S, et al. Fully deleted adenovirus persistently expressing GAA accomplishes long-term skelet al muscle glycogen correction in tolerant and nontolerant GSD-II mice. *Mol Ther.* 2006;13:127–134.

76. Palmer D, Ng P. Improved system for helper-dependent adenoviral vector production. *Mol Ther.* 2003;8:846–852.

77. Zaupa C, Revol-Guyot V, Epstein AL. Improved packaging system for generation of high-level noncytotoxic HSV-1 amplicon vectors using Cre-loxP site-specific recombination to delete the packaging signals of defective helper genomes. *Hum Gene Ther.* 2003;14:1049–1063.

78. Jiang H, Couto LB, Patarroyo-White S, et al. Effects of transient immunosuppression on adeno associated virus-mediated, liver-directed gene transfer in rhesus macaques and implications for human gene therapy. *Blood.* 2006;180:3321–3328.

79. Brunetti-Pierri N, Ng T, Iannitti DA, et al. Improved hepatic transduction, reduced systemic vector dissemination, and long-term transgene expression by delivering helper-dependent adenoviral vectors into the surgically isolated liver of nonhuman primates. *Hum Gene Ther.* 2006;17:391–404.

80. McCormack WM Jr, Seiler MP, Bertin TK, et al. Helper-dependent adenoviral gene therapy mediates long-term correction of the clotting defect in the canine hemophilia A model. *J Thromb Haemost.* 2006;4:1218–1225.

81. Xiong W, Goverdhana S, Sciascia SA, et al. Regulatable gutless adenovirus vectors sustain inducible transgene expression in the brain in the presence of an immune response against adenoviruses. *J Virol.* 2006;80:27–37.

15 Cancer Vaccines

RIMAS J. ORENTAS

Departments of Pediatrics, Medicine, Microbiology
and Molecular Genetics, Medical College
of Wisconsin, and the Children's Research
Institute of the Children's Hospital
of Wisconsin, Milwaukee, Wisconsin

Cancer vaccines can be produced from whole cancer cells, cancer-associated protein or peptide sequences, and adjuvants or cytokines that stimulate low-level immune activation that has already occurred (Figure 15.1). Cancer vaccines face a number of hurdles that antimicrobial vaccines do not. First, as currently employed, cancer vaccines are therapeutic and not preventive interventions. Second, a cancer vaccine must override immune tolerance mechanisms established during the initiation and growth of the malignancy. Finally, target antigen identification and presentation of those antigens in the appropriate immunostimulatory context is key to success. The identification of protective antigens has been approached from two directions. The most global is to use the entire transformed cell as a vaccine substrate. While including all possible antigens, the expression level of those antigens may be low within the cancer cell and carries the risk of autoimmunity. At the other end of the spectrum is the identification of tumor-associated proteins that provoke an immune response, or the peptide portions of those proteins presented by class I or class II major histocompatibility complex (MHC) molecules. Limitations here include a greater chance for immune evasion due to a more restricted repertoire of antigens used in the vaccine and that viral subunit vaccines are often not as good at inducing cellular immunity as whole viral vaccines. Many of the technological advances in recent years have featured unique ways of presenting both target antigens and immune stimulatory signals together. This has been accomplished most directly by viral vectors that express tumor antigens, stimulate innate immunity by the disruption of normal tissue architecture, and also encode either cytokines or immune co-stimulatory molecules.

Concepts in Genetic Medicine, Edited by Boro Dropulic and Barrie Carter
Copyright © 2008 John Wiley & Sons, Inc.

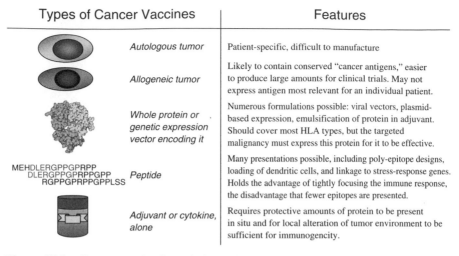

Types of Cancer Vaccines	Features
Autologous tumor	Patient-specific, difficult to manufacture
Allogeneic tumor	Likely to contain conserved "cancer antigens," easier to produce large amounts for clinical trials. May not express antigen most relevant for an individual patient.
Whole protein or genetic expression vector encoding it	Numerous formulations possible: viral vectors, plasmid-based expression, emulsification of protein in adjuvant. Should cover most HLA types, but the targeted malignancy must express this protein for it to be effective.
MEHDLERGPPGPRPP DLERGPPGPRPPGPP RGPPGPRPPGPPLSS Peptide	Many presentations possible, including poly-epitope designs, loading of dendritic cells, and linkage to stress-response genes. Holds the advantage of tightly focusing the immune response, the disadvantage that fewer epitopes are presented.
Adjuvant or cytokine, alone	Requires protective amounts of protein to be present in situ and for local alteration of tumor environment to be sufficient for immunogencity.

Figure 15.1 Cancer vaccine formulations. Cancer vaccine types are listed in hierarchical order corresponding to antigenic complexity, and features specific to each type are listed. Autologous and allogeneic tumor-based vaccines are usually engineered to express immune co-stimulatory molecules or cytokines, while whole proteins are usually expressed in the context of plasmid-based or viral vector-based vaccines. Adjuvants or cytokines administered on their own presume that some level of antigen-specific stimulation has already occurred, and merely seek to amplify these responses

IDENTIFICATION OF TUMOR ANTIGENS

The definitive identification of tumor antigens awaits both a standard mechanism to test those antigens and a validated immune assay that correlates to antitumor immunity. One of the most fruitful means of tumor antigen identification has been the screening of tumor cDNA libraries for the ability to transfer sensitivity to immune effector cells. This approach led to the identification of numerous tumor-associated antigens, such as the MAGE family and MART-1 [1,2]. Tumor antigens have also been identified by the elution of tumor-associated peptides from class I MHC and by use of patient-derived antibodies to screen tumor cDNA expression libraries (SEREX) [3–5]. Chromosomal translocations provide a direct means to map neoantigens expressed by cancer cells, as proteins transcribed from breakpoint regions serve as unique vaccine targets [6]. As the science of measuring peptide–MHC interactions has developed, so has the ability to predict specific epitopes that associate with different MHC alleles, and online algorithms are being developed to identify candidate peptide antigens (for an example, see www.syfpeithi.de). Nevertheless, the presentation of an entire protein coding sequence is preferable, as greater MHC coverage results. A novel way to purify antigenic peptides from tumor cells has been the purification of heat-shock proteins. These molecular chaperones are coated with tumor-derived peptides, are potent immune stimulators, and are currently being evaluated both in solid tumors and leukemia as vaccines [7,8].

The use of genomic tools to identify cancer-associated antigens has been complicated by the need for comparison to normal tissues. The careful stratification of tumors into higher-risk categories by gene expression analysis may prove to be how the next generation of cancer vaccine antigens are identified [9,10]. These approaches could be used to predict the best antigens to target as the malignancy progresses and expresses a more pathogenic transcriptome.

VACCINATION STRATEGIES

Vaccination is normally defined as the process of administering an antigen before the host is confronted by a challenge [11]. In the case of cancer, this remains only a hope, as vaccines are currently administered as a therapeutic modality. Cancer vaccines can take the form of proteins or peptides emulsified in adjuvant, and in some cases adjuvant has been directly introduced into the lesion. The need for an adjuvant is inversely proportional to the inflammatory response the immunizing agent is capable of provoking. If antigenic protein is expressed from plasmid DNA vectors, adjuvant is not required, as the transfected cells are transformed into efficient antigen-presenting cells (APCs). Subcellular targeting signals have been included in some plasmid vectors in order to promote better intracellular antigen processing [12]. The targets of plasmid-based or viral vectors can be dendritic cells infected ex vivo and then administered to the patient, or skin or muscle cells infected or transfected directly in vivo. When whole tumor cells are used as vaccines, usually upon genetic modification to express immunostimulatory proteins, they can be derived from a patient's own tumor (an autologous cell-based vaccine) or a single vaccine cell line can be administered to all patients with the same disease type (an allogeneic cell-based vaccine). Bacteria have also been engineered to express tumor-associated proteins and developed as vaccines [13,14]. The strong inflammatory response to the bacterial cell wall structures precludes the need for adjuvant.

Proteins or peptides emulsified in adjuvant are analogous to current subunit vaccines for infectious agents. The Th2-biased immune response to antigens emulsified in alum, the current clinic standard, and the granulomatous immune response induced by complete Freund's adjuvant has made the development of new adjuvants a necessity for cancer vaccines [15,16]. Due to the side effects of mineral oil–based adjuvants, more metabolizable products such as nonionic block copolymers have come into use and have been shown to influence the antibody isotypes produced. SAF-1 [threonyl-MDP (muramyl dipeptide) in a squalene–pluronic polymer emulsion] has been used to induce an immune response to B-cell lymphoma idiotype-KLH conjugates, and Montanide ISA 51 (mannide monooleate and mineral oil) is being used in a number of trials, including immunization with melanoma-specific peptides [17,18]. The precise signals required to steer an immune response toward a Th1-like response remains an active field of research, and numerous adjuvant additives are being evaluated. A partial list would include the lipid A component of lipopolysaccharide and MDP derivates to stimulate APCs, CpG oligonucleotides to activate Toll-like receptors, cell–cell interaction facilitators such as lysoecitin and Quil A, the focusing of antigen to leukocytes expressing Fc receptors by using zymosan or endotoxin, the inclusion of polyclonal T-cell activators such as tuberculin purified protein derivative, the use of detergents such as saponin to promote cross-presentation (presentation of endocytosed antigen, normally class II–associated, to the class I pathway), and the conjugation or engineering of proteins to contain epitopes that bind to molecules on the surface of APCs [12,19,20].

Maximization of vaccine effectiveness may also require focusing the immune response to the specific tissue where it is needed. For example, a vaccine known to induce expression of the $\alpha 4\beta 7$ integrin would target cells to the intestinal lamina propria, while $\alpha E\beta 7$ would cause cells to migrate deeper into intestinal epithelium and be retained by E-cadherin expressed on epithelial cells [21–24]. This need to recruit immune effectors to the appropriate tissue or mucosal surface may explain why intratumoral vaccination is superior to vaccination at a distant site [25].

CANCER VACCINES: INVESTIGATIONAL TOOLS BEING TRANSLATED TO CLINICAL REALITY

Positive clinical results with cancer vaccines have been modest. However, our view of vaccine trial outcomes may be skewed by the expectation of large effects on morbidity and mortality. As cancer vaccination remains a translational research enterprise, a more appropriate model may be an iterative view of vaccine trials wherein specific immune hypotheses are tested, and promising results followed with a restated or refined hypothesis that brings us a step closer to successful therapeutic treatment [26]. In this final section we highlight cancer vaccine approaches currently under clinical investigation. This is not a complete survey, but a look forward through the lens of some of the more effective or novel trials being pursued to date. A breakdown of vaccine trials by disease type is shown in Table 15.1.

Targeting Carcinomas

A resurgence of interest in cancer vaccines began approximately a decade ago when the retroviral transduction of autologous melanoma and renal carcinomas with a GM-CSF expression vector was proved feasible and safe in patients [27,28]. Although delayed-type hypersensitivity to the vaccine was noted, little clinical effect resulted. A newer generation of recombinant viral vaccines used to treat carcinoma is exemplified by the TRICOM system, wherein the immune system is primed by infection with a recombinant-attenuated vaccinia virus expressing the carcinoembryonic antigen (CEA) and a triad of the immune co-stimulatory molecules: CD80, CD54, and CD58. The immune response is subsequently boosted by treatment with nonreplicating fowlpox expressing the same set of transgenes [25]. The latest results in animal systems with TRICOM

TABLE 15.1   Current Cancer Vaccine Trials[a]

Cancer Type	Vaccine	Investigators
Bladder	Fowlpox TRICOM +/− GM-CSF	R. Weiss, University of Medicine and Dentistry, Newark, NJ
	NY-ESO-1 peptide vaccine, + BCG, +/− M-CSF	D. Bajorin and H. Herr, Memorial Sloan–Kettering Cancer Center, NY, NY
Breast	Allogeneic breast carcinoma cell lines, transduced to express the murine α (1,3)-galactosyl transferase antigen	C. Link, Jr., John Stoddard Cancer Center, Des Moines, IA
	Allogeneic breast cancer cell line producing GM-CSF in the context of immunodepletion	L. Emens, Johns Hopkins University
	Dendritic cells loaded with Her-2/neu peptide +/− chemotherapy or antibody therapy	J. Serody, University of North Carolina
	Vaccinia-MUC1-TRICOM	J. P. Elder, Dana Farber Cancer Institute
	Vaccinia/fowlpox-CEA-TRICOM + GM-CSF, followed by vaccination in the context of immunodepletion	C. Kasten-Sportes, National Cancer Institute, NIH
Colon/rectal	Excised tumor, IFNγ treated, given a vaccine + GM-CSF + immunodepletion	C. Wiseman, St. Vincent, Los Angeles, CA
	Vaccinia/fowlpox-CEA/MUC-1/ TRICOM + dendritic cells + GM-CSF	M. Morse, Duke University, Durham, NC
	Survivin peptides in adjuvant	J. Becker, Julius Maximillans University, Würzburg, Germany
Kidney (renal)	Excised tumor, IFNγ treated + dendritic cells	R. Dillman, Hoag Cancer Center, Newport Beach, CA
	Dendritic cells + autologous tumor cell lysate, + IL-2, + IFNα	M. Ernstoff, Norris Cotton Cancer Center, Lebanon, NH
	Peptides from fibroblast growth factor-5 in adjuvant	J. C.-Y. Yang, National Cancer Institute, NIH
Leukemia	Autologous CLL, + adenoviral IL-2 vector, + CD40L	M. Brenner, Baylor University, Waco, TX
	PR1 peptide in adjuvant	M. Qazilbash, M.D. Anderson Cancer Center

(continued overleaf)

TABLE 15.1   (*continued*)

Cancer Type	Vaccine	Investigators
	Autologous dendritic cells and leukemia cell fusion	A. Lerner, Cancer Research Center, Boston Medical Center
Lung	HSPPC-96, autologous heat-shock protein from autologous tumor (unique peptide signature)	Antigenics, Inc.
	Autologous tumor + adenoviral GM-CSF vector +/ − immunodepletion	Cell Genesys, Inc.
	Recombinant DNA for tumor protein (pVAX/L523S), followed by L523S adenovirus	Corixa, Inc.
Melanoma	gp100 protein/peptide, + adjuvant, + IL-2, w/IL-12, or w/IL-7	S. Rosenberg, National Cancer Institute; T. Gajewski, University of Chicago
	Peptides from tyrosinase, MART-1, and gp100 + GM-CSF	D. Lawson, ECOG; K. Margolin, SWOG
	Multipeptide vaccine + adjuvant (Montanide ISA-51) + CpG oligos	J. Weber, University of Southern California
Non-Hodgkin's lymphoma	Idiotype-KLH conjugate + GM-CSF	J. Gutheil, Favrille, Inc.
	Autologous tumor + GM-CSF/CD40L-expressing cell line + IL-2	S. Dessureault, H. Lee Moffitt Cancer Center
Pancreatic	Allogeneic line secreting GM-CSF	D. Laheru, Johns Hopkins University
	CEA peptide in adjuvant + GM-CSF	R. Whitehead, UTMB, Galveston, TX
Prostate	Vaccinia/fowlpox-PSA-TRICOM +/ − GM-CSF, or fowlpox GM-CSF	P. Arlen, National Cancer Institute, NIH
	PSA peptide in adjuvant	R. Alexander, University of Maryland
	EGFRvIII peptide + GM-CSF (or KLH, as adjuvant)	R. Montgomery, SWOG
Skin (nonmelanoma)	Imiquimod as topical adjuvant	Numerous

[a] All common cancers are listed (predicted incidence rate > 25,000 cases in 2005) with the exception of endometrial cancer, for which no trials are listed by the NIH. All data in this table are publicly available, www.cancer.gov. Vaccines chosen for this list do not represent all or even the best vaccine trial for each disease type; rather, trials were chosen to illustrate the current range of vaccine options available.

demonstrate that depletion of T-regulatory cells, inclusion of adjuvant therapy (external beam irradiation), and the timing and site of administration (intratumoral vs. subcutaneous) all affect outcomes in tumor-bearing animals [29].

A small percentage of *bladder cancer* patients initially present with superficial disease, termed carcinoma in situ (CIS). For CIS, treatment of choice is BCG (bacille Calmette-Guérin), as long-term durable remissions can be attained with this "adjuvant" treatment alone [30]. Although BCG has been tried in other settings with little success, bladder CIS is a powerful example of how a single vaccine-like treatment can reverse a neoplastic process.

Clinical trials with an allogeneic *breast cancer* cell line altered with a single co-stimulatory molecule were not effective. For example, a group led by Walter Urba developed a Her-2/*neu*+ allogeneic breast cancer cell line that expressed HLA-A2, CD54, CD58, and was permanently transfected with a CD80 plasmid-based expression vector. Patients with stage IV breast cancer received irradiated gene-modified tumor cells and GM-CSF or BCG. Prolonged disease stabilization was observed for four patients, but no objective tumor regression was seen [31]. Although T cells from some patients demonstrated production of intracellular cytokine (IFN-γ) upon stimulation with the vaccine cell line, these laboratory results could not be correlated to a clinical response. The recent availability of Her-2/*neu* transgenic mice has allowed rapid evaluation of cancer vaccine protocols in a tumor bearing model where the immune system is already tolerized by the presence of tumor. Studies by Quaglino et al. demonstrate that vaccination with a plasmid-based vector encoding a portion of Her-2/*neu* initiated at the onset of carcinoma in situ slightly delayed but could not stop tumor development. However, long-term prevention/cure was seen when the plasmids were electroporated intramuscularly (IM) every 10 weeks [32]. Positive correlates of successful vaccination included the induction of tumor-specific antibody and IFNγ-producing T cells. In this mouse model, B-cell responses were important and may reflect the biology of the cancer being studied. Human clinical trials with antibody to Her-2/*neu* (Herceptin) have shown clinical benefit. Thus, any tumor that is dependent on external growth signals may be inhibited by antibody production against specific cell-surface receptors.

In *colorectal carcinoma*, the tumor-associated antigen Ep-CAM (epithelial cell adhesion molecule) has been targeted by numerous vaccine strategies. Ep-CAM is an important vaccine target, as it is also expressed on a large number of other epithelial malignancies. In a recent study, anti-idiotypic antibody was used as the immunogen to induce an anti-Ep-CAM immune response in combination with GM-CSF, all administered as IM injections [33]. Although cellular and humoral immune responses were noted, patients still mounted a stronger response to the Ep-CAM protein itself. In small cell *lung cancer*, long-chain polysialic acid (polySA) has been used as an immunogen upon conjugation with KLH and administered in the saponin-based adjuvant QS-21 [34]. In patients who had successfully completed initial therapy, it was found that N-propionylation was required to overcome immune tolerance to polySA, and priopionylated polySA will be included in future polyvalent vaccine against small cell lung carcinoma that will also include GM2, fucosylated GM1, and Globo H [34]. Another cancer-specific saccharide being used as a vaccine target is the Thomasen–Friedenreich (TF) antigen, a core disaccharide of O-glycosylated proteins that is expressed in normal development, epithelial cells, and overexpressed on cancer cells. The TF antigen, linked to KLH and administered in QS-21, generated high-titer antibodies in *prostate cancer* patients [35]. Although a change in the log PSA (prostate-specific antigen over time) slopes was observed in a number of patients, the trial was too short to make outcomes conclusions. In all these malignancies, protein-based vaccine trials continue to be carried out. For example, it was recently demonstrated in prostate cancer patients who have biochemically relapsed that a regimen that features priming vaccinaton with a vaccina virus vector encoding PSA and CD80, followed by monthly boosts with fowlpox-PSA, given with local GM-CSF and low-dose systemic IL-2, generates a large increase in PSA-specific T cells [36]. These initial results are promising, but long-term outcomes have yet to be determined. In *pancreatic cancer*, the first trial with an alloegenic vaccine derived from a patient adenocarcinoma stably transfected to produce GM-CSF was published in 2001. Three of 14 patients appeared to have some benefit, surviving over two years after diagnosis [37]. *Renal carcinoma* also continues to be evaluated for responsiveness to autologous GM-CSF-transduced cell-based vaccines [38]. For ErbB2-positive cancer, which includes breast and renal carcinoma, a novel reagent, a chimeric CTLA-4-ErbB2 fusion protein, has been developed [19]. This reagent delivers the ErbB2 protein directly to APC, which express ligands for CTLA-4.

Hematologic Malignancies

The same principles of cancer vaccine production for solid tumors apply to hematologic malignancies. Already mentioned has been use of the chromosomal breakpoint encoded *bcr-abl* oncogene in CML as a vaccine target [6,39]. An overexpressed normal protein found in myeloid cells, PR1, has also been proposed as a vaccine target in CML [40]. Idiotype vaccines feature the presentation of the unique V-D-J rearranged sequences expressed by tumors of B- or T-cell origin. Extensive work has been done by Ron Levy's group on B-cell lymphoma, as mentioned above, and this model for vaccine development has extended to other hematologic malignancies, such as mutiple meyeloma, and has been used in the context of bone marrow transplantation to induce antitumor immunity in graft recipients [41].

With the continued progress in the identification of important premalignant biomarkers, cancer vaccines may soon hit their stride and be required to do only that which we require of antiviral vaccines: namely, prevent the onset of disease. Earlier targeting of antigens combined with new strategies to overcome the strong immune control mediated by T-regulatory cells will certainly play a role in the development of the next generation of more effective cancer vaccines [42,43].

REFERENCES

1. Van Pel A, van der Bruggen P, Coulie PG, et al. Genes coding for tumor antigens recognized by cytolytic T lymphocytes. *Immunol Rev.* 1995;145:229.

2. Heidecker L, Brasseur F, Probst-Kepper M, Boon T, Boon T, Van den Eynde BJ. Cytolytic T lymphocytes raised against a human bladder carcinoma recognize an antigen encoded by gene MAGE-A12. *J Immunol.* 2000;164:6041.

3. Hogan KT, Sutton JN, Chu KU, et al. Use of selected reaction monitoring mass spectrometry for the detection of specific MHC class I peptide antigens on A3 supertype family members. *Cancer Immunol Immunother.* 2005;54:359–371.

4. Scanlan MJ, Welt S, Gordon CM, et al. Cancer-related serological recognition of human colon cancer: identification of potential diagnostic and immunotherapeutic targets. *Cancer Res.* 2002;62:4041–4047.

5. Chen Y-T, Scanlan MJ, Sahin U, et al. A testicular antigen aberrantly expressed in human cancers detected by autologous antibody screening. *Proc Natl Acad Sci U S A.* 1997;94:1914–1918.

6. Cathcart K, Pinilla-Ibarz J, Korontsvit T, et al. A multivalent *bcr-abl* fusion peptide vaccination trial in patients with chronic myeloid leukemia. *Blood.* 2004;103(3):1037–1041.

7. Li Z, Qiao Y, Laska EJ, et al. Combination of imatinib mesylate with autologous leukocyte-derived heat shock protein and chronic myelogenous leukemia. *Clin Cancer Res.* 2005;11(12):4460–4468.

8. Belli F, Testori A, Rivoltini L, et al. Vaccination of metastatic melanoma patients with autologous tumor-derived heat shock protein gp96-peptide complexes: clinical and immunologic findings. *J Clin Oncol.* 2002;20(20):4169–4180.

9. Chen Y-T, Scanlan MJ, Vendetti CA, et al. Identification of cancer/testis-antigen genes by massively parallel signature sequencing. *Proc Natl Acad Sci U S A.* 2005;102(22):7940–7945.

10. Chen Q-R, Bilke S, Khan J. High-resolution cDNA microarray-based comparative genomic hybridization analysis in neuroblastoma. *Cancer Lett.* 2005;228:71–81.

11. Ada G, Ramsay A. Past achievements and future needs. In: *Vaccines, Vaccination and the Immune Response.* Philadelphia, PA: Lippincott-Raven; 1997:2–45.

12. Wu T-C, Guarnieri FG, Staveley-O'Carroll K, et al. Engineering an intracellular pathway for major histocompatibility complex class II presentation of antigens. *Proc Natl Acad Sci U S A.* 1995;92:11671–11675.

13. Hussain SF, Paterson Y. What is needed for effective antitumor immunotherapy? Lessons learned using *Listeria monocytogenes* as a live vector for HPV-associated tumors. *Cancer Immunol Immunother.* 2005;54:577–586.

14. Hussain SF, Paterson Y. CD4+CD25+regulatory T cells that secrete TGF-beta and IL-10 are preferentially induced by a vaccine vector. *J Immunother.* 2004;27:339–346.

15. Bomford R. Relative adjuvant efficacy of $Al(OH)_3$ and saponin is related to the immunogenicity of the antigen. *Int Arch Allergy Appl Immunol.* 1984;75:280–281.

16. Freund J, Casals J, Hosmer EP. Sensitization and antibody formation after injection of tubercle bacilli and paraffin oil. *Proc Soc Exp Biol and Med.* 1937;37(3):509–513.

17. Timmerman JM, Czerwinski DK, Davis TA, et al. Idiotype-pulsed dendritic cell vaccination for B-cell lymphoma: clinical and immune responses in 35 patients. *Blood*. 2002;99:1517–1526.

18. Sanderson K, Scotland R, Lee P, et al. Autoimmunity in a phase I trial of a fully human anti-cytotoxic T-lymphocyte antigen-4 monoclonal antibody with multiple melanoma peptides and Montanide ISA 51 for patients with resected stages III and IV melanoma. *J Clin Oncol.* 2005;23(4):741–750.

19. Rohrbach F, Weth R, Kursar M, Sloots A, Mittrucker H-W, Wels WS. Targeted delivery of the ErbB2/HER2 tumor antigen to professional APCs results in effective antitumor immunity. *J Immunol.* 2005;174:5481–5489.

20. Schnurr M, Chen Q, Shin A, et al. Tumor antigen processing and presentation depend critically on dendritic cell type and the mode of antigen delivery. *Blood*. 2005;105:2465–2472.

21. Sato S, Thorlacius H, Johnston B, et al. Role of CXCR6 in recruitment of activated CD8+lymphocytes to inflamed liver. *J Immunology*. 2005;174:277–283.

22. Chang C-J, Tai K-F, Roffler S, Hwang L-H. The immunization site of cytokine-secreting tumor cell vaccines influences the trafficking of tumor-specific T lymphocytes and antitumor efficacy against regional tumors. *J Immunol.* 2004;173:6025–60232.

23. Teraki Y, Picker LJ. Independent regulation of cutaneous lymphocyte-associated antigen expression and cytokine synthesis during human CD4+memory T cell differentiation. *J Immunol.* 1997;159:6018–6029.

24. Cepek KL, Shaw SK, Parker CM, et al. Adhesion between epithelial cells and T lymphocytes mediated by E-cadherin and the alpha-E beta-7 integrin. *Nature*. 1994;372:190–193.

25. Kudo-Saito C, Schlom J, Hodge JW. Intratumoral vaccination and diversified subcutaneous/intratumoral vaccination with recombinant poxviruses encoding a tumor antigen and multiple costimulatory molecules. *Clin Cancer Res.* 2004;10:1090–1099.

26. Piantadosi S. Translational clinical trials: an entropy-based approach to sample size. *Clin Trials*. 2005;2:182–192.

27. Simons JW, Jaffee EM, Weber CE, et al. Bioactivity of autologous irradiated renal cell carcinoma vaccines generated by ex vivo granulocyte–macrophage colony-stimulating factor gene transfer. *Cancer Res* 1997;57:1537.

28. Soiffer RJ, Lynch T, Mihm M, et al. Vaccination with irradiated autologous melanoma cells engineered to secrete human granulocyte–macrophage colony-stimulating factor generates potent antitumor immunity in patients with metastatic melanoma. *Proc Natl Acad Sci U S A.* 1998;95:13141–13146.

29. Kudo-Saito C, Schlom J, Camphausen K, Coleman CN, Hodge JW. The requirement of multimodal therapy (vaccine, local tumor radiation, and reduction of suppressor cells) to eliminate established tumors. *Clin Cancer Res.* 2005;11(12):4533–4544.

30. Sylvester RJ, van der Meijden APM, Witjes JA, Kurth K. Bacillus Calmette-Guerin versus chemotherapy for the intravesical treatment of patients with carcinoma in situ of the bladder: a meta-analysis of the published results of randomized clinical trials. *J Urol.* 2005;174:86–92.

31. Dols A, Smith JW, Meijer SL, et al. Vaccination of women with metastatic breast cancer, using a costimulatory gene (CD80)-modified, HLA-A2 matched, allogeneic, breast cancer cell line: clinical and immunological results. *Hum Gene Ther.* 2003;14:1117–1123.

32. Quaglino E, Rolla S, Iezzi M, et al. Concordant morphological and gene expression data show that a vaccine halts *HER-2/neu* preneoplastic lesions. *J Clin Invest.* 2004;113(5):709.

33. Mosolits S, Markovic K, Frodin J-E, et al. Vaccination with Ep-CAM protein or anti-idiotypic antibody induces Th1-biased response against MHC class I- and II-restricted Ep-CAM epitopes in colorectal carcinoma patients. *Clin Cancer Res.* 2004;10:5391–5402.

34. Krug LM, Ragupathi G, Ng KK, et al. Vaccination of small cell lung cancer patients with polysialic acid or N-propionylated polysialic acid conjugated to keyhole limpet hemocyanin. *Clin Cancer Res.* 2004;10:916–923.

35. Slovin SF, Ragupathi G, Musselli C, et al. Thomasen-Friedenreich (TF) antigen as a target for prostate cancer vaccine: clinical trial results with TF cluster (c)-KLH plus QS21 conjugate vaccine in patients with biochemically relapsed prostate cancer. *Cancer Immunol Immunother.* 2005;54:694–702.

36. Gulley JL, Arlen PM, Bastian A, et al. Combining a recombinant cancer vaccine with standard definitive radiotherapy in patients with localized prostate cancer. *Clin Cancer Res.* 2005;11(9):3353–3362.

37. Jaffee E, Hruban RH, Bierdrzycki B, et al. Novel allogeneic granulocyte–macrophage colony-stimulating factor-secreting tumor vaccine for pancreatic cancer: a phase I trial of safety and immune activation. *J Clin Oncol.* 2001;19:145–156.

38. Zhou X, Jun DY, Thomas AM, et al. Diverse CD8+ T-cell responses to renal cell carcinoma antigens in patients treated with an autologous granulocyte–macrophage colony-stimulating factor gene-transduced renal tumor cell vaccine. *Cancer Res.* 2005;65(3):1079–1088.

39. Mannering SI, McKenzie JL, Fearnley DB, Hart DNJ. HLA-DR1-restricted *bcr-abl* (*b3a2*)-specific CD4+ T lymphocytes respond to dendritic cells exposed to b3a2 containing cell lysates. *Blood.* 1997;90(1):290.

40. Molldrem JJ, Lee PP, Wang C, et al. Evidence the specific T lymphocytes may participate in the elimination of chronic myelogenous leukemia. *Nat Med.* 2000;6(8):1018.

41. Neelapu SS, Munshi NC, Jagannath S, et al. Tumor antigen immunization of sibling stem cell transplant donors in multiple myeloma. *Bone Marrow Transpl.* 2005;36:315–323.

42. Willimsky G, Blankenstein T. Sporadic immunogenic tumors avoid destruction by inducing T-cell tolerance. *Nature.* 2005;437:141–146.

43. Peng G, Guo Z, Kiniwa Y, et al. Toll-like receptor 8-mediated reversal of CD4+ regulatory T cell function. *Science* 2005;309:1380–1384.

16 Genetically Modified T Cells for Human Gene Therapy

JAMES L. RILEY and CARL H. JUNE
Abramson Family Cancer Research Institute, and
Department of Pathology and Laboratory Medicine,
School of Medicine, University of Pennsylvania,
Philadelphia, Pennsylvania

The idea that passive transfer of primed lymphocytes to generate immunity in the recipient of this transfer is a relatively old idea in the history of immunology. First proposed in 1954 by Billingham, Brent, and Medewar, who coined the term *adoptive immunity* (Billingham et al., 1954), numerous animal studies have demonstrated the effectiveness of this adoptive transfer of immunity toward cancer and infectious disease (for recent reviews, see June, 2005; Moss and Rickinson, 2005). Immunity has remarkable specificity toward its targets, and specificity can be controlled through strategies such as in vivo (Li et al., 1999) and ex vivo (Shu et al., 1986; Maus et al., 2002) priming and genetic engineering (Gross et al., 1989; Sadelain et al., 2003). Moreover, it has the potential to induce long-standing effects via the establishment of immunologic memory. However, despite many promising results from rodent studies with tumors and infections (reviewed in Melief, 1992; Riddell and Greenberg, 1995), there are no U.S. Food and Drug Administration (FDA)–approved forms of adoptive immunotherapy. T cells are particularly attractive targets for gene therapy because their cell cycle is well understood and they are long-lived cells. Below we review recent studies testing the safety and feasibility of adoptive transfer therapy with genetically engineered T cells.

RELATIVE SAFETY OF T CELLS AND HEMATOPOIETIC STEM CELLS

Over the past decade, the leading vectors used for human gene transfer research were derived from adenoviruses and gammaretroviruses. However, for

Concepts in Genetic Medicine, Edited by Boro Dropulic and Barrie Carter
Copyright © 2008 John Wiley & Sons, Inc.

T-cell-based therapies, murine oncoretrovirus-derived vectors have been more useful for long-term gene expression because of their ability to integrate into host DNA (Uchida et al., 1986). The use of this class of vector is somewhat cumbersome because it requires cell replication for integration. Lentivirus-derived vectors are more efficient in gene transfer because of their ability to integrate into nondividing cells (Naldini et al., 1996; Amado and Chen, 1999) and because under some circumstances they are less susceptible to silencing (Lois, et al., 2002; Pfeifer et al., 2002).

HIV-1 vectors expressing anti-HIV-1 genes have been described by several laboratories (Dropulic et al., 1996; Mautino and Morgan, 2002; Schroers et al., 2002; Qin et al., 2003). The advantages of using HIV-1-based vectors over other vector types are (1) that they can transduce primary nondividing CD4 T cells with high efficiency in less demanding cell culture conditions as opposed to with murine oncoretroviral vectors, and (2) that HIV has been studied extensively over the past 20 years, so another advantage of using HIV as a gene therapy vector is the wealth of knowledge available regarding its replication cycle and structure. The most important questions currently facing the field are whether lentiviral vectors are safe and under what conditions they are safe. Certainly, murine retrovirus vectors have been used in hundreds of persons and are generally safe. However, these vectors have been shown to induce lymphoma in animals when contaminated with replication competent virus, principally by means of insertional mutagenesis (Donahue et al., 1992); and T cell leukemia or clonal T-cell proliferation has complicated retrovirus CD34 cell gene therapy in 3 of 11 children treated for X-linked severe combined immunodeficiency disease [X-linked severe combined immunodeficiency disease SCID; Hacein-Bey-Abina et al., 2003]. Results from a second X-SCID trial using CD34 cells transduced with a GALV-pseudotyped gammaretrovirus in four patients were recently reported, and no adverse events were observed in follow-up of up to 29 months (Gaspar et al., 2004). The mechanism leading to T-cell leukemia in X-SCID appears to be the unfortunate "perfect storm" where the γc transgene contributes either additively or synergistically to LMO2-associated insertional mutagenesis leukemogenesis (Dave et al., 2004). At present, no malignancies have been reported in humans following adoptive transfer of genetically engineered T cells. Whether T cells continue to show a favorable safety profile over hematopoietic stem cells requires more experimentation and further observation.

Frederic Bushman and colleagues have shown that lentivirus vectors integrate into sites of active gene transcription (Mitchell et al., 2004; Schroder et al., 2002); however, the meaning of this in terms of determining risk for oncogenesis is unknown. T-cell leukemia is not a known risk factor in patients with HIV infection; and the increased rate of lymphoma in these patients is usually of B-cell origin and appears to be due more to immunodeficiency and infections with transforming herpesviruses than to HIV-1 integration events (Gates and Kaplan, 2003). Yet, provirus integration is known to occur in HIV-1-infected persons at rates that vary with progression of infection; and for advanced disease, provirus integration is seen in 1 per 700 to 3500 peripheral blood lymphoctyes

(Harper et al., 1986; Simmonds et al., 1990). Thus, considering the long, high, and continuous exposure to HIV-1 replication in patients, there is a lack of significant clinical problems due to insertional mutagenesis per se, suggesting that lentivirus vectors may have a superior safety profile to gammaretroviruses in this regard.

ENGINEERED VIRUSES FOR GENETIC MODIFICATION OF T CELLS FOR CANCER GENE THERAPY

Genetic modification of T cells ex vivo to engineer improved antitumor efficacy is an attractive strategy for many settings. Unlike hematopoietic stem cells, currently available vectors provide high-level expression of transgenes in T cells. The first use in humans of genetically modified T cells was to demonstrate that adoptively transferred cells could persist in the host and traffic to tumor, albeit with low efficiency (Rosenberg et al., 1990). A principal limitation of immunotherapy for some tumors is that the tumors are poorly antigenic, in that no T cells are available that have high avidity receptors for tumor-specific antigens, or that no T cells remain in the patient after chemotherapy that have the desired specificity. To address this problem, some clinical trials now in progress attempt to endow T cells with novel receptor constructs by introduction of *T bodies*, chimeric receptors that have antibody based external receptor structures and cytosolic domains that encode signal transduction modules of the T-cell receptor(TCR) (Eshhar et al., 1996). These constructs can function to retarget T cells in vitro in a major histocompatibity complex (MHC)-unrestricted manner. The major issues with the approach currently involve improved receptor design and the immunogenicity of the T-body construct. T cells are also being transduced to express natural TCR α,β heterodimers of known specificity and avidity for tumor antigens (Kessels et al., 2005; Xue et al., 2005). After transduction with these engineered TCRs, the T cells are rendered bispecific, in that the T cell retains its native antigenic specificity and acquires the new specificity of the retargeted TCR. Assuming that mispairing does not generate novel specificities that are harmful, this approach will be valuable to determine to what extent antitumor efficacy has been limited by insufficient T-cell numbers. However, this approach will probably be of limited general value for widespread clinical use because each TCR will be specific for a given MHC allele, such that each vector would be patient specific.

A major limitation to adoptive transfer of cytotoxic T cells (CTLs) is that they have short–term persistence in the host in the absence of antigen-specific T-helper cells. Greenberg and co-workers have transduced human CTLs with chimeric GM-CSF/IL-2 receptors that deliver an IL-2 signal on binding GM-CSF. Stimulation of the CTLs with antigen caused GM-CSF secretion and resulted in an autocrine growth loop such that the CTL clones proliferated in the absence of exogenous cytokines. This type of genetic modification has potential for increasing the circulating half-life and, by extension, the efficacy of ex vivo–expanded CTLs. A related strategy to rejuvenate T-cell function is to engineer T cells to ectopically express CD28 or the catalytic subunit of telomerase (Hooijberg et al., 2000; Topp, et al., 2003). To date, there is limited clinical experience with engineered T cells; however, in certain instances they have been shown to persist in lymphopenic humans after adoptive transfer for years (Blaese et al., 1995; Mitsuyasu et al., 2000).

Severe and potentially lethal graft versus host disease (GVHD) represents a frequent complication of allogeneic stem cell transplantation and adoptive transfer of allogeneic lymphocytes (Sullivan et al., 1989; Kolb et al., 1995). The promising results with allogeneic donor lymphocyte infusions (DLIs; Kolb et al., 1995; Lokhorst et al., 2004) have created increased interest in developing T cells with an inducible suicide phenotype. Expression of herpes simplex virus thymidine kinase (HSV TK) in T cells provides a means of ablating transduced T cells in vivo by the administration of acyclovir or ganciclovir (Helene et al., 1997). Using this strategy, Bordignon and colleagues infused donor lymphocytes into 12 patients who, after receiving allogeneic bone-marrow transplants, had suffered complications such as cancer relapse or virus-induced lymphomas (Bonini et al., 1997). The lymphocytes survived for up to a year, and complete or partial tumor remissions in five of the eight patients were achieved. Tumor regressions coincided with the onset of GVHD, and in most cases, the GVHD was abrogated when ganciclovir was given. Thus, GVHD associated with the therapeutic infusion of donor lymphocytes after allogeneic marrow transplantation could be controlled efficiently by these novel suicide gene strategies in allogeneic lymphocytes. However, subsequent studies have indicated problems with this approach, in that the HSV TK gene confers immunogenicity to the transfused cells in some patients, leading to impaired survival and the inability to re-treat a patient with DLI should the tumor recur. Future experiments will be required to develop vectors that are less immunogenic and able to confer even higher ganciclovir sensitivity to transduced human lymphocytes. Recently, investigators have developed suicide systems comprised of fusion proteins containing a fas or caspase death domain and a modified FKBP (Clackson et al., 1998; Straathof et al., 2003). These approaches have the advantage that the suicide switches are expected to be non-immunogenic. T cells expressing these modified chimeric proteins are induced to undergo apoptosis when exposed to a drug that dimerizes the modified FKBP (Berger et al., 2004; Thomis, et al., 2001). Finally, the advent of lentiviral vectors has greatly increased the efficiency of T-cell engineering (Cavalieri et al., 2003; Sadelain et al., 2003), so that at present, basic advances in cell culture technology and vector engineering are now in hand to permit meaningful clinical development of genetically engineered T cells so that this promising approach is poised to become a clinical reality.

T-CELL GENE THERAPY FOR HIV INFECTION

Gene transfer was originally proposed as a means of "intracellular immunization" for bolstering host resistance (Baltimore, 1988) and has been suggested as an alternative to antiretroviral drug regimes (Sarver and Rossi, 1993; Dropulic and

Jeang, 1994; Veres et al., 1998; Lori et al., 2002; Mautino and Morgan, 2002) Thus, if it is true that successful long-term suppression of disease progression will require nearly complete inhibition of virus replication, an efficient method of cell transfer therapy coupled with efficient gene transfer could supplement or replace conventional HIV antiviral chemotherapy (Bridges and Sarver, 1995). A number of different genetic vectors and accompanying genetic antiviral payloads are being studied to combat HIV-1, and these can be categorized into two types: protein-based and RNA-based strategies. Use of a therapeutic gene whose product is RNA rather than protein has an advantage, in that the gene delivered is not lost via an immune response (Riddell et al., 1996).

Transdominant Rev Trial

T cells have been the target of numerous immunogene therapy approaches because they (1) are major effectors of the immune system and (2) have the potential to engraft and survive in the host for extended periods of time provided that they are expanded ex vivo using optimal conditions. Nabel and colleagues (Ranga et al., 1998) tested the utility of an inhibitory Rev protein, Rev M10. Autologous cells separately transfected with either Rev M10 or a control protein were returned to each patient, and toxicity, gene expression, and survival of genetically modified cells were assessed. The engraftment of the gene-marked cells was poor, due to the low transduction efficiency and the CD3/IL-2 cell culture process. However, the cells that expressed Rev M10 were more resistant to HIV infection than those with Delta Rev M10 in vitro.

Infusions of CD4ζ-Modified T Cells

CD4ζ is a genetically engineered MHC-unrestricted receptor composed of the ζ subunit of the CD3 T-cell receptor, the cytoplasmic domain involved in signal transduction, fused to the transmembrane and extracellular domains of human CD4, which targets HIV *env* expressed on the surface of infected cells (Romeo and Seed, 1991). The MHC-unrestricted nature of this chimeric receptor allows for HIV-specific targeting of both CD4 + and CD8 + T cells. Upon binding to HIV envelope, CD8 + T cells engineered to express the CD4ζ fusion protein proliferate and initiate effector functions such as cytokine secretion and HIV-specific cytolytic activity (Roberts et al., 1994; Yang et al., 1997). In collaboration with K. Hege at Cell Genesys and others, the survival of co-stimulated gene-marked T cells was assessed in three recently completed studies (Mitsuyasu et al., 2000; Walker et al., 2000; Deeks et al., 2002). CD4ζ-modified T cells were detected by DNA polymerase chain reaction (PCR) in the peripheral blood of all patients following infusion, and sustained mean levels of 1 to 3% of T cells were detected at many time points after infusion. In extended follow-up, CD4ζ was detected in the blood of 17 of 18 patients one year following infusion. These high levels of sustained engraftment are several orders of magnitude higher than what has previously been observed following human T-cell infusions (Rosenberg et al., 1990; Riddell et al., 1996; Woffendin et al., 1996; Brodie et al.,

1999). In the only published phase II HIV gene therapy trial, 40 patients were randomized to receive an infusion of CD4ζ-modified T cells or nontransduced co-stimulated T cells. Evidence that the T-cell gene therapy was associated with a notable reduction (p value < 0.10 or less) in the levels of blood and tissue reservoirs of HIV-infected cells was obtained in two different assays. In patients receiving the gene-modified T cells, there was a mean 0.4 log decrease from baseline in the amount of HIV cultured from circulating blood cells at six months (p value $= 0.02$) and a mean 0.5 log decrease from baseline in HIV DNA detected in rectal tissue biopsies at six months (p value $= 0.007$). These were the first positive results, albeit modest in efficacy, from a randomized gene transfer trial in HIV (Deeks et al., 2002).

Lentiviral-Engineered T Cells for HIV Infection

The first clinical grade lentiviral vector to satisfy FDA cGMP manufacturing requirements was VRX496 (Dropulic, 2001). Briefly, VRX496 is an HIV-1-based lentiviral vector carrying a 937-nucleotide splice-independent antisense sequence targeted to the HIV-1 envelope (*env*) gene as payload. In vitro studies comparing antisense payloads derived from *pol, vif, and env* genes and the 3-long terminal repeat of HIV-1 found the *env* target region to provide the most efficient inhibition of HIV-1 replication (Veres et al., 1998). VRX496 is a fully gutted vector and does not encode any complete viral proteins. The vector retains the 5-and 3-long terminal repeats, the packaging sequence, cPPT/CTS, splice donor and splice acceptor, and rev response element (RRE). VRX496-transduced T cells can be distinguished from HIV-infected cells by virtue of a 186-base noncoding tag derived from the GFP gene, inserted to serve as a nonimmunogenic molecular marker for vector in HIV-infected patient cells.

The VRX496 antisense-based approach may provide several important advantages over other gene transfer approaches. First, the length of the antisense payload is over 900 nucleotides long, making it difficult for wild-type HIV to create resistant strains by deletion or multiple mutations of this region to result in a virus sufficiently fit to cause disease (Lu et al., 2004). Second, this vector is theoretically safer that the use of oncoretroviruses, since minimal new genetic sequences are introduced into an HIV-infected patient. All the sequences present in the HIV-based vector are derived from highly conserved regions of wt-HIV that would almost certainly be present in any given HIV-1-infected individual. The HIV sequences that are used to create VRX496 are derived solely from pNL4-3, a prototypic HIV-1 molecular clone that is derived from two North American strains of HIV-1 (Adachi et al., 1986). However, the vector is a lentivirus, and therefore the consequences of insertional mutagenesis must be considered carefully, as noted above.

Full regulatory approval to carry out the first lentiviral vector trial in humans was granted in 2003. In this protocol, clinical-grade VRX496 vector was produced, and the clinical-grade production of lentiviral-modified CD4 T cells was carried out at the University of Pennsylvania by Bruce Levine and colleagues.

The intent of this pilot trial was to test the safety and feasibility of a single infusion of 1×10^{10} lentiviral-modified CD4 T cells expressing the antisense *env* vector in five subjects. Eligibility criteria included failing two or more HAART regimens, ongoing HIV viremia > 5000 copies/mL, and > 150 CD4 cells/mL. To maximize safety, patient enrollment and treatment were serial. The first infusion was July 20, 2003, and the last patient was dosed September 27, 2004. Importantly, there have been no serious adverse events to date. ELISA tests to detect VSV-G antibodies were negative for all subjects tested, as were tests for VSV-G nucleic acids in plasma samples, so that there is no evidence for the generation of replication competent lentivirus in vivo. The T-cell repertoire has remained unchanged in the patients, with no evidence of clonal outgrowth, and early results from insertion-site analysis of the transduced cellular product by Frederic Bushman and colleagues are promising, indicating that the VRX496 vector inserts into the genome of HIV-infected patient CD4 cells in a similar fashion as wild-type HIV. Thus, to date there is no evidence of adverse events as a consequence of insertional mutagenesis.

The clinical-grade T-cell manufacturing and lentiviral transduction process in the pilot trial was successful, reaching target cell expansion with routine transduction efficiencies of > 90% in all patients. Persistence of the vector in vivo is being assessed by RT-PCR, and sustained lentiviral gene transfer has been demonstrated in the subjects. Furthermore, a single infusion of VRX496 cells does not appear to be immunogenic. All five subjects were engrafted at a frequency of about 0.1% of PBMC with vector containing cells 20 days after a single infusion of LV-modified CD4 cells; this is impressive considering their viral load and presumed high rate of CD4 cell turnover. The decay kinetics of the infused CD4 cells are encouraging compared to adoptive transfer of CD8 T cells in patients with advanced HIV infection (Brodie et al., 2000,1999) and are consistent with a selective advantage of the vector-modified CD4 cells in vivo, similar to the positive selection for transduced cells that we have observed in vitro (Lu et al., 2004). Thus, initial results with lentiviral-engineered T cells support the rationale for further testing in HIV infection and in patients with cancer.

HIT-AND-RUN STRATEGIES USING ENGINEERED ZINC-FINGER PROTEINS FOR T-CELL THERAPY

T cells are particularly amenable for gene therapy using retroviral and lentiviral vectors. However, for some diseases, particularly less severe disorders where the risk of insertional mutagenesis may not be tolerable, it is desirable to develop alternative nonviral gene therapies. Another approach to genetically altering T cells is gene correction or disruption of the host chromosome. Here, molecules are introduced into T cells that target specific regions with the chromosome, and once there, alter the T-cell DNA. Unlike viral strategies, this approach does not rely on integration into the genome and requires only transient expression, making it a potentially safer therapy with fewer off-target effects. Moreover, if successful, this approach will be permanent and has the potential to be curative in certain diseases since it repairs the genomic DNA. Multiple strategies have been described to alter the human genome, including homologous recombination and triplex-forming oligos (Koller and Smithies, 1992; Wang et al., 1996), but until recently the efficiency of gene correction has been too low to envision therapeutic uses. In a recent ground-breaking study scientists at Sangamo Biosciences demonstrated that gene correction could repair 18% of mutated IL-2 Rγ alleles (Urnov et al., 2005). The IL-2 Rγ locus was chosen as a model genetic disorder because mutations in this locus result in the most common severe combined immune deficiency (X-linked SCID) In these initial in vitro studies, zinc finger nucleases were designed specifically to bind the region surrounding an X-linked SCID hotspot, introduce double strand breaks, and repair the genetic region with a supplied donor DNA fragment that harbors the wild-type IL-2 Rγ sequence. The creation and use of these zinc finger nucleases are described below.

The modular nature of transcription factors, combined with the availability of detailed structural information, has allowed the design and synthesis of DNA-binding domains that can target nearly any sequence within the human genome with high specificity. The structural basis for this specificity is provided by the most abundant and versatile DNA-binding motif found in eukarya: the Cys_2-His_2 zinc-finger protein domain (Tupler et al., 2001). Naturally occurring zinc finger proteins contain multiple tandem fingers, each of which contacts a 3- or 4-bp subsite. Within each finger, the protein–DNA interface is established by a single α-helix that penetrates the major groove and establishes base-specific contacts. By linking these zinc fingers in tandem, zinc-finger proteins (ZFPs) with a high degree of sequence specificity have been engineered to bind any sequence up to 18 nucleotides in length (Snowden et al., 2003; Tan et al., 2003). By linking a nuclease to a sequence-specific ZFP, a zinc-finger nuclease (ZFN) is created. The bacterial restriction enzyme *Fok1* is often tethered to the zinc finger protein for applications regarding gene alteration. This enzyme is ideal because its nuclease activity can be separated from its DNA-binding activity (Kim and Chandrasegaran, 1994). When placed in the proximity of DNA the *Fok1* nuclease domain is able to induce a DSB efficiently in a non-sequence-specific manner (Kim, 1996). However, to cut DNA efficiently, *Fok1* must bind as a dimer (Vanamee et al., 2001), making the introduction of a DSB a highly specific event because ZFNs must bind both strands of DNA flanking the target region, resulting in up to 36 bases of specificity.

Introduced DSBs can be repaired either by homologous recombination or non-homologous end joining (van Gent et al., 2001). These two mechanisms differ in both fidelity and template requirements. Homologous recombination requires a DNA template and repairs the lesion without introducing errors. The DNA template can either be the sister chromatid or introduced with the ZFN as a plasmid. The efficiency of homologous recombination is increased in the presence of donor DNA templates (Urnov et al., 2005). This approach is used to correct mutations.

In contrast, nonhomologous endjoining does not employ a DNA template, is error prone, and routinely deletes or adds bases to the genome. This gene disruption approach would be useful when a cellular factor is contributing to the pathogenesis of infectious molecule, such as the case in HIV infection, where CCR5 is essential for viral transmission (Berger et al., 1999). Although the number of applications of this approach would be more limited than gene deletion, the absolute efficiency would be much higher than that for homologous recombination. Current studies in the laboratory are testing the feasibility of scaling up this process to test targeted gene disruption of CCR5 using engineered ZFNs in patients with HIV-1 infection who have wild-type alleles for CCR5 (Jouvenot, 2005).

CONCLUSIONS

It is our hypothesis that a number of deficiencies in vector and tissue culture technology have previously held back clinical success of T-cell genetic therapy. As the field of immunology has exploded, the potential for therapeutic manipulation of immunity through ex vivo culture and genetic manipulation of immune cells such as T cells holds great promise.

REFERENCES

Adachi A, Gendelman HE, Koenig S, et al. (1986). Production of acquired immunodeficiency syndrome-associated retrovirus in human and nonhuman cells transfected with an infectious molecular clone. *J Virol*. 59:284–291.

Amado RG, Chen IS (1999). Lentiviral vectors: the promise of gene therapy within reach? *Science*. 285:674–676.

Baltimore D (1988). Gene therapy. Intracellular immunization. *Nature*. 335:395–396.

Berger EA, Murphy PM, Farber JM (1999). Chemokine receptors as HIV-1 coreceptors: roles in viral entry, tropism, and disease. *Annu Rev Immunol*. 17:657–700.

Berger C, Blau CA, Huang ML, et al. (2004). Pharmacologically regulated Fas-mediated death of adoptively transferred T cells in a nonhuman primate model. *Blood*. 103: 1261–1269.

Billingham R, Brent L, Medawar P (1954). Quantitative studies on tissue transplantation immunity: the origin, strength and duration of actively and adoptively acquired immunity. *Proc R Soc Biol*. 143:58–80.

Blaese RM, Culver KW, Miller AD, et al. (1995). T lymphocyte-directed gene therapy for ADA-SCID: initial trial results after 4 years. *Science*. 270:475–480.

Bonini C, Ferrari G, Verzeletti S, et al. (1997). HSV-TK gene transfer into donor lymphocytes for control of allogeneic graft-versus-leukemia. *Science*. 276:1719–1724.

Bridges SH, Sarver N (1995). Gene therapy and immune restoration for HIV disease. *Lancet*. 345:427–432.

Brodie SJ, Lewinsohn DA, Patterson BK, et al. (1999). In vivo migration and function of transferred HIV-1-specific cytotoxic T cells. *Nat Med*. 5:34–41.

Brodie SJ, Patterson BK, Lewinsohn DA, et al. (2000). HIV-specific cytotoxic T lymphocytes traffic to lymph nodes and localize at sites of HIV replication and cell death. *J Clin Invest*. 105:1407–1417.

Cavalieri S, Cazzaniga S, Geuna M, et al. (2003). Human T lymphocytes transduced by lentiviral vectors in the absence of TCR activation maintain an intact immune competence. *Blood*. 102:497–505.

Clackson T, Yang W, Rozamus LW, et al. (1998). Redesigning an FKBP–ligand interface to generate chemical dimerizers with novel specificity. *Proc Natl Acad Sci U S A*. 95:10437–10442.

Dave UP, Jenkins NA, Copeland NG (2004). Gene therapy insertional mutagenesis insights. *Science*. 303:333.

Deeks S, Wagner B, Anton PA, et al. (2002). A phase II randomized study of HIV-specific T-cell gene therapy in subjects with undetectable plasma viremia on combination anti-retroviral therapy. *Mol Ther*. 5:788–797.

Donahue RE, Kessler SW, Bodine D, et al. (1992). Helper virus induced T cell lymphoma in nonhuman primates after retroviral mediated gene transfer. *J Exp Med*. 176:1125–1135.

Dropulic B (2001). Lentivirus in the clinic. *Mol Ther*. 4:511–512.

Dropulic B, Hermankova M, Pitha PM (1996). A conditionally replicating HIV-1 vector interferes with wild-type HIV-1 replication and spread. *Proc Natl Acad Sci U S A* 93:11103–11108.

Dropulic B, Jeang KT (1994). Gene therapy for human immunodeficiency virus infection: genetic antiviral strategies and targets for intervention. *Hum Gene Ther*. 5: 927–939.

Eshhar Z, Bach N, Fitzer-Attas CJ, et al. (1996). The T-body approach: potential for cancer immunotherapy. *Springer Semin Immunopathol*. 18:199-209.

Gaspar HB, Parsley KL, Howe S, et al. (2004). Gene therapy of X-linked severe combined immunodeficiency by use of a pseudotyped gammaretroviral vector. *Lancet*. 364:2181–2187.

Gates AE, Kaplan LD (2003). Biology and management of AIDS-associated non-Hodgkin's lymphoma. *Hematol Oncol Clin North Am*. 17:821–841.

Gross G, Waks T, Eshhar Z (1989). Expression of immunoglobulin-T-cell receptor chimeric molecules as functional receptors with antibody-type specificity. *Proc Natl Acad Sci U S A*. 86:10024–10028.

Hacein-Bey-Abina S, von Kalle C, Schmidt M, et al. (2003). A serious adverse event after successful gene therapy for X-linked severe combined immunodeficiency. *N Engl J Med*. 348:255–256.

Harper ME, Marselle LM, Gallo RC, Wong-Staal F (1986). Detection of lymphocytes expressing human T-lymphotropic virus type III in lymph nodes and peripheral blood from infected individuals by in situ hybridization. *Proc Natl Acad Sci U S A*. 83: 772–776.

Helene M, Lake-Bullock V, Bryson JS, Jennings CD, Kaplan AM (1997). Inhibition of graft-versus-host disease: use of a T cell-controlled suicide gene. *J Immunol*. 158:5079–5082.

Hooijberg E, Ruizendaal JJ, Snijders PJ, Kueter EW, Walboomers JM, Spits H (2000). Immortalization of human CD8(+) T cell clones by ectopic expression of telomerase reverse transcriptase. *J Immunol*. 165:4239–4245.

Jouvenot Y, Perez E, Urnov FD, et al. (2005). Towards gene knock out therapy for AIDS/HIV: targeted disruption of CCR5 using engineered zinc finger protein nucleases (ZFNs). *44th Interscience Conference on Antimicrobial Agents and Chemotherapy*, December 16; Abstract: 107.

June, CH (2005). Adoptive cellular therapies. In: Chabner B, Longo DL, ed. *Cancer Chemotherapy and Biotherapy: Principles and Practice*. Baltimore, MD: Lippincott Williams & Wilkins.

Kessels HW, Wolkers MC, Schumacher TN (2005). Gene transfer of MHC-restricted receptors. *Methods Mol Med*. 109:201–214.

Kim YG, Chandrasegaran S 1994. Chimeric restriction endonuclease. *Proc Natl Acad Sci U S A*. 91:883–887.

Kim YG, Cha J, Chandrasegaran S (1996). Hybrid restriction enzymes: zinc finger fusions to Fok I cleavage domain. *Proc Natl Acad Sci U S A* 93:1156–1160.

Kolb HJ, Schattenberg A, Goldman JM, et al. (1995). Graft-versus-leukemia effect of donor lymphocyte transfusions in marrow grafted patients. European Group for Blood and Marrow Transplantation Working Party Chronic Leukemia. *Blood*. 86: 2041–2050.

Koller BH, Smithies O (1992). Altering genes in animals by gene targeting. *Annu Rev Immunol*. 10:705–730.

Li Q, Furman SA, Bradford CR, Chang AE (1999). Expanded tumor-reactive CD4 + T-cell responses to human cancers induced by secondary anti-CD3/anti-CD28 activation. *Clin Cancer Res*. 5:461–469.

Lois C, Hong EJ, Pease S, Brown EJ, Baltimore D (2002). Germline transmission and tissue-specific expression of transgenes delivered by lentiviral vectors. *Science*. 295: 868–872.

Lokhorst HM, Wu K, Verdonck LF, et al. (2004). The occurrence of graft-versus-host disease is the major predictive factor for response to donor lymphocyte infusions in multiple myeloma. *Blood*. 103:4362–4364.

Lori F, Guallini P, Galluzzi L, Lisziewicz J (2002). Gene therapy approaches to HIV infection. *Am J Pharmacogenom*. 2:245–252.

Lu X, Yu Q, Binder GK, et al. (2004). Antisense-mediated inhibition of human immunodeficiency virus (HIV) replication by use of an HIV type 1-based vector results in severely attenuated mutants incapable of developing resistance. *J Virol*. 78: 7079–7088.

Maus MV, Thomas AK, Leonard DGB, et al. (2002). Ex vivo expansion of polyclonal and antigen-specific cytotoxic T lymphocytes by artificial APCs expressing ligands for the T-cell receptor, CD28 and 4-1BB. *Nat Biotechnol*. 20:143–148.

Mautino MR, and Morgan RA (2002). Enhanced inhibition of human immunodeficiency virus type 1 replication by novel lentiviral vectors expressing human immunodeficiency virus type 1 envelope antisense RNA. *Hum Gene Ther*. 13:1027–1037.

Melief CJ (1992). Tumor eradication by adoptive transfer of cytotoxic T lymphocytes. *Adv Cancer Res*. 58:143–175.

Mitchell RS, Beitzel BF, Schroder AR, et al. (2004). Retroviral DNA integration: ASLV, HIV, and MLV show distinct target site preferences. *PLoS Biol*. 2:E234.

Mitsuyasu RT, Anton PA, Deeks SG, et al. (2000). Prolonged survival and tissue trafficking following adoptive transfer of CD4zeta gene-modified autologous CD4(+) and CD8(+) T cells in human immunodeficiency virus-infected subjects. *Blood*. 96:785–793.

Moss P, Rickinson A (2005). Cellular immunotherapy for viral infection after Hsc transplantation. *Nat Rev Immunol*. 5:9–20.

Naldini L, Blomer U, Gallay P, et al. (1996). In vivo gene delivery and stable transduction of nondividing cells by a lentiviral vector. *Science*. 272:263–267.

Pfeifer A, Ikawa M, Dayn Y, Verma IM (2002). Transgenesis by lentiviral vectors: lack of gene silencing in mammalian embryonic stem cells and preimplantation embryos. *Proc Natl Acad Sci U S A*. 99:2140–2145.

Qin XF, An DS, Chen IS, Baltimore D (2003). Inhibiting HIV-1 infection in human T cells by lentiviral-mediated delivery of small interfering RNA against CCR5. *Proc Natl Acad Sci U S A*. 100:183–188.

Ranga U, Woffendin C, Verma S, et al. (1998). Retroviral delivery of an antiviral gene in HIV-infected individuals. *Proc Natl Acad Sci U S A*. 95:1201–1206.

Riddell SR, Greenberg PD (1995). Principles for adoptive T cell therapy of human viral diseases. *Annu Rev Immunol*. 13:545–586.

Riddell SR, Elliott M, Lewinsohn DA, et al. (1996). T-cell mediated rejection of gene-modified HIV-specific cytotoxic T lymphocytes in HIV-infected patients. *Nat Med*. 2:216–223.

Roberts MR, Qin L, Zhang D, et al. (1994). Targeting of human immunodeficiency virus-infected cells by CD8 + T lymphocytes armed with universal T-cell receptors. *Blood*. 84:2878–2889.

Romeo C, Seed B (1991). Cellular immunity to HIV activated by CD4 fused to T cell or Fc receptor polypeptides. *Cell*. 64:1037–1046.

Rosenberg SA, Aebersold P, Cornetta K, et al. (1990). Gene transfer into humans: immunotherapy of patients with advanced melanoma, using tumor-infiltrating lymphocytes modified by retroviral gene transduction. *N Engl J Med*. 323:570–578.

Sadelain M, Riviere I, Brentjens R (2003). Targeting tumours with genetically enhanced T lymphocytes. *Nat Rev Cancer*. 3:35–45.

Sarver N, Rossi J (1993). Gene therapy: a bold direction for HIV-1 treatment. *AIDS Res Hum Retroviruses*. 9:483–487.

Schroder AR, Shinn P, Chen H, Berry C, Ecker JR, Bushman F (2002). HIV-1 integration in the human genome favors active genes and local hotspots. *Cell*. 110:521–529.

Schroers R, Davis CM, Wagner HJ, Chen SY (2002). Lentiviral transduction of human T-lymphocytes with a RANTES intrakine inhibits human immunodeficiency virus type 1 infection. *Gene Ther*. 9:889–897.

Shu S, Chou T, Rosenberg SA (1986). In vitro sensitization and expansion with viable tumor cells and Il-2 in the generation of specific therapeutic effector cells. *J Immunol*. 136:3891–3898.

Simmonds P, Balfe P, Peutherer JF, Ludlam CA., Bishop JO, Brown AJ (1990). Human immunodeficiency virus–infected individuals contain provirus in small numbers of peripheral mononuclear cells and at low copy numbers. *J Virol*. 64:864–872.

Snowden AW, Zhang L, Urnov F, et al. (2003). Repression of vascular endothelial growth factor A in glioblastoma cells using engineered zinc finger transcription factors. *Cancer Res*. 63:8968–8976.

Straathof KC, Spencer DM, Sutton RE, Rooney CM (2003). Suicide genes as safety switches in T lymphocytes. *Cytotherapy*. 5:227–230.

Sullivan KM, Storb R, Buckner CD, et al. (1989). Graft-versus-host disease as adoptive immunotherapy in patients with advanced hematologic neoplasms. *N Engl J Med*. 320:828–834.

Tan S, Guschin D, Davalos A, et al. (2003). Zinc-finger protein-targeted gene regulation: genomewide single-gene specificity. *Proc Natl Acad Sci U S A*. 100:11997–12002.

Thomis DC, Marktel S, Bonini C, Traversari C, Gilman M, Bordignon C, Clackson T (2001). A Fas-based suicide switch in human T cells for the treatment of graft-versus-host disease. *Blood* 97:1249–1257.

Topp MS, Riddell SR, Akatsuka Y, Jensen MC, Blattman JN, Greenberg PD (2003). Restoration of CD28 expression in CD28- CD8 + memory effector T cells reconstitutes antigen-induced IL-2 production. *J Exp Med*. 198:947–955.

Tupler R, Perini G, Green MR (2001). Expressing the human genome. *Nature*. 409: 832–833.

Uchida N, Cone RD, Freeman GJ, Mulligan RC, Cantor H (1986). High efficiency gene transfer into murine T cell clones using a retroviral vector. *J Immunol*. 136:1876–1879.

Urnov FD, Miller JC, Lee YL, et al. (2005). Highly efficient endogenous human gene correction using designed zinc-finger nucleases. *Nature*. 435:646–651.

Vanamee ES, Santagata S, Aggarwal AK (2001). FokI requires two specific DNA sites for cleavage. *J Mol Biol*. 309:69–78.

van Gent DC, Hoeijmakers JHJ, Kanaar R (2001). Chromosomal stability and the DNA double-stranded break connection. *Nat Rev Genet*. 2:196–206.

Veres G, Junker U, Baker J, et al. (1998). Comparative analyses of intracellularly expressed antisense RNAs as inhibitors of human immunodeficiency virus type 1 replication. *J Virol*. 72:1894–1901.

Walker RE, Bechtel CM, Natarajan V, et al. (2000). Long-term in vivo survival of receptor-modified syngeneic T cells in patients with human immunodeficiency virus infection. *Blood*. 96:467–474.

Wang G, Seidman MM, Glazer PM (1996). Mutagenesis in mammalian cells induced by triple helix formation and transcription-coupled repair. *Science*. 271:802–805.

Woffendin C, Ranga U, Yang ZY, Xu L, Nabel GJ (1996). Expression of a protective gene prolongs survival of T cells in human immunodeficiency virus–infected patients. *Proc Natl Acad Sci U S A*. 93:2889–2894.

Xue S, Gillmore R, Downs A, et al. (2005). Exploiting T cell receptor genes for cancer immunotherapy. *Clin Exp Immunol*. 139:167–172.

Yang OO, Tran AC, Kalams SA, Johnson RP, Roberts MR, Walker BD (1997). Lysis of HIV-1-infected cells and inhibition of viral replication by universal receptor T cells. *Proc Natl Acad Sci U S A*. 94:11478–11483.

17 Lentiviral Vector Delivery of RNAi for the Treatment of HIV-1 Infection

KEVIN V. MORRIS

Department of Molecular and Experimental Medicine,
The Scripps Research Institute, La Jolla, California

JOHN J. ROSSI

Department of Molecular Biology, Beckman Research
Institute of the City of Hope, Duarte, California

RNA interference (RNAi) was first described as an antiviral mechanism to protect organisms from RNA viruses and integration events induced by transposable elements (Waterhouse et al., 2001). RNAi has been described in human cells and is a process in which double-stranded RNA induces homology-dependent degradation of mRNA, termed *posttranscriptional gene silencing* (PTGS) (Montgomery et al., 1998; Nishikura, 2001; Sharp, 2001), or directed epigenetic modifications of DNA, termed *transcriptional gene silencing* (TGS) (Sijen et al., 2001; Pal-Bhadra, 2002).

The generation of simianRNA and subsequent PTGS is the result of a multistep process that involves the action of RNase III endonuclease Dicer (Bernstein et al., 2001) (Figure 17.1). PTGS involves small interfering double-stranded RNAs (siRNAs) 21 to 22 bp in length with $3'$ overhanging ends that can induce a homology-dependent degradation of cognate mRNA (Nishikura, 2001). The siRNAs are introduced into the cell either as synthetic siRNAs or expressed within the cell from the context of a vector in the form of short hairpin RNAs (shRNAs). The shRNAs are exported by exportin 5 from the nucleus to the cytoplasm (Lee et al., 2003; Lund et al., 2004), where they are then processed by Dicer (reviewed in Tomari and Zamore, 2005) to 19 to 21-bp duplexes with two base, $3'$ single-stranded overhangs. Following the action of the Dicer, the product 21-nt siRNAs are incorporated into the RNA-induced silencing complex

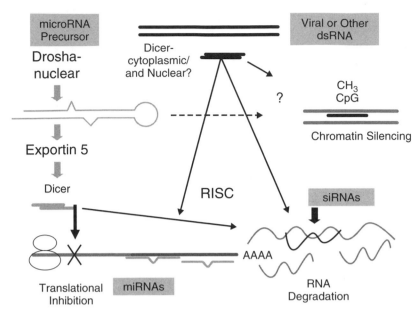

Figure 17.1   RNAi includes several different mechanisms for sequence-specific inhibition of gene expression. The endogenous microRNA pathway begins with transcription of primary micro-RNA transcripts that are processed in the nucleus into pre-micro RNA hairpins. These are exported to the cytoplasm by exportin 5 and processed further by Dicer into miRNAs. One of the two strands is selected for incorporation into RISC. The normal inhibitory mechanism for miRNAs is via partial Watson–Crick binding to sequences in the 3′ untranslated region (UTR) of target transcripts. This binding results in inhibition of translatin. In contrast, the small interfering RNAs (siRNAs) are processed from double-stranded precursors (either viral or cellular in origin). One of the two strands is selected in RISC to serve as the guide strand, which forms fully Watson–Crick base-paired duplexes with target sequences in any portion of the transcript. A component of RISC, the Argonaute 2 protein, acts as a sequence-specific endonuclease which cleaves the target mRNA, resulting in its destruction. These two pathways (miRNA and siRNA) are completely interchangeable, depending on the extent of Watson–Crick base pairing with the target, although for translational inhibition, the pairing most often takes place in the 3′ UTR. The third RNAi pathway involves transcriptional gene silencing (TGS). This involves siRNA pairing to promoter regions either via interaction with promoter-specific RNAs or via RNA/DNA pairing. The siRNA–promoter interaction results in histone methylation and ultimately, DNA methylation and gene silencing.

(RISC), which identifies and silences by slicing the mRNAs complementary to the antisense strand of the siRNA through interactions with Argonaute 2 in the cytoplasm (Hammond et al., 2001; Zeng and Cullen, 2002; Liu et al., 2004; Song et al., 2004). The siRNAs provide much of the target specificity in the silencing process.

RNAi AND HIV THERAPEUTICS

HIV was the first infectious agent targeted by RNAi, perhaps because the life cycle and patterns of gene expression of HIV are well understood. Synthetic siRNAs and expressed shRNAs have been used to target virtually all of the HIV-encoded RNAs in cell lines, including *tat, rev, gag, pol, nef, vif, env, vpr*, and the long terminal repeat (LTR) (Coburn and Cullen, 2002; Jacque et al., 2002; Lee et al., 2002; Martinez et al., 2002; Novina et al., 2002). Subsequent work showed that a host of other viruses, including hepatitis B virus (HBV), hepatitis C virus (HCV), poliovirus, Rous sarcoma virus (RSV), and others, were targetable by RNAi (reviewed in Leonard and Schaffer, 2006).

Despite the early successes of RNAi-mediated inhibition of HIV-encoded RNAs in cell lines, targeting the virus directly represents a substantial challenge for clinical applications because the high viral mutation rate will lead to mutants that can escape being targeted (Boden et al., 2003; Das et al., 2004; Westerhout et al., 2005; Sabariegos et al., 2006), although a clever recent strategy takes advantage of escape mutants in critical genes by targeting the mutants directly (Brake and Berkhout, 2005). The problem of viral-resistant mutants to RNAi is not limited to HIV, as other RNA viruses with RNA-dependent RNA polymerases or reverse transcriptases share this propensity to produce populations of mutants during replicative cycles (Das et al., 2004; De Francesco and Migliaccio, 2005; Xu et al., 2005; Zheng et al., 2005). An alternative approach to avoid this problem is to target cellular transcripts that encode functions required for HIV 1 entry and replication. To this end, cellular cofactors such as NF $\kappa\beta$, the HIV receptor CD4, and the co-receptors CCR5 and CXCR4 have all been down-regulated, with the result of blocking viral replication or entry (Martinez et al., 2002; Novina et al., 2002; Surabhi and Gaynor, 2002; Cordelier et al., 2003; Anderson and Akkina, 2005). The macrophage-tropic CCR5 co-receptor holds particular promise as a target. This receptor is not essential for normal immune function, and individuals homozygous for a 32-bp deletion in this gene are resistant to HIV infection, whereas individuals who are heterozygous for this deletion have delayed progression to AIDS (Samson et al., 1996; Eugen-Olsen et al., 1997; Garred et al., 1997). Andersen and Akkina 2005 used a lentiviral vector to transduce a combination of anti-CCR5 and CXCR4 shRNAs in human lymphocytes. Down-regulation of these receptors resulted in virtually complete inhibition of viral infectivity relative to controls. However, since CXCR4 is essential for hematopoietic stem cell homing to marrow and subsequent T-cell differentiation (Lapidot, 2001; Lapidot and Kollet, 2002; Kahn et al., 2004), targeting this receptor is not a good choice for an anti-HIV therapy, nor is targeting the essential CD4 receptor, with the exception of dendritic cells, where the DC-SIGN receptor can be targeted by siRNAs to prevent infection (Nair et al., 2005). Targeting only the CCR5 co-receptor may also present problems since HIV-1 switches to CXCR4 tropism during the course of AIDS, creating a more virulent infection (Arien et al., 2006). Thus, there are drawbacks in targeting cellular HIV cofactors, and viral targets will need to be included in any successful strategy using RNAi. A possible solution to using shRNAs against essential cellular targets is to incorporate them into a Tat-inducible promoter system (Unwalla et al., 2004). This strategy is yet to be applied to cellular targets essential for HIV replication, but should be used in the future. Finally, it may be possible to use RNAi to prevent viral transmission in by employing siRNAs as microbicides (Palliser et al., 2006).

Viral targets should be sequences that are highly conserved throughout the various clades to ensure efficacy against all viral strains and to minimize emergence of viral mutants resistant to RNAi. Multiplexing shRNAs targeting several sites in the virus is an option that should be fully explored and examined carefully for efficacy, inhibition of viral mutants, and potential toxicity. Since the shRNA pathway impinges on the endogenous microRNA pathway, there is ample opportunity for off-target effects and competition with miRNAs for loading into the RNA-induced silencing complex (RISC). An additional potential concern is the putative inhibition of RNAi via HIV Tat and trans-activation responce (TAR) element. HIV-1 Tat has been demonstrated to bind and inhibit Dicer (Bennasser et al., 2005), although most investigators do not see inhibition of RNAi in targeting HIV, suggesting that this is a minor concern for therapeutic applications. TAR also binds TAR RNA binding protein (TRBP), which is a Dicer cofactor and is a component of RISC (Gatignol et al., 2005). Moreover, unlike other components of RISC, TRBP is made in limited amounts in the cell, and hence binding to the TAR RNA could sequester TRBP from interacting with RISC and perhaps limit the effectiveness of an RNAi-based therapy. Binding of TRBP by TAR may also be a factor in the observed changes in miRNA profiles in HIV-infected cells (Yeung et al., 2005). A few early reports showed that both siRNAs and shRNAs induced type I interferons and interferon-regulated gene expression, suggesting that small RNAs could activate proteins such as protein kinase resource (PKR) and $2'$ to $5'$ oligoadenylate synthetase (OAS) (Bridge et al., 2003; Sledz et al., 2003). Other potential toxicity issues reside around the ability of some siRNAs to activate the Toll-like receptors in immune cells. This is a sequence-specific effect (Hornung et al., 2005; Judge et al., 2005), and clearly a problem when siRNAs are delivered by lipid vehicles, but has not yet been shown to be a problem with expressed shRNAs (Robbins et al., 2006).

An alternative approach to relying solely on RNAi as an anti-HIV approach is mixing a single shRNA with other antiviral genes to provide a potent combinatorial approach. This has been accomplished successfully by coexpressing an anti *tat/rev* shRNA, a nucleolar localizing TAR decoy, and an anti-CCR5 ribozyme in a single vector backbone (Li et al., 2005). A somewhat different combination used an shRNA with a dominant negative Rev M10 protein in a coexpression system (Unwalla et al., 2006). Perhaps other, more potent combinations of shRNAs with mixtures of non-shRNA antivirals will be developed in the near future for testing in preclinical settings.

TRANSCRIPTIONAL GENE SILENCING

Certainly, the majority of siRNAs targeted to genes has been carried out by targeting siRNAs to the cognate mRNAs in a posttranscriptional gene silencing (PTGS)-based manner. However, a few groups have been able to develop and target genes at the promoter [i.e., upstream of the transcribed messenger ribonucleic acid target]. This form of RNA interference, transcriptional gene silencing (TGS), was first observed when doubly transformed tobacco plants exhibited a suppressed phenotype of the transformed transgene. Further analysis denoted that methylation of the targeted gene was involved in the suppression (Matzke et al., 1989) (reviewed in Sijen et al., 2001; Matzke et al., 2004). TGS mediated by double-stranded RNAs was further substantiated in viroid-infected plants (Wassenegger et al., 1994) and was shown to be due to RNA-dependent methylation of DNA (RdDM). The RNA-directed DNA methylation of DNA requires a dsRNA that is processed to yield short RNAs (Wassenegger et al., 1994; Mette et al., 2000). These short RNAs included sequences that are identical to promoter regions, and they are capable of inducing methylation of the homologous promoter and subsequent transcriptional gene silencing (i.e., RNA provides the specificity for the promoter-targeted suppression).

In *S. pombe* RNAi-mediated TGS has been implicated in regulating heterochromatic silencing through histone 3–lysine 9 methylation (H3K9) (Volpe et al., 2002). In human cells TGS has been reported (Morris et al., 2004a; Buhler et al., 2005; Castanotto et al., 2005; Janowski et al., 2005; Suzuki et al., 2005; Ting et al., 2005; Zhang et al., 2005) and reviewed in (Morris, 2005), but the underlying mechanism is not yet completely clear but appears to involve chromatin remodeling complexes and specifically the methylation of histone 3 and lysines 9 and 27 (Buhler et al., 2005; Ting et al., 2005; Weinberg et al., 2006).

With the advent of small interfering RNA-mediated TGS in human cells, one can envision a plethora of new targets that are (1) in conserved genomic regions (i.e., viral promoters), (2) susceptible to epigenetic changes that could result in long-term suppression (i.e., DNA and histone methylation mediated by siRNA-directed TGS), and (3) may operate in a fundamentally different pathway than Dicer and RISC and thus avoid saturation of the endogenous RNAi components. Currently, the pathway involved in small interfering RNA-mediated TGS in human cells remains to be determined but appears to involve one or more RISC components (Kim et al., 2006).

DIVERSITY OF VIRAL TARGETS

Unfortunately, despite the excitement and the early proofs of principle in the literature, there are important issues and concerns about therapeutic application of this technology, including difficulties with efficient delivery, uncertainty about potential toxicity, and the emergence of siRNA-resistant viruses. Indeed, resistance to siRNAs occurs rather rapidly and often can be achieved by a single nucleotide substitution (Gitlin et al., 2002). The use of alternative splice variants has also been observed in eluding the pressures of RNAi on HIV-1 replication (Westerhout et al., 2005).

A possible way to circumvent the emergence of viral variants capable of eluding the pressures of RNAi might be to design siRNAs to best fit targets from an extensive database of the variants in the particular target virus (Morris et al., 2004c) and place these best-fit candidates in a long-hairpin-based expression cassette (Akashi et al., 2005), potentially generating various siRNAs targeted to the most conserved regions of HIV-1. Alternatively, the combining of siRNAs targeted to both the transcript and promoter regions of the virus might provide for a potential target that is overall less capable of accumulating mutations capable of supporting viral replication. Finally, the targeting of essential genes involved in the viral life cycle and/or genes known to suppress RNAi could prove efficacious in successful targeting of HIV-1. The ability of HIV-1 to elude therapeutic interventions suggests that multiplexing of several different siRNAs targeting multiple sites in the HIV genome along with nonessential cellular targets such as CCR5 should be utilized to harness the full potential of this mechanism in treating HIV-1 with siRNA technology. Alternatively, siRNAs designed for more conserved regions such as intron/exon splice junctions might also prove to be more effective at inhibiting the emergence of variant viral strains.

GENE THERAPY APPROACHES FOR TREATMENT OF HIV-1

The idea of using gene therapy for the treatment of HIV infection is certainly not new. Several clinical trials involving gene therapy of T-lymphocytes or hematopoietic stem cells have been initiated over the past 12 years (Fanning et al., 2003; Michienzi et al., 2003; van Griensven et al., 2005). To date, there have been only limited reports of efficacy, since most of the trials have been either safety studies or proof of principal. A limitation for hematopoietic stem cell (HSC)–based gene therapy has been inefficient transduction of transgenes into pluripotent hematopoietic progenitor cells, resulting in a very small population of protected cells (Fanning et al., 2003; Michienzi et al., 2003; van Griensven et al., 2005). All previous clinical trials in HSCs have utilized murine-based retroviral vectors to deliver the therapeutic genes. Since these vectors are best at transducing actively dividing cells, they most often transduce committed progenitor cells, which are not self-renewing. Within the past several years there has been a tremendous amount of progress in the development of lentiviral vectors for gene delivery (Uchida et al., 1998; Engel and Kohn, 1999; Miyoshi et al., 1999; Chen et al., 2000; Follenzi et al., 2000; Guenechea et al., 2000; Sirven et al., 2000; Hanazono et al., 2001; Trono, 2001). These vectors have the distinct advantage of being capable of infecting cells in G0, or slowly dividing cell populations. Self-renewing pluripotent stem cells fall into the category of nondividing or slowly dividing cells. Although no lentiviral vector-mediated transductions of HSCs have been used clinically to date, has an ongoing clinical trial using lentiviral vector-transduced CD4+ lymphocytes (MacGregor, 2001). This trial represents the first FDA approved use of a lentiviral vector for gene therapy.

Unlike retroviruses such as Moloney murine leukemia virus (MoMLV), lentiviruses tend not to integrate in close proximity to active promoters but often within introns of an active transcriptional units, potentially limiting their overall oncogenicity (Wu et al., 2003). Moreover, lentiviral-based vectors are capable of transducing nondividing cells and specifically targeting the nucleus (Greber and Fassati, 2003). Lentiviral vectors have been constructed from HIV-1, HIV-2/SIV, or feline immunodeficiency virus (FIV) and are capable of stably transducing many cell types, including hematopoietic stem cells (Gervaix et al., 1997; Yam et al., 2002), integrating into the target genome, and expressing desired transgenes (Poeschla, 1996; Price et al., 2002; Quinonez and Satton, 2002; Yam et al., 2002). Lentiviruses have also been shown to cross-package one another (White et al., 1999; Browning et al., 2001; Goujon et al., 2003). This observation has been carried over experimentally with HIV-1 and HIV-2 vectors being cross-packaged by FIV and capable of stably transducing and protecting human primary blood mononuclear cells from HIV-1 infection (Morris et al., 2004b). The cross-packaging of lentiviral vectors such as HIV-1 with an FIV packaging system offers a unique and possibly safer method for delivering antiviral vectors to target cells in HIV-1-infected individuals. For instance, FIV packaged HIV-1 or HIV-2 vectors reduce the likelihood of immune recognition, or seroconversion, due to exposure to HIV-1 structural proteins. Finally, lentiviral vectors can be specifically pseudotyped (Kobinger, 2001; Sandrin et al., 2003) or designed with a receptor–ligand bridge to target specific cell types (Boerger et al., 1999).

Therapeutically, the use of lentiviral or other stable integrating vector systems may prove useful in protecting those cells generally infected by HIV-1, but to target cells actually infected by HIV-1 may require the use of conditionally replicating lentiviral-based vectors. Conditionally replicating HIV-based vectors (crHIV) have intrinsic antiviral effects due to competition with wild-type viral RNAs for regulatory proteins such as Tat and Rev (Bukovsky et al., 1999), as well as encapsidation (Corbeau and Wong-Staal, 1998), leading ultimately to the targeting of the vectors to those cells that are naturally infected by the virus (Dropulic et al., 1996; Bukovsky et al., 1999). Conditionally replicating vectors might prove to be a useful method for selectively targeting therapuetic RNAi-based cassettes to reservoirs susceptible to HIV-1 infection. To date, work with a conditionally replicating shRNA-expressing lentiviral vector system has not yet been performed but could prove an effective method for delivering the therapuetic siRNAs to those cells infected with wildtype HIV-1.

CHALLENGES TO THE EFFECTIVE USE OF RNAi IN ANTI-HIV APPLICATIONS

The advantage of using RNAi to treat infectious agents such as HIV-1 is the relative ease of design, construction, and testing. The emerging field of RNAi and siRNA therapeutics in particular provides a potentially cost-effective and relatively quick methodology for treating HIV-1 infection. Although the future looks bright for RNAi as a therapuetic, there most certainly will be problems that require attention. These include the potential for siRNA-mediated off-target effects, the sometimes variable effectiveness of certain siRNAs to suppress gene expression, and most important, delivery of the therapeutic siRNAs to target cells. At this time, effective delivery of siRNAs in vivo is the major challenge. Lentiviral-based vectors offer one methodology that is particularly attractive with regard to using therapeutic siRNAs to treat HIV-1. Lentiviral vectors could be envisioned to be used either to protect the cell from incoming virus, or crHIV vectors could be used to spread the vector and subsequent siRNA-mediated antiviral effect to target cells. Indeed, crHIV vectors could be used to augment current drug regimens. However, before crHIV-based vectors can be used in a therapeutic setting some issues remain to be addressed, one being recombination with wild-type HIV. Although crHIV vectors are designed to be replication defective, unless co-infected into cells with replication-competent virus, there is a theoretical chance that a recombination event could occur between the vector and the wild-type virus, creating recombinant virus with more pathogenic qualities. However, even a crHIV vector lacking any antiviral modalities has been shown to add negative pressure to HIV-1 (Corbeau and Wong-Staal, 1998). Furthermore, it would be difficult to envision a recombinant mutant that is more pathogenic when it derives from a defective lentivirus.

The most potent anti-HIV strategies employ combinations of inhibitory agents, yet resistance to three or more drugs has been observed. This is due largely to the fact that these drugs target very specific regions of viral proteins. Mutations within the targets as well as outside the drug-targeted domains can lead to resistance. SiRNAs are also susceptible to point mutations within and outside the targeted regions (Westerhout et al., 2005). Thus, it is going to be important to multiplex either the shRNAs in a single vector, or to use combinations of different RNA-based inhibitors (Li et al., 2005). A somewhat different shRNA approach is to avoid targeting the virus and target cellular messages required for HIV infection. The problem with the latter approach is that all cells expressing these shRNAs will be affected regardless of whether they are infected by HIV-1. To circumvent this problem, it may be possible to use HIV inducible expression of shRNAs (Unwalla et al., 2004) and to target both cellular and viral sequences.

The final consideration for siRNA/lentiviral-mediated gene therapy in the treatment of HIV infection is that of the target cells. Ideally, one would like to protect all the hematopoietic cell lineages that are infectible by HIV-1, which includes CD4+ T-lymphocytes, monocytes, macrophages, dendritic cells, and microglial cells. This type of protection is best accomplished via transducing hematopoietic progenitor cells, which have the potential to differentiate into all of these lineages (Banerjea et al., 2003; Li et al., 2005). Indeed, this strategy has been used for ribozyme-mediated gene therapy, and is now an attractive possibility for shRNA

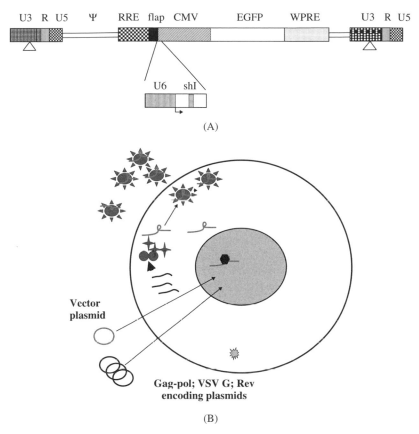

| U3 | R | U5 | Ψ | | RRE | flap | CMV | EGFP | WPRE | | U3 | R | U5 |

(A)

Vector
plasmid

Gag-pol; VSV G; Rev
encoding plasmids

(B)

Figure 17.2 Lentiviral-mediated delivery of shRNAs. (A) A typical lentiviral vector harboring an shRNA gene. The vector shown is a third-generation vector with a deletion in the U3 region of the LTR, which prevents transcription from this promoter. The various parts of HIV remaining in the vector, including the packaging signal Ψ, the polypurine tract (ppt), and the rev response element (RRE) are indicated. (B) A typical four-plasmid packaging scheme used to produce lentiviral vectors. A plasmid encoding the lentiviral vector is cotransfected into HEK 293-T cells along with plasmids encoding HIV *rev*, HIV *gag-pol*, and the VSV-G protein, which replaces the HIV envelope, and allows pseudo-typing of the vectors. Viral particles are secreted into the media, collected, concentrated, and used to transduce target cells. For purposes of tracking transduction, the EGFP gene is included in the vector.

gene therapy (Figure 17.2) (Bauer et al., 1997; Michienzi et al., 2003). Regardless of the approach, the most important question is: How much selective pressure is enough to block the onset of T-cell loss and immunodeficiency? Only clinical trials using lentiviral vector–mediated transduction of hematopoietic cells will address this challenge.

CONCLUSIONS

RNA interference was first described in *Caenorhabditis elegans* in 1998 and shown to be active in mammals in 2001. During the relatively short time span from 1998 to the present there has been rapid progress from concept to deployment of RNAi as a therapeutic agent. Since this is such a powerful mechanism for target-specific inhibition of gene expression, it has rapidly caught on as a potential therapeutic approach for the treatment viral infection, including HIV. Demonstrations that RNAi can be a potent inhibitor of HIV replication has prompted investigations into optimizing its use for clinical treatment of HIV infection. To date, the most logical approach for using RNAi as an anti-HIV agent is via gene therapy, wherein short-hairpin RNAs that can be processed into anti-HIV siRNAs are delivered to hematopoietic cells via lentiviral vectors. These vectors can be engineered to express multiple hairpins targeting both viral and cellular RNAs, thereby minimizing the emergence of viral escape mutants. The cellular tropism of these vectors can be altered such that they can be used to transduce hematopoietic progenitor cells ex vivo. The idea of using a stem cell–based approach for anti-HIV gene therapy has merit in that these cells give rise to all the lineages that HIV can infect, including T-lymphocytes, monocytes, macrophages, dendritic cells, and microglial cells. Despite the great potential for using RNAi-based gene therapy, there are potential safety issues that still need to be considered. These include the possibility of "off-target" effects of siRNAs, potential stimulation of the innate immune system, and competition with endogenous microRNAs for nuclear to cytoplasmic export and incorporation into RISC. Understanding the biology of RNAi will aid in the development of safer shRNA design. Learning how to achieve maximal target inhibition with minimal perturbation of the microRNA pathway is also a challenge. Despite the potential problems, the power of RNAi as a therapeutic should lead to clinical trials and new therapeutics for HIV treatment within the near future.

Acknowledgments

This work was supported by grants from the National Institutes of Health (AI29329, AI42552, and HL07470 to J.J.R. and HL83473 to K.V.M.) and the National Cancer Institute (5P30 CA33572 to J.J.R. and K.V.M.).

REFERENCES

Akashi H, Miyagishi M, Yokota T, et al. (2005). Escape from the interferon response associated wtih RNA inference using vectors that encode long modified hairpin-RNA. *Mol BioSyst*. 1:382–390.

Anderson J, Akkina R. (2005). CXCR4 and CCR5 shRNA transgenic CD34 + cell derived macrophages are functionally normal and resist HIV-1 infection. *Retrovirology*. 2:53.

Arien KK, Gali Y, El-Abdellati A, Heyndrickx L, Janssens W, Vanham G. (2006). Replicative fitness of CCR5-using and CXCR4-using human immunodeficiency virus type 1 biological clones. *Virology*. 347(1):65–74.

Banerjea A, Li MJ, Bauer G, et al. (2003). Inhibition of HIV-1 by lentiviral vector-transduced siRNAs in T lymphocytes differentiated in SCID-hu mice and CD34 + progenitor cell-derived macrophages. *Mol Ther*. 8:62–71.

Bauer G, Valdez P, Kearns K, et al. (1997). Inhibition of human immunodeficiency virus-1 (HIV-1) replication after transduction of granulocyte colony–stimulating factor-mobilized CD34 + cells from HIV-1-infected donors using retroviral vectors containing anti-HIV-1 genes. *Blood*. 89:2259–2267.

Bennasser Y, Le SY, Benkirane M, Jeang KT (2005). Evidence that HIV-1 encodes an siRNA and a suppressor of RNA silencing. *Immunity*. 22:607–619.

Bernstein E, Caudy AA, Hammond SM, and Hannon GJ (2001). Role for a bidentate ribonuclease in the initiation step of RNA interference. *Nature*. 409:363–366.

Boden D, Pusch O, Lee F, Tucker L, Ramratnam B (2003). Human immunodeficiency virus type 1 escape from RNA interference. *J Virol*. 77:11531–11535.

Boerger AL, Snitkovsky S, Young JAT (1999). Retroviral vectors preloaded wtih a viral receptor–ligand bridge protein are targeted to specific cell types. *Proc Natl Acad Sci U S A*. 96:9867–9872.

Brake O, Berkhout B. (2005). A novel approach for inhibition of HIV-1 by RNA interference: counteracting viral escape with a second generation of siRNAs. *J RNAi Gene Silenc*. 1:56–65.

Bridge AJ, Pebernard S, Ducraux A, Nicoulaz AL, Iggo R (2003). Induction of an interferon response by RNAi vectors in mammalian cells. *Nat Genet*. 34:263–264.

Browning MT, Schmidt RD, Lew KA, Rizvi TA (2001). Primate and feline lentivirus vector RNA packaging and propagation by heterologous lentivirus virions. *J Virol*. 75:5129–5140.

Buhler M, Mohn F, Stalder L, Muhlemann O (2005). Transcriptional silencing of nonsense codon-containing immunoglobulin minigenes. *Mol Cell*. 18:307–317.

Bukovsky AA, Song J, Naldini L (1999). Interaction of human immunodeficiency virus-derived vectors with wild-type virus in transduced cells. *J Virol*. 73:7987–7092.

Castanotto D, Tommasi S, Li M, et al. (2005). Short hairpin RNA-directed cytosine (CpG) methylation of the RASSF1A gene promoter in HeLa cells. *Mol Ther*. 12:179–183.

Chen W, Wu X, Levasseur DN, et al. (2000). Lentiviral vector transduction of hematopoietic stem cells that mediate long-term reconstitution of lethally irradiated mice. *Stem Cells*. 18:352–359.

Coburn GA, Cullen BR (2002). Potent and specific inhibition of human immunodeficiency virus type 1 replication by RNA interference. *J Virol*. 76:9225–9231.

Corbeau P, Wong-Staal F (1998). Anti-HIV effects of HIV vectors. *Virology*. 243:268–274.

Cordelier P, Morse B, Strayer DS. (2003). Targeting CCR5 with siRNAs: using recombinant SV40-derived vectors to protect macrophages and microglia from R5-tropic HIV. *Oligonucleotides*. 13:281–294.

Das AT, Brummelkamp TR, Westerhout EM, et al. (2004). Human immunodeficiency virus type 1 escapes from RNA interference-mediated inhibition. *J Virol*. 78:2601–2605.

De Francesco R, Migliaccio G (2005). Challenges and successes in developing new therapies for hepatitis C. *Nature*. 436:953–960.

Dropulic BMH, Pitha PM (1996). A conditionally replicating HIV-1 vector interferes with wild-type HIV-1 replication and spread. *Proc Natl Acad Sci U S A*. 93:11103–11108.

Engel BC, Kohn DB (1999). Stem cell directed gene therapy. *Front Biosci*. 4:e26–33.

Eugen-Olsen J, Iversen AK, Garred P, et al. (1997). Heterozygosity for a deletion in the CKR-5 gene leads to prolonged AIDS-free survival and slower CD4T-cell decline in a cohort of HIV-seropositive individuals. *AIDS*. 11:305–310.

Fanning G, Amado R, Symonds G (2003). Gene therapy for HIV/AIDS: the potential for a new therapeutic regimen. *J Gene Med*. 5:645–653.

Follenzi A, Ailles LE, Bakovic S, Geuna M, Naldini L (2000). Gene transfer by lentiviral vectors is limited by nuclear translocation and rescued by HIV-1 pol sequences. *Nat Genet*. 25:217–222.

Garred P, Eugen-Olsen J, Iversen AK, Benfield TL, Svejgaard A, Hofmann B (1997). Dual effect of CCR5 delta 32 gene deletion in HIV-1-infected patients. Copenhagen AIDS Study Group. *Lancet*. 349:1884.

Gatignol A, Laine S, Clerzius G (2005). Dual role of TRBP in HIV replication and RNA interference: viral diversion of a cellular pathway or evasion from antiviral immunity? *Retrovirology*. 2:65.

Gervaix A, West D, Leoni LM, Richman DD, Wong-Staal F, Corbeil J (1997). A new reporter cell line to monitor HIV infection and drug susceptibility in vitro. *Proc Natl Acad Sci U S A*. 94:4653–4658.

Gitlin L, Karelsky S, Andino R (2002). Short interfering RNA confers intracellular antiviral immunity in human cells. *Nature* June 26:1–5.

Goujon C, Jarrosson-Wuilleme L, Bernaud J, Rigal D, Darlix J, Cimarelli A (2003). Heterologous human immunodeficiency virus type 1 lentiviral vectors packaging a simian immunodeficiency virus–derived genome display a specific postentry transduction defect in dendritic cells. *J Virol*. 787:9295–9304.

Greber UF, Fassati A (2003). Nuclear import of viral DNA genomes. *Traffic*. 4:136–143.

Guenechea G, Gan OI, Inamitsu T, et al. (2000). Transduction of human CD34 + CD38-bone marrow and cord blood–derived SCID-repopulating cells with third-generation lentiviral vectors. *Mol Ther*. 1:566–573.

Hammond SM, Boettcher S, Caudy AA, Kobayashi R, Hannon GJ (2001). Argonaute2, a link between genetic and biochemical analyses of RNAi. *Science*. 293:1146–1150.

Hanazono Y, Terao K, Ozawa K (2001). Gene transfer into nonhuman primate hematopoietic stem cells: implications for gene therapy. *Stem Cells*. 19:12–23.

Hornung V, Guenthner-Biller M, Bourquin C, et al. (2005). Sequence-specific potent induction of IFN-alpha by short interfering RNA in plasmacytoid dendritic cells through TLR7. *Nat Med*. 11:263–270.

Jacque JM, Triques K, Stevenson M. (2002). Modulation of HIV-1 replication by RNA interference. *Nature*. 418:435–438.

Janowski BA, Huffman KE, Schwartz JC, et al. (2005). Inhibiting gene expression at transcription start sites in chromosomal DNA with antigene RNAs. *Nat Chem Biol*. 1:210–215.

Judge AD, Sood V, Shaw JR, et al. (2005). Sequence-dependent stimulation of the mammalian innate immune response by synthetic siRNA. *Nat Biotechnol*. 23:457–462.

Kahn J, Byk T, Jansson-Sjostrand L, et al. (2004). Overexpression of CXCR4 on human CD34+ progenitors increases their proliferation, migration, and NOD/SCID repopulation. *Blood*. 103:2942–2949.

Kim D, Villeneuve L, Morris K, et al. (2006). Argonaute 1 directs siRNA-mediated transcriptional gene silencing in human cells. *Nat Struct Mol Biol*. 13:793–797.

Kobinger GP, Weiner DJ, Yu Q, Wilson JM (2001). Filovirus-psuedotyped lentiviral vector can efficiently and stably transduce airway epithelia in vivo. *Nat Biotechnol*. 19:225–230.

Lapidot T. (2001). Mechanism of human stem cell migration and repopulation of NOD/SCID and B2mnull NOD/SCID mice: the role of SDF-1/CXCR4 interactions. *Ann N Y Acad Sci*. 938:83–95.

Lapidot T, Kollet O. (2002). The essential roles of the chemokine SDF-1 and its receptor CXCR4 in human stem cell homing and repopulation of transplanted immune-deficient NOD/SCID and NOD/SCID/B2m(null) mice. *Leukemia*. 16:1992–2003.

Lee NS, Dohjima T, Bauer G, et al. (2002). Expression of small interfering RNAs targeted against HIV-1 rev transcripts in human cells. *Nat Biotechnol*. 20:500–505.

Lee Y, Ahn C, Han J, et al. (2003). The nuclear RNase III Drosha initiates microRNA processing. *Nature*. 425:415–419.

Leonard JN, Schaffer DV (2006). Antiviral RNAi therapy: emerging approaches for hitting a moving target. *Gene Ther*. 13(6):532–540.

Li MJ, Kim J, Li S, et al. (2005). Long-term inhibition of HIV-1 infection in primary hematopoietic cells by lentiviral vector delivery of a triple combination of anti-HIV shRNA, anti-CCR5 ribozyme, and a nucleolar-localizing TAR decoy. *Mol Ther*. 12:900–909.

Liu J, Carmell MA, Rivas FV, et al. (2004). Argonaute 2 is the catalytic engine of mammalian RNAi. *Science*. 305(5689):1437–1441.

Lund E, Guttinger S, Calado A, Dahlberg JE, Kutay U (2004). Nuclear export of microRNA precursors. *Science*. 303:95–98.

MacGregor RR (2001). Clinical protocol: a phase I open-label clinical trial of the safety and tolerability of single escalating doses of autologous CD4T cells transduced with VRX496 in HIV-positive subjects. *Hum Gene Ther*. 12:2028–2029.

Martinez MA, Clotet B, Este JA (2002). RNA interference of HIV replication. *Trends Immunol*. 23:559–561.

Matzke MA, Primig M, Trnovsky J, Matzke AJM (1989). Reversible methylation and inactivation of marker genes in sequentially transformed tobacco plants. *EMBO J*. 8:643–649.

Matzke M, Aufsatz W, Kanno T, et al. (2004). Genetic analysis of RNA-mediated transcriptional gene silencing. *Biochim Biophys Acta*. 1677:129–141.

Mette MF, Aufsatz W, Van Der Winden J, Matzke AJM, Matzke MA (2000). Transcriptional silencing and promoter methylation triggered by double-stranded RNA. *EMBO J*. 19:5194–5201.

Michienzi A, Castanotto D, Lee N, Li S, Zaia JA, Rossi JJ (2003). RNA-mediated inhibition of HIV in a gene therapy setting. *Ann N Y Acad Sci*. 1002:63–71.

Miyoshi H, Smith KA, Mosier DE, Verma IM, Torbett BE. (1999). Transduction of human CD34+ cells that mediate long-term engraftment of NOD/SCID mice by HIV vectors. *Science*. 283:682–686.

Montgomery MK, Xu S, Fire A (1998). RNA as a target of double-stranded RNA-mediated genetic interference in *Caenorhabditis elegans*. *Proc Natl Acad Sci U S A*. 95:15502–15507.

Morris KV (2005). siRNA-mediated transcriptional gene silencing: the potential mechanism and a possible role in the histone code. *Cell Mol Life Sci*. 62:3057–3066.

Morris KV, Chan SW, Jacobsen SE, Looney DJ (2004a). Small interfering RNA-induced transcriptional gene silencing in human cells. *Science* 305:1289–1292.

Morris KV, Gilbert J, Wong-Staal F, Gasmi M, Looney DJ (2004b). Transduction of cell lines and primary cells by FIV-packaged HIV vectors. *Mol Ther*. 10:181–190.

Morris KV, Chung C, Witke W, Looney DJ (2004c). Inhibition of HIV-1 Replication by siRNA Targeting Conserved Regions of *gag/pol*. *RNA Biol*. 1:114–117.

Nair MP, Reynolds JL, Mahajan SD, et al. (2005). RNAi-directed inhibition of DC-SIGN by dendritic cells: prospects for HIV-1 therapy. *Aaps J*. 7:E572–E578.

Nishikura K (2001). A short primer on RNAi: RNA-directed RNA polymerase acts as a key catalyst. *Cell*. 107:415–418.

Novina CD, Murray MF, Dykxhoorn DM, et al. (2002). siRNA-directed inhibition of HIV-1 infection. *Nat Med*. 8:681–686.

Pal-Bhadra M, Bhadra U, Birchler JA (2002). RNAi related mechanisms affect both transcriptional and posttranscriptional transgene silencing in *Drosophila*. *Mol Cell*. 9:315–327.

Palliser D, Chowdhury D, Wang QY, et al. (2006). An siRNA-based microbicide protects mice from lethal herpes simplex virus 2 infection. *Nature*. 439:89–94.

Poeschla E, Corbeau P, Wong-Staal F (1996). Development of HIV vectors for anti-HIV gene therapy. *Proc Natl Acad Sci U S A*. 93:11395–11399.

Price MA, Case SS, Carbonaro DA, et al. (2002). Expression from second-generation feline immunodeficiency virus vectors is impaired in human hematopoietic cells. *Mol Ther*. 6:645–652.

Quinonez R, Sutton RE (2002). Lentiviral vectors for gene delivery into cells. *DNA Cell Biol*. 12:937–951.

Robbins MA, Li M, Leung I, et al. (2006). Stable expression of shRNAs in human CD34+ progenitor cells can evade triggering interferon responses to siRNAs in vitro. *Nat Biotechnol*. 24(5):566–571.

Sabariegos R, Gimenez-Barcons M, Tapia N, Clotet B, Martinez MA (2006). Sequence homology required by human immunodeficiency virus type 1 to escape from short interfering RNAs. *J Virol*. 80:571–577.

Samson M, Libert F, Doranz BJ, et al. (1996). Resistance to HIV-1 infection in Caucasian individuals bearing mutant alleles of the CCR-5 chemokine receptor gene. *Nature*. 382:722–725.

Sandrin V, Russell SJ, Cosset FL (2003). Targeting retroviral and lentiviral vectors. *Curr Top Microbiol Immunol*. 281:137–178.

Sharp PA (2001). RNA interference. *Genes Dev*. 15:485–490.

Sijen T, Fleenor J, Simmer F, et al. (2001). On the role of RNA amplification in dsRNA-triggered gene silencing. *Cell*. 107:465–476.

Sirven A, Pflumio F, Zennou V, et al. (2000). The human immunodeficiency virus type-1 central DNA flap is a crucial determinant for lentiviral vector nuclear import and gene transduction of human hematopoietic stem cells. *Blood*. 96:4103–4110.

Sledz CA, Holko M, De Veer MJ, Silverman RH, Williams BR (2003). Activation of the interferon system by short-interfering RNAs. *Nat Cell Biol*. 5:834–839.

Song JJ, Smith SK, Hannon GJ, Joshua-Tor L (2004). Crystal structure of Argonaute and its implications for RISC slicer activity. *Science*. 305:1434–1437.

Surabhi RM, Gaynor RB (2002). RNA interference directed against viral and cellular targets inhibits human immunodeficiency virus type 1 replication. *J Virol*. 76:12963–12973.

Suzuki K, Shijuuku T, Fukamachi T, et al. (2005). Prolonged transcriptional silencing and CpG methylation induced by siRNAs targeted to the HIV-1 promoter region. *J RNAi Gene Silenc*. 1:66–78.

Ting AH, Schuebel KE, Herman JG, and Baylin SB (2005). Short double-stranded RNA induces transcriptional gene silencing in human cancer cells in the absence of DNA methylation. *Nat Genet*. 37(8):906–910.

Tomari Y, Zamore PD (2005). Perspective: machines for RNAi. *Genes Dev*. 19:517–529.

Trono D (2001). Lentiviral vectors for the genetic modification of hematopoietic stem cells. *Ernst Schering Research Foundation Workshop*. (33):19–28.

Uchida N, Sutton RE, Friera AM, et al. (1998). HIV, but not murine leukemia virus, vectors mediate high efficiency gene transfer into freshly isolated G0/G1 human hematopoietic stem cells. *Proc Natl Acad Sci U S A*. 95:11939–11944.

Unwalla HJ, Li MJ, Kim JD, et al. (2004). Negative feedback inhibition of HIV-1 by TAT-inducible expression of siRNA. *Nat Biotechnol*. 22:1573–1578.

Unwalla HJ, Li HT, Bahner I, Li MJ, Kohn D, Rossi JJ (2006). Novel pol II fusion promoter directs human immunodeficiency virus type 1–inducible coexpression of a short hairpin RNA and protein. *J Virol*. 80:1863–1873.

Van Griensven J, De Clercq E, Debyser Z (2005). Hematopoietic stem cell–based gene therapy against HIV infection: promises and caveats. *AIDS Rev*. 7:44–55.

Volpe TA, Kidner C, Hall IM, Teng G, Grewal SIS, Martienssen RA (2002). Regulation of heterchromatic silencing and histone-3 lysine-9 methylation by RNAi. *Science*. 297:1833–1837.

Wassenegger M, Graham MW, Wang MD. (1994). RNA-directed de novo methylation of genomic sequences in plants. *Cell*. 76:567–576.

Waterhouse PM, Wang MB, Lough T (2001). Gene silencing as an adaptive defence against viruses. *Nature*. 411:834–842.

Weinberg MS, Villeneuve LM, Ehsani A, et al. (2006). The antisense strand of small interfering RNAs directs histone methylation and transcriptional gene silencing in human cells. *RNA*. (2):256–262.

Westerhout EM, Ooms M, Vink M, Das AT, Berkhout B (2005). HIV-1 can escape from RNA interference by evolving an alternative structure in its RNA genome. *Nucleic Acids Res*. 33:796–804.

White SM, Renda M, Nam NY, et al. (1999). Lentivirus vectors using human and simian immunodeficiency virus elements. *J Virol*. 73:2832–2840.

Wu X, Li Y, Crise B, Burgess SM (2003). Transcription start regions in the human genome are favored targets for MLV integration. *Science*. 300:1749–1751.

Xu D, McCarty D, Fernandes A, Fisher M, Samulski RJ, Juliano RL (2005). Delivery of MDR1 small interfering RNA by self-complementary recombinant adeno-associated virus vector. *Mol Ther*. 11:523–530.

Yam PY, Li S, Wu JU, Hu J, Zaia JA, Yee J (2002). Design of HIV vectors for efficient gene delivery into human hematopoietic cells. *Mol Ther*. 5:479–484.

Yeung ML, Bennasser Y, Myers TG, Jiang G, Benkirane M, Jeang KT (2005). Changes in microRNA expression profiles in HIV-1-transfected human cells. *Retrovirology*. 2:81.

Zeng Y, Cullen BR. (2002). RNA interference in human cells is restricted to the cytoplasm. *RNA*. July 8:855–860.

Zhang M, Ou H, Shen YH, et al. (2005). Regulation of endothelial nitric oxide synthase by small RNA. *Proc Natl Acad Sci U S A*. 102:16967–16972.

Zheng ZM, Tang S, Tao M (2005). Development of resistance to RNAi in mammalian cells. *Ann N Y Acad Sci*. 1058:105–118.

18 Vector Targeting

QIANA L. MATTHEWS and DAVID T. CURIEL

Division of Human Gene Therapy, Gene Therapy Center,
University of Alabama at Birmingham, Birmingham, Alabama

Over the past few decades it has become increasingly accepted that genetic diseases and cancer can be corrected through a process of gene transfer, *gene therapy*. The success of gene therapy depends largely on the suitability of vehicles, or *vectors*, to transfer a particular transgene to diseased tissues and avoid healthy organs, thus limiting toxicity (Wolff and Lederberg, 1994). Currently, there are a variety of vectors available for utilization, which are classified as either viral or nonviral vectors. Some nonviral vectors have limitations, such as low transduction efficiencies, but viral vectors such as adenoviruses (Ads) have shown encouraging results in vitro and in vivo.

ADENOVIRUSES AS A VECTOR SYSTEM

Adenoviral vectors are attractive as gene delivery vehicles for several reasons. First, they can provide efficient in vivo gene transfer in both nondividing and dividing cells (Kay et al., 2001; Barnett et al., 2002). Second, they possess high in vivo stability and can be produced in high titers. Third and most important, adenovirus (Ad) vectors do not integrate into the human genome and are not oncogenic; their pathology is limited primarily to mild upper respiratory tract infections (Curiel, 1999; Barnett et al., 2002). Unfortunately, adenoviral vectors are not without their shortcomings; preclinical and clinical trials have demonstrated limited efficacy, partly because of preexisting antivector immunity. Another contributing factor limiting efficacy of Ad infection has been shown to be the paucity of expression of the coxsackie–adenovirus receptor (CAR) on some target cells, such as hematopoietic (Wickham, 2000), smooth muscle, and some advanced cancer cells (Barnett et al., 2002; Kim et al., 2002). Since CAR is the primary cellular receptor for Ad serotype 5, the most commonly used Ad for

Concepts in Genetic Medicine, Edited by Boro Dropulic and Barrie Carter
Copyright © 2008 John Wiley & Sons, Inc.

gene therapy, in this chapter we focus on strategies that allow for better targeting of Ads, thus overcoming this obstacle for successful gene therapy.

TRANSDUCTIONAL TARGETING

There are multiple avenues by which Ad targeting can be improved; one such improvement is transductional targeting. Transductional targeting enhances or modifies tropism via interaction of viruses and cells. There are two approaches to transductional targeting: adaptor-based targeting and genetic capsid modifications. These approaches can be used to target Ads to an alternative receptor other than the native CAR. The first approach, *adaptor-based targeting*, is based on the configuration of a "molecular bridge" between an Ad vector and a cell surface receptor (Glasgow et al., 2004). The adaptor molecule is a bifunctional protein, where one domain binds to the Ad vector while the other domain of the molecule redirects the Ad to a new target receptor. The predominant principle of adaptor-based Ad targeting is twofold: ablation of CAR-dependent entry pathways and the formation of novel receptor target specificity. One early example of in vitro Ad targeting via adapter based modalities was endeavored with a bispecific conjugate consisting of an antiknob neutralizing Fab fragment chemically conjugated to folate (Douglas et al., 1996). Although there have been a variety of adaptor-based conjugates made since then with successful retargeting demonstrated both in vitro an in vivo (Everts et al., 2005), there are drawbacks to this approach. For instance one-component systems are more easily approved by the U. S. Food and Drug Administration as compared to multiple component systems.

The second approach to transductional targeting is *genetic capsid modifications*, one objective of which is to incorporate receptor ligands into capsid proteins. Targeting via genetic capsid modifications utilizes Ad fiber. There are several innovative approaches which have incorporated the genetic capsid modification strategies. One of the first approaches to accomplishing this goal was that of Michael and colleagues in 1995. This group genetically incorporated gastrin-releasing peptide (GRP) into the C terminus of fiber protein. This study demonstrated that incorporation of heterologous ligands was not detrimental to fiber trimerization, which is necessary for virus assembly (Michael et al., 1995). In addition to C-terminus incorporations, the HI loop has been exploited for peptide insertions. The HI loop is exposed on the knob surface; therefore, incorporated ligands will be readily accessible for receptor binding (Krasnykh et al., 1998). Belousova and colleagues incorporated 83 amino acid residues in the HI loop without any major reduction in production and infectivity of the virus (Belousova et al., 2002). The limits of fiber incorporations have been examined strenuously with the incorporation of molecules ranging from peptide sequences such as polylysines, Arg-Gly-Asp (RGD) motifs (Wickham et al., 1997), or large ligands such as CD40L (Belousova et al., 2003). Although approaches with transductional targeting have the ability to increase target specificity to a group of target cells, further Ad modifications such as transcriptional modifications are necessary to improve Ad efficacy.

TRANSCRIPTIONAL TARGETING

Ad targeting can also be improved via transcriptional targeting. Transcriptional targeting of Ad utilizes spatially controlled, inducible, or physiological regulated therapy by incorporating DNA sequences, such as promoters, enhancers, and/or silencers to facilitate target gene expression in a target tissue (Nettlebeck et al., 2002). A number of candidate tumor/tissue-specific promoters (TSPs) have been identified for cancer gene therapy. The TSPs vary based on activity, specificity, disease target, and many other factors (Glasgow et al., 2004). One of the first TSPs to be utilized for adequate gene therapy applications was the carinoembryonic antigen (CEA) promoter. CEA is overexpressed in pancreatic, gastric, lung cancers (Tanaka et al., 1996), and adenocarcinomas (Richards et al., 1995). Proof of principle has been shown in in vitro experiments, where CEA-driven herpes simplex virus *thymidine kinase* (HSVtk) transgene expression resulted in a 1000-fold increase in gancyclovir (GCV) sensitivity in CEA-positive A549 cells compared to CEA-negative control cells (Osaki et al., 1994).

COMBINATION APPROACHES

Currently, most genetic retargeting strategies utilize a single modification or combination approach. Altering a single component of Ad is frequently inadequate in achieving true selective Ad targeting. Combination approaches of Ad targeting can employ a variety of paradigms. Two such paradigms are complex mosaics and double targeting. *Complex mosaics* build on the concept of the aforementioned genetic modifications. There are multiple goals of *complex mosaics*; one tactic can be to ablate native Ad tropism while redirecting Ad to a novel pathway. The concept of complex mosaics was first demonstrated with a virion containing a CAR-ablated knob which contains an endothelial cell-binding peptide SIGYLPL; this strategy illustrates untargeting as well as retargeting (Nicklin et al., 2001). Another innovative combination approach is *double targeting*, which increases Ad specificity by means of both transcriptional and transductional control. These two approaches can be combined in a multitude of ways to create the next generation of Ads. Recently, Okada and colleagues illustrated a very effective combination approach. This group produced Ads containing HSVtk as a suicide gene with fiber that contained RGD, which enhances αv-integrin tropism under the control of melanoma-specific tyrosinase (Tyr) or tumor-specific telomerase reverse transcriptase (TERT) promoter. Okada's findings were that AdRGD-TERT/HSVtk and AdRGD-Tyr/HSVtk induced ganciclovir (GCV) sensitivity only in tumor and melanoma cells, respectively, while transduction with AdRGD-CMV/HSVtk followed by GCV treatment led to cytotoxicity in normal cells as well as in melanoma and nonmelanoma tumor cells (Okada et al., 2005).

IMAGING AND OTHER TARGETING APPLICATIONS

Ad targeting can be improved if adenoviral location can be better validated after virion infection. There have been multiple methods developed to assess adenovirus replication and virion location. An early advance in sophisticated adenovirus labeling was the incorporation of enhanced green fluorescent protein (EGFP) at the carboxyl terminus of protein IX (pIX) (Le et al., 2004; Meulenbroek et al., 2004). This data illustrated that fluorescent labeling of Ad at pIX had minimal effects on virion function; it was also demonstrated that these viral particles can be exploited for either in vitro and in situ studies (Le et al., 2004). Finally, pIX has been a candidate site for other useful molecules such as HSVtk. Using a [^{3}H]thymidine kinase phosphorylation assay, Li and colleagues demonstrated that the kinase activity of the pIX-HSVtk fusion was functional (Li et al., 2005). In addition, a cell-killing assay demonstrated that pIX-HSVtk could serve as a therapeutic gene rendering transduced cells sensitive to GCV (Li et al., 2005).

CONCLUSIONS

The ability to deliver therapeutic genes effectively is the most important requirement for successful gene therapy interventions. Gene therapy can be achieved by utilizing targeted Ad vectors. Ad vectors have native properties which make them attractive gene delivery vectors, but these adenoviral vectors also have limitations. To improve Ad efficacy and ultimately, gene therapy, it is necessary to create vectors that encompass multiple targeting paradigms, such as transductional targeting, transcriptional targeting, and combination approaches.

Acknowledgments

This work was supported by grants from the National Institutes of Health: R01 CA083821, R01 CA094084, and 1 R01 CA111569-01A1; the National Institutes of Health/National Institute of Allergy and Infectious Disease: 2T32AI07493-11; and DOD Idea Development Award: 3000394. The authors gratefully acknowledge Drs. M. Everts, M. A. Stoff-Khalili, and R. Wachler for their assistance.

REFERENCES

Barnett BG, Crews CJ, Douglas JT (2002). Targeted adenoviral vectors. *Biochim Biophys Acta*. 1575:1–14.

Belousova N, Krendelchtchikova V, Curiel DT, Krasnykh V (2002). Modulation of adenovirus vector tropism via incorporation of polypeptide ligands into the fiber protein. *J Virol*. 76:8621–8631.

Belousova N, Korokhov N, Krendelshchikova V, et al. (2003). Genetically targeted adenovirus vector directed to CD40-expressing cells. *J Virol*. 77:11367–11377.

Curiel DT (1999). Strategies to adapt adenoviral vectors for targeted delivery. *Ann N Y Acad Sci*. 886:158–171.

Douglas JT, Rogers BE, Rosenfeld ME, Michael SI, Feng M, Curiel DT (1996). Targeted gene delivery by tropism-modified adenoviral vectors. *Nat Biotechnol*. 14:1574–1578.

Everts M, Kim-Park SA, Preuss MA, et al. (2005). Selective induction of tumor-associated antigens in murine pulmonary vasculature using double-targeted adenoviral vectors. *Gene Ther*. 12:1042–1048.

Glasgow JN, Bauerschmitz GJ, Curiel DT, Hemminki A (2004). Transductional and transcriptional targeting of adenovirus for clinical applications. *Curr Gene Ther*. 4:1–14.

Kay MA, Glorioso JC, Naldini L (2001). Viral vectors for gene therapy: the art of turning infectious agents into vehicles of therapeutics. *Nat Med*. 7:33–40.

Kim M, Zinn KR, Barnett BG, et al. (2002). The therapeutic efficacy of adenoviral vectors for cancer gene therapy is limited by a low level of primary adenovirus receptors on tumour cells. *Eur J Cancer*. 38:1917–1926.

Krasnykh V, Dmitriev I, Mikheeva G, Miller CR, Belousova N, Curiel DT (1998). Characterization of an adenovirus vector containing a heterologous peptide epitope in the HI loop of the fiber knob. *J Virol*. 72:1844–1852.

Le LP, Everts M, Dmitriev IP, Davydova JG, Yamamoto M, Curiel DT (2004). Fluorescently labeled adenovirus with pIX-EGFP for vector detection. *Mol Imag*. 3:105–116.

Li J, Le L, Sibley DA, Mathis JM, Curiel DT (2005). Genetic incorporation of HSV-1 thymidine kinase into the adenovirus protein IX for functional display on the virion. *Virology*. 338:247–258.

Meulenbroek RA, Sargent KL, Lunde J, Jasmin BJ, Parks RJ (2004). Use of adenovirus protein IX (pIX) to display large polypeptides on the virion: generation of fluorescent virus through the incorporation of pIX-GFP. *Mol Ther*. 9:617–624.

Michael SI, Hong JS, Curiel DT, Engler JA (1995). Addition of a short peptide ligand to the adenovirus fiber protein. *Gene Ther*. 2:660–668.

Nettlebeck DM, Curiel DT, Müller R (2002). Promoter optimization and artificial promoters for transcriptional targeting in gene therapy. In: *Vector Targeting for Therapeutic Gene Delivery*. Hoboken, NJ: Wiley; 484–503.

Nicklin SA, Von Seggern DJ, Work LM, et al. (2001). Ablating adenovirus type 5 fiber-CAR binding and HI loop insertion of the SIGYPLP peptide generate an endothelial cell-selective adenovirus. *Mol Ther*. 4:534–542.

Okada Y, Okada N, Mizuguchi H, Hayakawa T, Nakagawa S, Mayumi T (2005). Transcriptional targeting of RGD fiber-mutant adenovirus vectors can improve the safety of suicide gene therapy for murine melanoma. *Cancer Gene Ther*. 12:608–616.

Osaki T, Tanio Y, Tachibana I, et al. (1994). Gene therapy for carcinoembryonic antigen-producing human lung cancer cells by cell type-specific expression of herpes simplex virus thymidine kinase gene. *Cancer Res*. 54:5258–5261.

Richards CA, Austin EA, Huber BE (1995). Transcriptional regulatory sequences of carcinoembryonic antigen: identification and use with cytosine deaminase for tumor-specific gene therapy. *Hum Gene Ther*. 6:881–893.

Tanaka T, Kanai F, Okabe S, et al. (1996). Adenovirus-mediated prodrug gene therapy for carcinoembryonic antigen-producing human gastric carcinoma cells in vitro. *Cancer Res*. 56:1341–1345.

Wickham TJ (2000). Targeting adenovirus. *Gene Ther*. 7:110–114.

Wickham TJ, Tzeng E, Shears LL, et al. (1997). Increased in vitro and in vivo gene transfer by adenovirus vectors containing chimeric fiber proteins. *J Virol*. 71:8221–8229.

Wolff JA, Lederberg J (1994). An early history of gene transfer and therapy. *Hum Gene Ther*. 5:469–480.

19 The Manufacture of Genetic Viral Vector Products

DOUGLAS J. JOLLY

Advantagene, Inc., Encinitas, California

ESTUARDO AGUILAR-CORDOVA

Advantagene, Inc., Waban, Massachusetts

Viral vectors for clinical gene transfer are complicated multicomponent molecular structures. Preparing batches of such vectors so that the properties are consistent from batch to batch is a central challenge that must be met for these entities to be evaluated, and used. Without an understanding of the quality and consistency of the products, it is impossible to expect consistent data from preclinical and clinical experiments. This challenge has confounded interpretation of early-stage research with viral vectors. Currently, this is true to a greater or lesser extent, depending on the system being used. For example, first-generation adenoviral vectors have a reasonably well-defined set of manufacturing methods, assays, and requirements for manufacturing, based on extensive preclinical and clinical data.[1] On this basis it is quite possible to use a contract manufacturer successfully for these types of agents. On the other hand, alphaviral vectors such as those based on Sindbis or Venezuelan equine encephalitis (VEE) virus have limited experience and have only recently entered the clinic (http://www.alphavax.com/products/pipeline.aspx, viewed April 2006). These vectors are most likely to be developed by the groups working with them, and standardization of characterization assays across groups may take awhile.

This highlights the difference between process development, which is the research associated with figuring out how to make vectors, and actual production or manufacturing. For the latter to be robust, a particular process has to be chosen, run multiple times to make sure that it works repeatably, and then used with as little variation as possible, and with a standardized set of assays, to produce consistent batches of clinical material. In the manufacture of gene delivery vehicles, these activities may well overlap, and at some point a process that still incorporates obvious limitations has to be "frozen" and characterized.

Concepts in Genetic Medicine, Edited by Boro Dropulic and Barrie Carter
Copyright © 2008 John Wiley & Sons, Inc.

While this is going on, it is inevitable that further possible improvements (both large and small) will be identified. The tension between including or excluding these, and whether this involves going back to the beginning in characterization of the manufacturing process, will be recognized by anyone who has developed early-stage manufacturing technology. This tension has been investigated in the context of production of recombinant proteins, and the general answer in terms of time and cost turns out to be roughly in accord with intuition.[2] With early-stage technology it is best to forge ahead and adjust as you go along, whereas with more characterized technology, it makes sense to choose a process and stick with it. The real dilemmas for early-stage development and manufacture are when the process is "good enough," and because the process development researchers are usually (and rightly) involved in the manufacturing, how the management group limits inappropriate modifications in the process that may lead to inconsistent clinical material. It should be noted that in the context of good manufacturing practice (GMP) of biologicals at an early stage, the regulatory criteria for good enough may not be identical in Europe and the United States[3] (see below). In this chapter we discuss generally various aspects of developing and implementing manufacturing methods, then consider briefly most of the systems for which there is clinical manufacturing experience.

PRECEDENTS AND EXPERIENCE SO FAR

There are two main types of precedents for manufacturing viral vectors as licensed prescription drugs: products on the market in China, and live viral vaccines, marketed widely for several viral diseases, including MMR (measles mumps rubella) and the chickenpox vaccine Varivax.[4] The two products in China are Gendicine[5,6] (Ad-p53) and H101[7] (previously, Onyx-015).[8] There is some information[9] as to the manufacturing of these agents in terms of methods, scale, and efficiency of production, and further estimates can be made based on the Onyx experience in the United States and the production entities equivalent to Gendicine by Introgen (Houston, Texas).

The viral vaccine precedents should be treated cautiously. For example, the smallpox vaccine Dryvax, made by Wyeth until 1983 and still stored for use by the U.S. government, was made by scraping viral pustules from the skin of live calves infected with vaccinia. The well-known example of the annual trivalent influenza vaccine made in fertilized hen's eggs is another outmoded procedure that should not be used as a model. More useful are the newer vaccines, such as Varivax (attenuated varicella zoster for chickenpox from Merck) grown in MRC-5 diploid human cells, and the cell culture–based cloned smallpox vaccines (vaccinia or derivatives) grown in Vero cells from Baxter and Acambis.[10] However, these vaccines are usually potent enough (see Table 19.1) that little downstream processing is required, unlike most uses for viral vectors in general. The low dose and lack of processing may limit their value as models for viral vector manufacture.

TABLE 19.1 Examples of Viral Vectors and Doses in Clinical Use^a

Vector	Route	Indication	Human Dose	Status	Yield/mLCulture	Ref.
Ad Gen1/2	Intratumoral	Various solid tumors	$2 \times 10^{11} - 2 \times 10^{13}$ vp	Phase III, licensed in China	10^{11} vp/mL	5, 24, 25
AdGen2	Intraocular	Macular degeneration	$10^{9.5}$ vp	Phase I	10^{11} vp/mL	59
Rep Ad	Intratumoral	Various solid tumors head and neck	$10^{12} - 2 \times 10^{14}$ vp	Phase II, licensed in China	10^{11} vp/mL	51, 31
AAV2	Aerosol	Cystic fibrosis	10^{13} vg	Phase II	$10^{10} - 10^{12}$ vg/mL	32
	Intracerebral	Parkinson's disease, Alzheimer's	8×10^{11} vg	Phase I	$10^{10} - 10^{12}$ vg/mL	GeMCRIS 0104-469, 0307-593, 0401-623, 0501-689
AAV1	Intramuscular.	α1-Antitrypsin deficiency	Up to 7×10^{13} vg	Phase 1	$10^{10} - 10^{12}$ vg/mL	GeMCRIS 0404-638
Retrovirus	Ex vivo	SCIDS, CGD	1.5×10^8 TU	Phase I	$10^6 - 10^3$ TU/mL	38, 40
	In vivo, intravenous	Hemophilia A	8×10^{10} TU	Phase I	$10^6 - 10^7$ TU/mL	36
Lentivirus	Ex vivo T cells	HIV infection	5×10^9 TU (used to transduce T cells)	Phase I	10^7 TU/mL	42, 43
Alphavirus	Intracerebral	Parkinson's disease	10^7 TU	Preclinical (chimps)	10^7 TU/mL	44
	Subcutaneous	HIV vaccine	$10^7 - 10^9$ IU	Phase 1	10^7 IU/mL	Clinicaltrialsgov, NCT0097838
Poxviruses	Intradermal	Smallpox vaccine	1.5×10^6 pfu	BLA submitted	10^7 pfu/mL	10
	Intradermal	HIV vaccine		Phase III	10^7 mL^{-1}	61
NR herpes	Intratumoral	Cancer (glioblastoma)	Up to 10^9 pfu	Phase I	$10^7 - 10^8$ pfu/mL	Gemcris 0201-505
Rep herpes	Intratumor	Cancer (glioblastoma)	3×10^9 pfu	Phase1	$10^7 - 10^9$ pfu/mL	51
Measles	Subcutaneous	Measles vaccine	1000 TCID50	Market	10^7 TCID 50/mL	http://www.fda.gov/cber/label/mmrvmer, 090605 LB.pdf
	Intratumoral	Cancer	Up to 10^9 pfu	Phase I	10^7 pfu/mL	GeMCRIS, 0204-523

^{a}Examples, where information is available, of the human dose (or estimated human dose) and the productivity of the manufacturing system used, given as the number of bulk harvestable vector units per volume of fermentation. References are given where there is published information; otherwise, the Gemcris (www.gemcris.od.nih.gov/) protocol number or the clinical trials.gov (www.clinicaltrials.gov/) protocol numbers are given. Also shown for comparison are data for attenuated live viral vaccines for measles. Abbreviations: AdGen1/2, AAV 1 and 2, adeno-associated virus, serotypes 1 and 2; adenoviral vector generation 1or 2; AdGen2 adenoviral vector generation 2; Rep, replicative; NR, nonreplicative; SCIDS, severe combined immuno deficiency syndrome; TCID50, tissue culture infections dose; vp, viral particles; vg, viral genomes; pfu, plaque-forming units; TU, transducing units.

231

KEY ISSUES

There are many issues in designing production methods for viral vectors. However, two in particular are key in practice. These are the estimated human dose, as that dictates the scale of production, and the development of appropriate assays to characterize the vector, Without the latter, it is difficult to be sure what the real dose is, how that compares from lot to lot, and even that the material is safe to use.

Dose Requirement

Table 19.1 lists a number of different vector types, some of the applications for which there is significant data and the productivity of the systems used to produce them. This list is meant to be illustrative and not exhaustive. For indications where vector is administered locally, such as various Central Nervous System indications, the dose is often two orders of magnitude less than for more systemic applications. In general, viral vectors have an enormous production advantage over other biologics, such as mononclonal antibodies or even clotting factor proteins, in terms of the mass of material necessary for therapy and hence the required manufacturing scale. Doses for monoclonals tend to be in the hundreds to thousands of milligrams (Herceptin for metastatic breast cancer has an initial dose of 4 mg/kg), clotting factors in the hundreds of micrograms, and viral vectors in the hundreds of nanograms [10^{12} vector genome equivalents (vg) of adenovirus is about 300 ng]. Clinical indications and vectors that allow thousands of doses to be produced from tens of liters have clear advantages over indications and vectors requiring even a tenfold increase, because scale-up of biological production is seldom easy or straightforward. For some indications and vectors, manufacturing for the market could occur at scales of 10 to 100L, normally thought of as useful only for pilot production in phase I or II. This relatively small production scale has also allowed the intense involvement of academic researchers in clinical gene delivery and vector process development research.

Assays

A second key issue is the set of assays used to assess what has been made. Assays are used to qualify components (such as raw materials, master cell banks, or master viral stocks), to monitor the manufacturing process and to release the final product. The general list[11] of these includes safety (i.e., freedom from adventitious agents or deleterious contaminants), identity, potency, functionality, purity, titer, and stability. A minimal set of release assays is listed in Table 19.2. An example of qualification assays for cell banks and viral stocks are in the posted Certificates for Analysis for the Adenovirus Reference Material (ARM, ATCC VR 1516) at www.wilbio.com, viewed April 2006). All vectors with genomes under 40 kb are required to be sequenced in their entirety, but this is usually performed as a qualification assay at the master bank stage, not as a release assay for product.

TABLE 19.2 Minimal Release Assays for a Viral Gene Vector Product

Category	Assay[a]
Safety	Sterility
	Mycoplasma
	Endotoxin
	Adventitious viral contaminants (PCR panel, or microarray)
	Replication competent virus (corresponding to parent of vector system)
	pH
	Osmolality
	Appearance
Identity	Restriction analysis/Southern/PCR
	Transgene expression
Purity	Host cell protein
	Host cell DNA
	Residual BSA
	Residual benzonase (DNAase)
Potency	Titer (viral particle number)
	Bioactivity/functionality
	Particle to infectious titer ratio

[a]Some assays have preset, generally acceptable pass/fail criteria (e.g., endotoxin and sterility); others, in particular potency-related assays, will have acceptable ranges based on the expected performance of the manufacturing system.

Many of the assays are standard assays used for many different products and are very often performed by an outside contractor with specific experience and validated assays. For example, it is rare to conduct in-house sterility, endotoxin, mycoplasma, or in vitro viral testing for individual viruses. Nevertheless, careful thought is always required, as automatic application of preexisting tests can lead to embarrassing undesirable results for trivial reasons. For example, standard viral testing panels applied to the human cell line 293 T (used for transient transfection manufacturing procedures) can give be positive for simian virus 40 (SV40), because it carries about half of the SV40 viral genome. Finally, the level of assurance that assays give valid results can vary depending on where, in the incremental development of the manufacturing process, the vector happens to be. Assays considered key normally receive the earliest and most exact attention, but by the time a product is ready for market, all such assays should be validated.

TITERING ASSAYS

Titering assays for the vectors should be, in principle, comparable for different vectors in the same class and are an important element of potency testing. These assays should be standardized and used for correlation with dosing in animals and clinical trials. Conventional titering for bioactivity, by measurement of tissue culture infectious dose (TCID50) or plaque-forming unit (pfu), where target cells are infected with a dilution series of vector and the cells then scored for vector uptake, can be useful. However, these tend to be laboratory and operator specific[12] and do not register all the infectious particles in a sample, because of diffusion-limited access to the target cells.[13,14] This effect can be calculated to yield more reliable assay results (see "Adenovirus Reference Material Standard Operating Procedure for Determination of Infectious Titer in 293 Cells in a 96-Well Format" at www.wilbio.com[15]).

The problems with using the more limited pfu assays with adenoviral vectors was highlighted by the examination of issues for adenoviral vectors after the Gelsinger incident.[12] If measurements of potency and/or titer are not easily replicated from laboratory to laboratory, toxicities may appear at different apparent doses. Another situation where a commonly used potency assay can give unreliable results is the use of polymerase chain reaction (PCR) to measure the number of vector genomes in crude or partially purified retroviral, lentiviral, and adeno-associated virus (AAV) preparations or even in target cells after transduction. If transient transfection production methods have been used, there is typically leftover DNA from the transient transfection that registers in the PCR test of target genomic material.[16] The same type of caveat is relevant for the A260 absorbance measurements for viral particle number measurements for adenoviral vectors.[17] Standard stocks of first-generation adenoviral vectors[17] and oncoretroviruses (ATCC VR1450) are available for use as standards in potency assays. In general, it appears that generating standard preparation of other vectors, such as adeno-associated virus (AAV) and lentiviral vectors,[18] only becomes worthwhile once a delivery system has been developed to a point where the vector format has been well defined, based on experimental data.

Individual potency/activity/functionality assays for different vectors are the most vector-specific aspect of vector characterization. Here again, thought is required. It is very undesirable to end up with assays that involve animal testing, because such tests are much harder to standardize and validate. The activity/functionality test should relate to the mechanism of action of the vector, so for vectors carrying genes where the mechanism of action is disputed, unclear, or quite complex, this can present extra problems. Examples are agents that modulate immunity (such as CD28 agonists, to quote a recent disastrous example[19]) and products where further processing of the therapeutic entity takes place (such as vectors encoding antigens to induce cytotoxic T-cell responses, where complex antigen processing to allow antigen presentation via the major histocompatibility complex (MHC) class must take place to produce a biological effect).

REGULATORY FRAMEWORK

The overall regulatory considerations are quite standard in different regulatory regimes, but there are significant finer-grain differences. The following discussion is U.S.-centric.

The overall legal regulations governing the development of viral vectors are written into the U.S. *Code of Federal Regulations*, Title 21 (chapters 210, 211, and 600–680 (21CFR210,211,600–680). These are then expanded on and made more explicit in a series of guidance documents from the Food and Drug Administration (FDA). The regulation of biological entities has undergone several changes over the last few years. Until 1996–1997 and the FDA Modernization Act, biologics (including recombinant proteins, vaccines, blood-derived products, and gene therapy agents) were regulated by the FDA Center for Biologics Evaluation and Research (CBER) and defined by how they were made rather than just by characterization assays. Licensing was accomplished through a PLA (product license application) and an ELA (establishment licence application) that were held by the same entity. This effectively prevented contract manufacturing and meant that the phase III trial material needed to be made at the marketing manufacturing site. After 1997, a single application, a BLA (biologics licensing application) was all that was needed, and contract manufacturing for phase II and III trials became possible, as a process was now not tied to a single facility. In addition in October 2003 "well-characterized" biologics (i.e., recombinant proteins) were transferred to regulation by the CDER (Center for Drug Evaluation and Research) at the FDA. In 2004 the *critical path initiative* was launched by FDA (www.fda.gov/oc/initiatives/criticalpath/). This initiative has a number of facets and one important goal is to encourage and require more rapid adoption of scientific advances and methods in pharmaceutical manufacturing. A significant aspect of this effort is to encourage continuous development of process analytical technology (PAT)[20] for the manufacturing process. In plain language this involves monitoring the manufacturing process closely and in real time, using new or improved assays, and incorporating scientifically justified modifications. The critical path manufacturing initiative was stimulated by the well-known conservatism in biologics manufacturing that, for example, famously led Amgen to manufacture the blockbuster drug EPO by mammalian cell fermentation in outmoded roller-bottle technology. Although it is not clear exactly where this will lead, it seems fair to assume that it will allow more flexibility in upgrading or improving manufacturing methods as technology advances, provided that an equivalency between the product made in the old and new ways can be demonstrated. Indications are that many such equivalency demonstrations may not need to be onerous or involve extra clinical trials. This, in turn, may make it simpler to upgrade a process to full GMP manufacturing in a more graduated fashion and as the phase III trial is taking place.

The FDA has long recognized the logic of an incremental approach to GMP implementation as a biologic passes through the clinical trial stages (see, e.g., a presentation by J. L. Frey in 2001: (www.asgt.org/member_resources/recent _course_materials/vector_production_conference/index.shtml), and recently published draft guidelines formally describing an incremental approach to implementing GMP processes. In Europe the path toward vector manufacturing seems less well defined at present[3]. The EMEA directive 2003/94/EC requires that "manufacturing operations are carried out in accordance with good manufacturing practice" without differentiating manufacture for phase I trials from those for market. This seems to restrict the incremental approach to GMP implementation endorsed by FDA. It still seems unclear how this will be handled.

PROGRESSION FROM BENCH TO PIVOTAL TRIALS, SCALE CONSIDERATIONS, AND GMP IMPLEMENTATION

A typical vector development process goes as follows: (1) research material is made in a research laboratory and used in small-animal models; (2) some form of scalable process is developed with limited characterization to make material for large animals or larger experiments; (3) the process and the key characterization assays are further optimized and a pilot GMP process used to make material for toxicology and clinical use; and (4) final scale-up, with process and assay validation for pivotal phase III trials and marketing. In terms of manufacturing, this process is markedly less painful, time consuming, and expensive where there is preexisting experience. However, there are often short-term incentives and priorities at the beginning of a program that can cause problems or at least require significant changes as the process scales up and matures. A typical process using (adenoviral) vector production as an example is shown in Figure 19.1. Several processes that resemble this have been described.[21,22]

SUMMARIES OF INDIVIDUAL VECTOR SYSTEMS IN TABLE 1

For descriptions of the properties of the parent viruses, the reader is referred to ref.[23]

Adenovirus Vectors

Adenoviruses are double-stranded 36-kb DNA viruses that replicate in the nucleus. These vectors, usually based on adenovirus 5, have deletions in the *E1a*, *E1b*, and *E3* regions (generation 1) or in addition in the *E4* region (generation 2) and are grown batchwise in cells that trans-complement the *E1* and *E4* functions.[24] The archetype cell line 293HEK carries 11% of the genome of serotype 5 adenovirus, from the 5' end region. These sequences overlap the complementing adenoviral vector sequences, often leading to the generation of replication competent adenovirus (RCA). Alternative lines have been generated that minimize recombination. The recently licensed Chinese products appear to be grown in derivatives of the 293 cell line.[9]

Adenoviral vectors have the most scale-up and production experience and have been grown at scales up to at least 300 L.[25] They account for about 25% of clinical trials with therapeutic gene delivery vectors, and several large U.S. companies have invested considerable effort to develop manufacturing processes, most notably Merck (as a component of an HIV prophylactic vaccine),[26] but also Berlex (Schering AG, cardiovascular disease[27]), Genzyme (cardiovascular

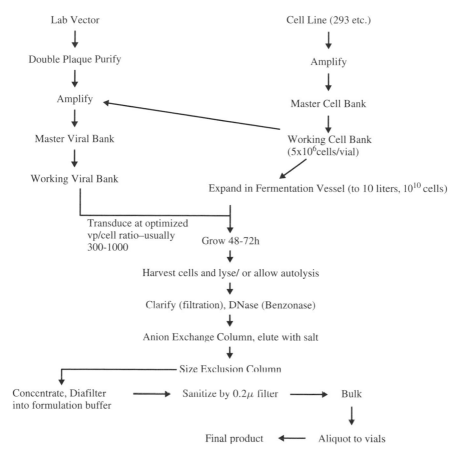

Figure 19.1 Typical adenoviral vector production process. The quantities and number given are typical but are optimized for individual processes. The general scheme models most vector preparation methods, with working and master cell stocks that have been qualified for clinical use by testing, and scalable processes such as chromatography rather than centrifugation steps. In process, bulk and final product testing is conducted to document that the process is performing within preset limits and to gurantee the reproducibility of the process and the consistency of the product. (From refs. 21 and 22.)

disease) and Schering Plough (cancer[28]). In addition, several biotech companies (e.g., GenVec, Introgen, Crucell) have used and manufactured these vectors scaled for phase II and III trials. The most clinical experience with such manufactured products lies with Gendicine, where over 3500 patients have been treated as of March 2006.[6]

High capacity (HC) Ad [also known as helper dependent (HD)Ad, "gutless" Ad, mini-Ad, or maxi-Ad][29] are produced in a similar way[30] but with an *E1* to *E3* negative helper, which is in some way attenuated for packaging to minimize helper contamination. Replication competent Ad vectors (including H101, the descendant of Onyx-015 on the market in China[7]) are also usually made in 293 cells or other cell lines commonly used to propagate adenoviruses (A549, HeLa) or derivatives.[31]

Adeno-Associated Virus Vectors

AAVs are parvoviruses that are also "dependoviruses"— that is, they are not capable of autonomous replication but need the presence of another virus. They replicate in the nucleus and have a 4.7-kb single-stranded DNA genome with terminal hairpin sequences that becomes double-stranded upon productive infection. The vectors (as opposed to the virus) do not appear to integrate actively into the host genome. AAV serotype 2 has been used extensively in clinical trials[32,34] but has presented a manufacturing challenge because the viral replication proteins (rep proteins) are toxic to most cells, and the production needs helper functions from another virus (usually, adenovirus). The production methods vary[33,34] from transient transfection of 293 cells to HeLa cell–based systems where the vector production occurs in a producer cell line carrying viral vector and AAV viral rep and capsid genes that is triggered to produce by adenoviral infection. This process appears to be the most scalable method (up to 100 L so far[35]). Recently, baculovirus production systems in insect cells have been shown to have manufacturing potential.[34]

A key issue has also been the apparent large particle to infectivity ratio (up to 1/10,000). This seems to be improved to around 1/100 with recent process improvements. However, these numbers are not easy to interpret in the absence of a reference for comparison. A working group to produce standards for this vector type, similar to that accomplished for adenoviruses, is in progress. Recently, the properties of other AAV strains (AAV1 through 9) have been investigated.[34] AAV2 genomes pseudotyped by capsids from these strains show promise in terms of in vivo transduction efficiencies of various different tissue types. It seems likely that AAV serotypes will benefit from the AAV2 experience but may also have process development issues of their own.

Retrovirus Vectors

Retroviruses are positive-stranded RNA viruses with a genome of approximately 8.5 kb that integrates a double-stranded DNA form of the virus into the DNA of a dividing target cell, usually without killing the cell. The vectors, based mainly on murine leukemia virus (MLV), have been scaled up and used as a purified agent for in vivo delivery[36,37] but appear now to be seen primarily as useful for ex vivo transduction of stem cells. In this mode only moderate doses and purification seem to be needed. These vectors are generally made in a highly engineered producer cell lines that essentially leak vector slowly but continuously into the media. Vector can be made in production runs that last up to two weeks or more. One of the most successful gene therapy protocols was with retrovirus transduction of hematopietic stem cells in children with severe combined immunodeficiency syndrome (SCIDS). Introduction of a functional gene copy of the γ-chain interleukin receptor led to a cure in nine of 10 children treated. However, four of the children subsequently developed leukemia. The experience with successful therapy for SCIDS followed by leukemia side effects[38] has made investigators cautious with these vectors. However, there is now strong evidence that it was probably the transgene that contributed most significantly to leukemogenesis.[39] Other clinical data continue to support the utility of these vectors for hematopoietic stem cell transduction.[40]

Lentivirus Vectors

These are a type of retroviruses that carry "accessory" viral genes and can infect and integrate genes into nondividing cells. Several varieties of vector based on human (HIV), simian (SIV), feline (FIV), equine (EIAV), and bovine (BIV) viruses have been developed.[41] HIV-based vectors have shown some promise in the clinic as an anti-HIV agent[42,43] and the vectors in general are seen as potentially useful for other indications, including neurological disease.[44] The vectors are usually made by transient transfection of 293 or 293 T cells and are stripped of most viral functions, mostly for safety reasons. Typically, the envelope protein is derived from a heterologous virus, most often from vesicular stomatitis virus (VSVg). Useful packaging cell lines have been difficult to make, as the VSVg protein is toxic to mammalian cells, and expression of some lentiviral proteins can inhibit growth in some cells. Nonintegrating versions of these vectors appear to be feasible,[45] but there is, as yet, little experience with these.

Alphavirus Vectors

Alphaviruses are positive-stranded RNA cytoplasmic viruses that amplify their structural protein message using a viral polymerase. They include Sindbis, Semliki Forest, and Venezuelan equine encephalitis (VEE) viruses. In the vectors the genes desired are substituted for the structural proteins and in general they are delivered as nonreplicative particles.[46] The U.S. army uses a live attenuated vaccine to VEE virus.[47] They are seen primarily as vehicles for heterologous vaccines, and the current versions are eventually toxic to the transduced cells. Functional producer cell lines capable of continuous production can be made from BHK cells,[48] but the clinical material for a current HIV vaccine trial (ClinicalTrials.gov identifier: NCT00097838) is made by in vitro RNA transcription followed by transient transfection of Vero cells and purification by ultracentrifugation (www.alphavax.com/technology/system.aspx).[49]

Poxvirus Vectors

Poxvirus Vectors are double-stranded DNA viruses that replicate in the cytoplasm. Vaccinia is the archetype but attenuated versions (MVA, NYVAC), and other members of the family, including fowlpox and canarypox (ALVAC), have been used clinically.[50] Vaccinia has a linear genome of about 180 kb, and genes can be substituted at a number of sites. Manufacturing these vectors has benefited from the effort to update smallpox vaccine production (e.g., by Baxter and Acambis) and this has taken place at scales up to 1200 L in serum-free medium in Vero cells.[10] In general, these vectors are grown as lytic viruses with limited downstream processing.

Herpesvirus Vectors

Herpesviruses are large double-stranded DNA viruses with genome sizes in excess of 150 kb. Most current vectors are based mainly on herpes simplex virus 1 or 2. They replicate in the nucleus and are capable of latent persistence in neurons. There are three basic types of vectors: (1) attenuated replication competent[51] (e.g., G207[52]) grown as lytic viruses on Vero or BHK cells; (2) replication incompetent with several deletions, usually grown on Vero cells with complementing functions to allow production[53]; and (3) replicon vectors,[54] which incorporate only the packaging signal at the ends of the viral genome, and all the viral helper function are supplied in trans by a defective helper delivered as a virus or as a DNA molecule. A major hurdle for the clinical use of these vectors has been balancing the attenuation of function to minimize toxicity against the vector production efficiency. In general, the more deletion, the lower the productivity. Until now the replicon version of the vector has not produced enough titer to allow progress into clinical trials. Interestingly, a recent addition to the attenuated live viral vaccine repertoire is Varivax, an attenuated varicella zoster (a herpesvirus) as vaccine for chickenpox (www.fda.gov/CBER/sba/varmer031795sba.pdf virus), but manufacturing details for this product are difficult to ascertain.

Measles Virus Vectors

Measles virus is a negative stranded nonsegmented RNA virus that replicates in the cytoplasm of target cells. The vector in clinical trial use is derived form the Edmonston vaccine strain and carries a marker encoding soluble human carcinoembryonic antigen (hsCEA).[55] It replicates preferentially in tumor cells, kills them by fusion induced by the viral H and F proteins, and is in phase I trial for ovarian cancer.[56] The vector is produced by replicative growth on Vero cells. The starter particles are generated from plasmid DNA transfected onto a cell line derived from 293 cells that expresses the measles N and P proteins plus T7 polymerase. Vero cells are collected and the viral vector is released by freeze–thaw. It does not appear at present that much downstream processing has been attempted.

CHALLENGES MOVING FORWARD

The basic challenge for viral vector manufacturing is to make it as routine as recombinant protein production. However, the systems are not as mature as protein production, and although once a process for a specific kind of vector has been developed, the results tend to be portable for another vector in the same class, each vector system is different. There are, however, at least three generic issues that will become more important and relevant in the next few years. The first is to increase the efficiency of production, and a major component of this is to learn to grow cells efficiently at high densities while maintaining the number of virions per cell. A second issue is the development of production systems that avoid the use of animal products (e.g., serum) and the consequent risk of contamination with adventitious agents. Several examples of such methods have recently been published[21,57] and are currently in use. The usual problem is maintaining the productivity of the system in serum-free procedures. A third generic issue that could be very useful is the advent and common use of disposable equipment (including bioreactors) in manufacturing.[58] The follow-on implications include a modular manufacturing capability where standardized processes can be performed in a low-cost manner at different sites. Because of the scale advantage of viral vector manufacture over, for example, monoclonal antibody manufacture, this has a strong appeal for vector manufacturing.

REFERENCES

1. Lusky M. Good manufacturing practice production of adenoviral vectors for clinical trials. *Hum Gene Ther*. 2005;16:281–291.
2. Pisano GP. Learning-before-doing in the development of new process technology. *Res Policy*. 1996;25:1097–1119.
3. Jones SD, Levine HL. Impact of the EU Clinical Trials Directive and other recent regulatory changes on the manufacture of biopharmaceuticals. *Preclinica* 2004;2:301–304.
4. Kuter BJ, Ngai A, Patterson CM, et al. Safety, tolerability, and immunogenicity of two regimens of Oka/Merck varicella vaccine (Varivax) in healthy adolescents and adults. Oka/Merck Varicella Vaccine Study Group. *Vaccine*. 1995;13:967–972.
5. Peng Z. Current status of gendicine in China: recombinant human Ad-p53 agent for treatment of cancers. *Hum Gene Ther*. 2005;16:1016–1027.
6. Jia H. Controversial Chines gene-therapy drug entering unfamiliar territory. *Nat Rev Drug Discov*. 2006;5:269–270.
7. Garber K. China approves world's first oncolytic virus therapy for cancer treatment. *J Natl Cancer Inst*. 2005;98:298–300.
8. Reid T, Galanis E, Abbruzzese J, et al. Hepatic arterial infusion of a replication-selective oncolytic adenovirus (dl1520): phase II viral, immunologic, and clinical endpoints. *Cancer Res*. 2002;62:6070–6079.
9. Peng Z. The genesis of gendicine: the story behind the first gene therapy. *Biopharm Int*. 2004;17:42–45.
10. Monath TP, Caldwell JR, Mundt W, et al. ACAM2000 clonal Vero cell culture vaccinia virus (New York City Board of Health strain): a second-generation smallpox vaccine for biological defense. *Int J Infect Dis*. 2004;8S2: S31–S44.
11. Gombold J, Peden K, Gavin D, et al. Lot release and characterization testing of live-virus based vaccines and gene therapy products part1. *Bioprocess Int*. 2006;4:46–56.

242   THE MANUFACTURE OF GENETIC VIRAL VECTOR PRODUCTS

12. NIH Recombinant DNA Advisory Committee. Assessment of adsenoviral vector safety and toxicity: report of the National Institutes of Health Recombinant DNA Advisory Committee. *Hum Gene Ther* 2002;13:3–13.
13. Nyberg-Hoffman C, Shabram P, Li W, Giroux D, Aguilar-Cordova E. Sensitivity and reproducibility in adenoviral infectious titer determination. *Nat Med*. 1997;3:808–811.
14. Chuck AS, Clarke MF, Palsson BO. Retroviral infection is limited by Brownian motion. *Hum Gene Ther*. 1996;7:1527–1534.
15. Andreadis S, Lavery T, Davis HE, Le Doux JM, Yarmush ML, Morgan JR. Toward a more accurate quantitation of the activity of recombinant retroviruses: alternatives to titer and multiplicity of infection. *J Virol*. 2000;74:3431–3439.
16. Sastry L, Xu Y, Cooper R, Pollok K, Cornetta K. Evaluation of plasmid DNA removal from lentiviral vectors by benzonase treatment. *Hum Gene Ther*. 2004;15:221–226.
17. Sweeney JA, Hennessey JPJr. Evaluation of accuracy and precision of adenovirus absorptivity at 260nm under conditions of complete DNA disruption. *Virology* 2002;295: 284–288.
18. Kiermer V, Borellini F, Lu X, et al. Report form the Lentivirus Working Group. *Bioprocess J*. 2005;4:39–42.
19. Wadman M. London's disastrous drug trial has serious side effects for research. *Nature* 2006;440:388–389.
20. Restivo G. The PAT Initiative. *Bioprocess Int*. 2005;3:24–26.
21. Kamen A, Henry O. Development and optimization of an adenovirus production process. *J Gene Med*. 2004;6:S184–S192.
22. Burova E, Ioffe E. Chromatographic purification of recombinant adenoviral and adeno-associated viral vectors: methods and implications *Gene Ther*. 2005;12,S5–S17.
23. Howley PM, Griffin DE, Martin MA, Roizman B, Straus SE, Knipe DM, eds. *Fields Virology*. 4th ed. Philadelphia, PA: Lippincott Williams, & Wilkins; 2001.
24. Hackett NR, Crystal RG Adenovirus vectors for gene therapy. In: Templeton NS, ed., *Gene and Cell Therapy*. New York: Marcel Dekker; 2004.
25. Altaras NE, Aunins JG, Evans RK, Kamen A, Konz JO, Wolf JJ. Production and formulation of adenovirus vectors. *Adv Biochem Eng Biotechnol*. 2005;99:193–260.
26. Shiver JW, Emilio A, Emini EA, Recent advances in the development of HIV-1 vaccines using replication incompetyent adenovirus vectors. *Annu Rev Med*. 2004;55:355–372.
27. Grines CL, Watkins MW, Helmer G, et al. Angiogenic gene therapy (AGENT) trial in patients with stable angina pectoris. *Circulation*. 2002;105:1291–1297.
28. Howe JA, Pelka P, Antelman D, et al. Matching complementing functions of transformed cells with stable expression of selected viral genes for production of *E1*-deleted adenovirus vectors. *Virology* 2006;345:220–230.
29. Palmer DJ, Ng P. Helper–dependent adenoviral vectors for gene therapy. *Hum Gene Ther*. 2005;16:1–16.
30. Palmer D, Ng P. Improved system for helper-dependent adenoviral vector production. *Mol Ther*. 2003;8:846–852.
31. Working PK, Lin A, Borellini F. Meeting product development challenges in manufacturing clinical grade oncolytic adenoviruses. *Oncogene* 2005;24:7792–7801.

32. Carter BJ. Adeno-associated virus vector in clinical trials. *Hum Gene Ther*. 2005;16:541–550.

33. Merten O-W, Geny-Fiamma C, Douar AM. Current issues in adeno-associated viral vector production. *Genet Ther*. 2005;12:S51–S61.

34. Grieger JC, Samulski RJ. Adeno-associated virus as a gene therapy vector: vector development, production and clinical applications. *Adv Biochem Eng Biotechnol*. 2005;99:119–145.

35. Carter BJ. Presentation at Phacilitate Cell and Gene Therapy Forum, Washington, DC, January 2005.

36. Sheridan PL, Bodner M, Lynn A, et al. Generation of retroviral packaging and producer cell lines for large-scale vector production and clinical application: improved safety and high titer. *Mol Ther*. 2000;2:262–275.

37. Cornetta K, Matheson L, Ballas C. Retroviral vector production in the National Gene Vector Laboratory at Indiana University. *Genet Ther* 2005;12:28–35.

38. Hacein-Bey-Abina S, Von Kalle C, Schmidt M, et al. LMO2-associated clonal T cell proliferation in two patients after gene therapy for SCID-X1. *Science*. 2003;302:415–419.

39. Woods NB, Bottero V, Schmidt M, von Kalle C, Verma IM. Gene therapy: therapeutic gene causing lymphoma. *Nature*. 2006;440:1123.

40. Ott MG, Schmidt M, Schwarzwaelder K, et al. Correction of X-linked chronic granulomatous disease by gene therapy, augmented by insertional activation of *MDS1-EVI1*, *PRDM16 or SETBP1*. *Nat Med*. 2006;12:401–409.

41. Jolly DJ. Lentiviral vector. In: Templeton NS, *Gene and Cell Therapy*. 2nd ed. New York: Marcel Dekkers.

42. Manilla P, Rebello T, Afable C, et al. Regulatory considerations for novel gene therapy products: a review of the process leading to the first clinical lentiviral vector. *Hum Gene Ther*. 2005;16:17–25.

43. Lu X. Presentation at Phacilitate Cell and Gene Therapy Forum, Washington, DC, January 2005.

44. Kordower JH, Emborg ME, Bloch J, et al. Neurodegeneration prevented by lentiviral vector delivery of GDNF in primate models of Parkinson's disease. *Science*. 2000;290:767–773.

45. Yanez-Munoz RJ, Balaggan KS, Macneil A, et al. Effective gene therapy with nonintegrating lentiviral vectors. *Nat Med*. 2006;12:348–353.

46. Dubensky TW, Polo JM, Jolly DJ. Alpha-virus based vectors. In: Templeton NS, Lasic DD, eds. *Gene Therapy, Therapeutic Mechanisms and Strategies*. New York: Marcel Dekker; 2000.

47. Rao V, Hinz ME, Roberts BA, Fine D. Toxicity assessment of Venezuelan equine encephalitis virus vaccine candidate strain V3526. *Vaccine*. 2006;24:1710–1715.

48. Polo JM, Belli BA, Driver DA, et al. Stable alphavirus packaging cell lines for Sindbis virus and Semliki forest virus-derived vectors. *Proc Natl Acad Sci U S A*. April 13; 1999;96(8):4598–4603.

49. Davis NL, Caley IJ, Brown KW, et al. Vaccination of macaques against pathogenic simian immunodeficiency virus with Venezuelan equine encephalitis virus replicon particles. *J Virol*. 2000;74:371–378.

50. Moroziewicz D, Kaufman HL. Gene therapy with poxvirus vectors. *Curr Opin Mol Ther*. 2005;7:317–325.

51. Aghi M, Martuza ML. Oncolytic viral therapies: the clinical experience. *Oncogene*. 2005;24:7802–7816.

52. Markert JM, Medlock MD, Rabkin SD, et al. Conditionally replicating herpes simplex virus mutant, G207 for the treatment of malignant glioma: results of a phase I trial. *Gene Ther*. 2000;7:867–874.

53. Jiang C, Wechuck JB, Goins WF, et al. Immobilized cobalt affinity chromatography provides a novel, efficient method for herpes simplex virus type 1 gene vector purification. *J Virol* 2004;78:8994–9006.

54. Epstein AL. HSV-1-based amplicon vectors: design and applications. *Gene Ther*. 2005;12 (Suppl 1):S154–S158.

55. Peng K-W, Facteau S, Wegman T, O'Kane D, Russell SJ. Non-invasive in vivo monitoring of trackable viruses expressing soluble marker peptides. *Nat Med*. 2002;8:527–531.

56. Myers R, Greiner S, Harvey M, et al. Oncolytic activities of approved mumps and measles vaccines for therapy of ovarian cancer. *Cancer Gene Ther*. 2005;12:593–599.

57. Farson D, Harding TC, Tao L, et al. Development and characterization of a cell line for large-scale, serum-free production of recombinant adeno-associated viral vectors. *J Gene Med*. 2004;6:1369–1381.

58. Montgomery SA. An evolving technology. *Bioprocess Int*. October 2005;Suppl: 4–8.

59. Campochiaro PA, Nguyen QD, Shah SM, et al. Adenoviral vector– delivered pigment epithelium-derived factor for neovascular age-related macular degeneration: results of a phase I clinical trial. *Hum Gene Ther*. 2006;17:167–176.

60. Powell JS, Ragni MV, White GC 2nd, et al. Phase 1 trial of FVIII gene transfer for severe hemophilia A using a retroviral construct administered by peripheral intravenous infusion. *Blood*. 2003;102:2038–2045.

61. Excler J-L. AIDS vaccine development: perspectives, challenges and hopes. *Indian J Med Res*. 2005;121:568–581.

20 The Manufacture of Adeno-Associated Viral Vectors

RICHARD PELUSO

Targeted Genetics Corporation, Seattle, Washington

This chapter is intended to provide the reader with an up-to-date understanding of the manufacture of recombinant adeno-associated virus (rAAV)–based vectors for early research and proof-of-concept studies up to later-stage product development and clinical use. Most rAAV vectors in the clinic are based on the capsid of serotype 2 AAV, but there is increased interest in exploring the advantages that alternative serotypes of AAV may be able to provide: namely, the ability to more effectively transduce a specific cell/tissue/organ system, thereby lowering the dose of vector needed and/or increasing the safety of the therapy (Hildinger and Auricchio, 2004). Any of the manufacturing systems discussed here is capable of generating vectors from any serotype. In practice, most vectors based on capsids other than AAV2 are pseudotyped vectors, containing AAV2 inverted repeat sequences flanking an expression cassette packaged in a capsid from a different serotype. Separate scalable purification methods will need to be developed for any new serotype envisioned to move to the clinic.

There is a misconception in the minds of some not closely involved with rAAV manufacture that scalable processes needed for eventual commercial manufacture of these vectors is problematic and difficult. It is the intent of this short communication to dispel this misconception by reviewing the progress that has been made in developing scalable production methods for the commercial manufacture of AAV-based vectors.

PROPERTIES OF AAV

AAV is a member of the dependo group of parvoviruses, and as such is replication defective and must be supplied with helper functions for a productive infection cycle. The helper functions usually come from adenovirus or herpes viruses, and the genes necessary are known in each case. AAV itself is quite a simple animal

Concepts in Genetic Medicine, Edited by Boro Dropulic and Barrie Carter
Copyright © 2008 John Wiley & Sons, Inc.

virus, possessing just two genes, *rep* and *cap*. The *rep* gene encodes four proteins from two promoters, and the *cap* gene encodes three proteins from a single promoter. The *rep* gene products are involved in replication and packaging of the viral ssDNA genome, and the *cap* gene products assemble into the icosahedral viral capsid, the substrate for virus and vector assembly (Myers and Carter, 1980; King et al., 2001). The ends of the viral genome are flanked by short (~145 to 150 nt, depending on serotype), inverted terminal repeat sequences (ITRs) that fold into a T-shaped structure. The ITRs are the only AAV-specific sequences needed in vectors, since they contain all of the information needed for replication and packaging of the DNA into capsids. Therefore, to make an AAV-based vector, one needs to bring together into a cell the *rep* and *cap* genes, the vector construct flanked by AAV ITRs, and the necessary helper functions. Wild-type AAV is approximately 4.7 kb; although it is possible to package DNA larger than this into a particle, the efficiency drops as the size increases much beyond 4.8 to 5.0 kb (Dong et al., 1996; Grieger and Samulski, 2005).

PLASMID TRANSFECTION-BASED MANUFACTURE

The earliest vector production systems were based on plasmid transfection and are still useful for manufacture of vector for research studies (Grimm et al., 1998; Matsushita et al., 1998; Salvetti et al., 1998; Xiao et al., 1998). A widely used system utilizes three plasmids; one (the *cis* plasmid) contains the rAAV vector that is to be packaged (i.e., the expression cassette flanked by AAV ITRs), a second (the *trans* plasmid) contains the AAV *rep* and *cap* genes, and a third (the *helper* plasmid) contains the necessary helper functions, usually the adenovirus *E2a*, *E4*, and *VA* genes, with the *E1* gene provided by the cell. These plasmids are mixed and co-transfected into 293 cells (Figure 20.1). After three days the cells are harvested and vector is purified. This method of vector manufacture can be highly productive, generating up to 50,000 to 100,000 genome-containing vector particles per cell. In this approach to vector production the cis plasmid is construct specific (meaning that it contains the DNA sequences to be packaged into vector particles), and the trans plasmid contains the cap gene from the serotype of AAV being manufactured. Although this method can be high yielding, it is limited in terms of scalability, due to the fact that it uses cells in attached mode coupled with DNA transfection. In addition, plasmid supply for large-scale manufacturing can be difficult and expensive to generate. This production method is limited in scalability, limiting its ultimate utility for large-scale commercial manufacture. However, it has been used to generate clinical-grade vectors for small phase I trials.

SCALABLE PRODUCTION SYSTEMS

Alternatives to plasmid transfection for vector manufacture have been developed around industry-standard scalable unit operations, including stirred tank

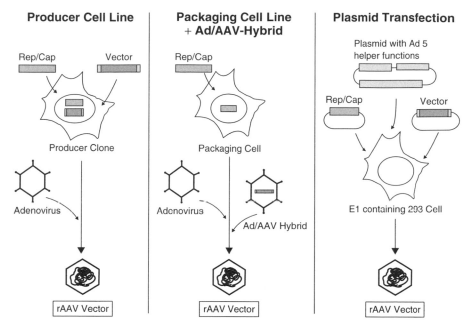

Figure 20.1   Three approaches to the manufacture of AAV vectors used most often. In the left panel, a producer cell clone containing the AAV *rep* and *cap* genes along with the vector genome construct is made and infected with adenovirus to generate AAV vectors. The center panel depicts the use of a packaging cell line containing the AAV *rep* and *cap* genes. The packaging cell is infected with adenovirus, then superinfected with an Ad/AAV hybrid virus to generate AAV vectors. The third panel depicts vector manufacture using triple-plasmid transfection. Details on each method of vector manufacture are provided in the text

bioreactors and automated chromatographic purification systems, using cells in suspension culture. These systems are scalable and have thus far been carried out at 2-, 10-, and 100-L scales with no limitations foreseen up to 2000-L reactors. Although little space is spent here discussing vector purification, it is worth pointing out that scalable automated column chromatography-based purification systems are in place or are being developed for each of the large-scale manufacturing systems that are discussed using industry-standard ion-exchange resins and other chromatography substrates (see below).

A number of investigators have attempted to develop vector production systems that delivered the *rep* and *cap* genes as part of a recombinant adenovirus, and all ultimately have failed, most often due to the instability of the *rep* gene in adenovirus. Rep protein is toxic to cells and also to adenovirus (Fisher et al., 1996; Saudan et al., 2000; Schmidt et al., 2000; Zhang et al., 2001), so most scalable manufacturing methods have been based on engineered HeLa cells orA549 cells, which appear to be more resistant to the toxic effects of rep proteins and use adenovirus to provide helper functions or to deliver the rAAV genome to the cell (Clark et al., 1995; Gao et al., 1998,2002; Farson et al., 2004; Zolotukhin, 2005).

There are two general systems in use, a producer clone-based system and an adenovirus Ad/AAV hybrid-based system (Figure 20.1). In the producer clone method, a cell is engineered to contain the *rep* and *cap* genes of AAV and the vector genome of interest. One can start with a generic *rep/cap*-containing packaging cell line as a substrate for introduction of the product-specific rAAV construct, or a single plasmid containing *rep, cap*, and rAAV sequences can be introduced into a naive cell. In either case, candidate clones are screened and a clone is selected based on productivity and growth characteristics. Screening, as well as vector production, is carried out by infection of the cell clone with wild-type adenovirus, which provides helper functions for replication of rAAV as well as inducing the synthesis of the AAV *rep* and *cap* proteins. A new producer cell clone is generated for each product. Productivity is clone dependent and can be as high or higher as that from the best transfection-based methods. Yields of over 100,000 genome-containing particles per cell have been achieved in bioreactor cultures.

In the Ad/AAV-hybrid method, a serotype-specific "generic" packaging cell line is made that contains the AAV *rep* and *cap* genes. This packaging cell line can be used to manufacture any vector of interest, and one can be made for each AAV capsid serotype. The product-specific component in this system is a recombinant adenovirus that harbors the rAAV genome, usually in the position normally occupied by the adenovirus E1 gene (Gao et al., 1998; Liu et al., 1999). It is a simple, efficient, and short task to generate a recombinant Ad/AAV hybrid, and there are a number of plasmid-based systems that can be used for this (He et al., 1998; Mizuguchi and Kay, 1999). To manufacture rAAV vectors, the packaging cell line is infected with wild-type adenovirus to induce the synthesis of the AAV *rep* and *cap* gene products and provide the helper functions for rAAV replication from adenovirus (Gao et al., 1998; Liu et al., 1999). The infected cells are then superinfected with the (Ad)/AAV hybrid virus. Vector particles are purified from the cells at the end of the production, and adenoviruses are removed by chromatographic separation methods used in vector purification and easily inactivated by heat. The multiplicity of infection of each of the adenoviruses and the timing of superinfection are critical parameters that need to be optimized for each packaging cell line. Productivity is packaging cell dependent, is somewhat independent of Ad/AAV hybrid construct, and is as high or higher as that seen from the best transfection-based methods. Yields of over 100,000 genome-containing particles per cell have been achieved in bioreactor cultures.

There are separate advantages of each of these two scalable, adenovirus-based manufacturing methods. In the Ad/AAV hybrid method, one can engineer, select, and bank generic, serotype-specific but "product-general" packaging cell lines and use them in conjunction with any Ad/AAV hybrid. GMP-tested and released cell banks can be made, their growth in suspension bioreactors can be optimized, and these cells and optimal growth conditions can be used for the manufacture of any rAAV vector in a given packaging cell line by using a product-specific Ad/AAV hybrid. Generation of the Ad/AAV hybrid is easier, faster, and less expensive than screening, banking, and testing a cell bank. In addition, the productivity is dependent on properties of the packaging cell used as opposed to the Ad/AAV hybrid, making the vector yields predictable from product to product within a cell line.

Product-specific producer clones for vector manufacture are most useful when a product has been chosen for later-stage clinical development, a stage where it is worth the time, effort, and expense needed to generate a high-yield clone with favorable growth and yield characteristics. The advantage is an overall reduced cost of goods since manufacture of a product-specific AAV/Ad hybrid is not needed. It is possible to begin a clinical development program using vector generated from the Ad/AAV hybrid manufacturing method because of its speed to the clinic and change to a producer clone method in phase III trials, when there is a commitment to a product, if it is felt to be worth the effort needed to engineer an optimal product-specific cell clone.

Potentially scalable and high-yielding systems are being developed using herpes viruses to provide helper functions, and most recently, vector has been generated in insect cells using recombinant baculoviruses.

Unlike adenovirus, herpes simplex viruses (HSVs) carrying *rep* genes are stable, and the *rep* protein does not hinder production of the recombinant HSV. A system has been described that combined a recombinant HSV (rHSV, containing the *rep* and *cap* genes) with a deletion in an essential HSV gene (ICP27) with an engineered cell line containing the rAAV construct stably integrated (Conway et al., 1999). Infection of the cell with the rHSV resulted in apparently high levels of vector production. Several groups are working to develop all HSV-based manufacturing systems by combining *rep* and *cap* in one rHSV vector and the rAAV construct in a second rHSV vector, and HSV mutants were screened to evaluate productivity (Booth et al., 2004; Toublanc et al., 2004). At this point, all of these approaches use cells in attached mode, but there is the possibility that further work will yield suspension systems that could be adapted to bioreactors.

A recent report describes the use of insect cells and recombinant baculoviruses for potentially scalable vector production (Urabe et al., 2002). Additional work on this system is being carried out in a number of laboratories, with efforts aimed at understanding the critical components of this insect cell–based vector manufacturing system, the stability of the components, and the properties of the vectors that are produced, focused on determining how this approach can best be used for generating high-quality potent clinical-grade vectors for product development.

PURIFICATION

A detailed description of all of the vector purification methods that have been reported is beyond the scope of this short overview. However, a number of scalable purification schemes, using industry-standard chromatographic separation methods and resins, have been reported (Clark et al., 1999; Gao et al.,

2000; O'Riordan et al., 2000; Drittanti et al., 2001; Anderson et al., 2000; Brument et al., 2002; Kaludov et al., 2002; Zolotukhin et al., 2002; Smith et al., 2003; Blankinship et al., 2004; Davidoff et al., 2004), mostly for AAV2 vectors, although there have been reports of purification of AAV1, 4, 5, 6, and 8. Any purification scheme designed to yield vector suitable for product development/clinical use must not only achieve vector in reasonable yields, but must accomplish removal of process-related impurities, including serum components, cellular proteins and DNA, helper viruses, and helper virus proteins, and demonstrate the ability to remove or inactivate adventitious viruses, resulting in vectors with adequate purity and safety for use in human subjects. Therefore, although potentially suitable for research studies, it is unlikely that a single-step purification scheme would be suitable for vector of sufficient quality for use in a clinical trial.

CONCLUSIONS

It is hoped that the reader of this brief chapter understands the state of the art in scalable rAAV manufacturing and sees that there are few impediments to commercial manufacture of vectors in industry-standard stirred-tank bioreactors. Coupled with scalable chromatographic purification methodology that is in place or being developed for many serotypes of AAV, the development of rAAV as a gene therapy or vaccine vector system will not be held back by manufacturing considerations.

REFERENCES

Anderson R, MacDonald I, Corbett T, Whiteway A, Prentice GH (2000). A method for the preparation of highly purified adeno-associated virus using affinity column chromatography, protease digestion and solvent extraction. *J Virol Methods*. 85:23–34.

Blankinship MJ, Gregorevic P, Allen JM, et al. (2004). Efficient transduction of skeletal muscle using vectors based on adeno-associated virus serotype 6. *Mol Ther.* 10: 671–678.

Booth MJ, Mistry A, Li X, Thrasher A, Coffin RS (2004). Transfection-free and scaleable recombinant AAV vector production using HSV/AAV hybrids. *Gene Ther.* 11:829–837.

Brument N, Morenweiser R, Blouin V, et al. (2002). A versatile and scalable two-step ion-exchange chromatography process for the purification of recombinant adeno-associated virus serotypes-2 and -5. *Mol Ther.* 6:678–686.

Clark KR, Voulgaropoulou F, Fraley DM, Johnson PR (1995). Cell lines for the production of recombinant adeno-associated virus. *Hum Gene Ther.* 6:1329–1341.

Clark KR, Liu X, McGrath JP, Johnson PR (1999). Highly purified recombinant adeno-associated virus vectors are biologically active and free of detectable helper and wild-type viruses. *Hum Gene Ther.* 10:1031–1039.

Conway JE, Rhys CM, Zolotukhin I, et al. (1999). High-titer recombinant adeno-associated virus production utilizing a recombinant herpes simplex virus type 1 vector expressing AAV-2 Rep and Cap. *Gene Ther.* 9:986–993.

Davidoff AM, Ng CYC, Sleep S, et al. (2004). Purification of recombinant adeno-associated virus type 8 vectors by ion exchange chromatography generates clinical grade vector stocks. *J Virol Methods.* 121:209–215.

Dong JY, Fan PD, Frizzell RA (1996). Quantitative analysis of the packaging capacity of recombinant adeno-associated virus. *Hum Gene Ther.* 7:2101–2112.

Drittanti L, Jenny C, Poulard K, et al. (2001). Optimised helper virus-free production of high-quality adeno-associated virus vectors. *J Gene Med.* 3:59–71.

Farson D, Harding TC, Tao L, et al. (2004). Development and characterization of a cell line for large-scale, serum-free production of recombinant adeno-associated viral vectors. *J Gene Med.* 6:1369–1381.

Fisher KJ, Kelley WM, Burda JF, Wilson JM (1996). A novel adenovirus-adeno-associated virus hybrid vector that displays efficient rescue and delivery of the AAV genome. *Hum Gene Ther.* 7:2079–2087.

Gao GP, Qu G, Faust LZ, et al. (1998). High-titer adeno-associated viral vectors from a Rep/Cap cell line and hybrid shuttle virus. *Hum Gene Ther.* 9:2353–2362.

Gao GP, Qu G, Burnham MS, et al. (2000). Purification of recombinant adeno-associated virus vectors by column chromatography and its performance in vivo. *Hum Gene Ther.* 11:2079–2091.

Gao GP, Lu F, Sanmiguel JC, et al. (2002). Rep/Cap gene amplification and high-yield production of AAV in an A549 cell line expressing Rep/Cap. *Mol Ther.* 5:644–649.

Grieger JC, Samulski RJ (2005). Packaging capacity of adeno-associated virus serotypes: impact of larger genomes on infectivity and post entry steps. *J Virol.* 79:9933–9944.

Grimm D, Kern A, Rittner K, Kleinschmidt JA (1998). Novel tools for production and purification of recombinant adeno-associated virus vectors. *Hum Gene Ther.* 9: 2745–2760.

He TC, Zhou S, daCosta LT, Yu J, Kinzler KW, Vogelstein B (1998). A simplified system for generating recombinant adenoviruses. *Proc Natl Acad Sci U S A.* 95:2509–2514.

Hildinger M, Auricchio A (2004). Advances in AAV-mediated gene transfer for the treatment of inherited disorders. *Eur J Hum Genet.* 12:263–271.

Kaludov N, Handelman B, Chiorini JA (2002). Scalable purification of adeno-associated virus type 2, 4, or 5 using ion-exchange chromatography. *Hum Gene Ther.* 13: 1235–1243.

King JA, Dubielzig R, Grimm D, Kleinschmidt JA (2001). DNA helicase-mediated packaging of adeno-associated virus type 2 genomes into preformed capsids. *EMBO J.* 20:3282–3291.

Liu XL, Clark KR, Johnson PR (1999). Production of recombinant adeno-associated virus vectors using a packaging cell line and a hybrid recombinant adenovirus. *Gene Ther.* 6:293–299.

Matsushita T, Elliger S, Elliger C, et al. (1998). Adeno-associated virus vectors can be efficiently produced without helper virus. *Gene Ther.* 5:938–945.

Mizuguchi H, Kay MA (1999). A simple method for constructing *E1*-and *E1/E4*-deleted recombinant adenoviral vectors. *Hum Gene Ther.* 10:2013–2017.

Myers MW, Carter BJ (1980). Assembly of adeno-associated virus. *Virology.* 102:71–82.

O'Riordan CR, Lachapelle AL, Vincent KA, Wadsworth SC (2000). Scalable chromatographic purification process for recombinant adeno-associated virus (rAAV). *J Gene Med.* 2:444–454.

Salvetti A, Oreve S, Chadeuf G, et al. (1998). Factors influencing recombinant adenoassociated virus production. *Hum Gene Ther.* 9:695–706.

Saudan P, Vlach J, Beard P (2000). Inhibition of S-phase progression by adeno-associated virus Rep78 protein is mediated by hypophosphorylated pRb. *EMBO J.* 19:4351–4361.

Schmidt M, Afione S, Kotin RM (2000). Adeno-associated virus type 2 Rep78 induces apoptosis through caspase activation independently of p53. *J Virol.* 74:9441–9450.

Smith RH, Ding C, Kotin RM (2003). Serum-free production and column purification of adeno-associated virus type 5. *J Virol Methods.* 114:115–124.

Toublanc E, Benraiss A, Bonnin D, et al. (2004). Identification of a replication-defective herpes simplex virus for recombinant adeno-associated virus type 2 (rAAV2) particle assembly using stable producer cell lines. *J Gene Med.* 6:555–564.

Urabe M, Ding C, Kotin RM (2002). Insect cells as a factory to produce adeno-associated virus type 2 vectors. *Hum Gene Ther.* 13:1935–1943.

Xiao X, Li J, Samulski RJ (1998). Production of high-titer adeno-associated virus vectors in the absence of helper virus. *J Virol.* 72:2224–2232.

Zhang HG, Wang YM, Xie JF, et al. (2001). Recombinant adenovirus expressing adenoassociated virus Cap and Rep proteins supports production of high-titer recombinant adeno-associated virus. *Gene Ther.* 8:704–712.

Zolotukhin S (2005). Production of recombinant adeno-associated virus vectors. *Hum Gene Ther.* 16:551–557.

Zolotukhin S, Potter M, Zolotukhin I, et al. (2002). Production and purification of serotype 1, 2, and 5 recombinant adeno-associated viral vectors. *Methods.* 28:158–167.

21 Lentivirus Vector Manufacturing

GWENDOLYN K. BINDER

Abramson Family Cancer Research Institute,
School of Medicine, University of Pennsylvania,
Philadelphia, Pennsylvania

BORO DROPULIC

Lentigen Corporation, Baltimore, Maryland

Lentiviral vector manufacture is technically challenging. Even small-scale vector production, although reasonably straightforward on paper, often results in a frustrating unpredictable titer variation. Over the past decade, researchers have sought to identify factors at each production step that optimize production and preserve titer, in particular to enable production scale-up. Courtesy of the lessons learned from retroviral vectors, the lentiviral vector field has experienced a notably rapid advancement.

Manufacture of vector that is suitable for application in clinical trials, otherwise called *clinical grade*, present further challenges in scalability, purity, and cost. The first lentiviral vector clinical trials are under way, and the method for virus manufacture in these first trials has been published by the Williamsburg Bioprocessing Foundation.[1] The purification methods used for clinical-grade manufacture have been drawn largely from existing technology for virus and protein purification as well as previously reported optimized retroviral vector production data.

Vector manufacture comprises upstream and downstream processes, and release testing. Upstream processes include DNA production and purification, transfection of cells for virus production and associated culture conditions, and vector collection. Alternatively, it includes establishment of a packaging/producer cell line, production and associated culture conditions, and collection. Downstream processes include the clarification (removal of gross cellular debris), concentration, and optionally purification of the vector. Release testing involves titration and optional testing for a replication-competent lentivirus (RCL). For clinical-grade vector, the release testing is far more vigorous and includes testing for

Concepts in Genetic Medicine, Edited by Boro Dropulic and Barrie Carter
Copyright © 2008 John Wiley & Sons, Inc.

potency, identity, purity, and safety (including RCL), which are on a sliding scale of GMP (good manufacturing practice) compliance from phase I through phase III trials and onto product registration. Current release testing of clinical-grade vector has been reported only for phase I and II production.[2]

Various methods exist for lentiviral vector manufacture. The optimal method for a given application depends on the flexibility needed in the system, the scale desired, and the purity warranted by its application. As examples, in the experimental setting, high flexibility, small scale, and lower purity is acceptable. Therefore small-scale transient transfection followed by concentration by centrifugation is typically sufficient.[3] For animal experiments, higher purity is required to avoid robust immunogenicity, and thus small-scale production by transient transfection might be followed by sucrose gradient ultracentrifugation.[4] Clinical application requires larger-scale production, preferably in the absence of serum, by transient transfection or by a producer cell line in cell factories (or other large-scale cell culture system, such as a cell cube[5,6]), followed by extensive concentration, purification, and release testing.[7] As clinical-grade vector is made on a larger scale when trials advance into later phases with more patients, a producer cell line that can be grown at industry scale, such as in a bioreactor, must be developed. Purification methods are limited by their scalability, and preservation of vector potency is a challenge with scalable purification.

In this chapter we present an overview of elements in upstream manufacture that lead to optimized vector production, and current options for downstream purification are discussed. Unique aspects of release testing, in particular for detection of a replication-competent lentivirus, and optimal titer assays are given.

UPSTREAM PROCESSES

Viral vector can be produced by transient transfection or by a stable packaging cell line. In the past, retroviral vectors were made primarily by stable cell lines, as the packaging components were not toxic to the cells, and therefore these cells yielded high titers. In contrast, lentiviral vectors have several proteins that are toxic to cells, the protease (in *gag*),[8] *env*,[9] *tat*,[10] *rev*,[11] and *vpr* (although *vpr* is not used in current generation vectors).[12] In addition, constitutive expression of the VSV-G protein is also toxic to cells.[13] Due to this, lentiviral vectors were first produced in the laboratory by transient transfection in order to achieve high-enough titers. Over the years, packaging cell lines have evolved for regulated expression of packaging genes and have achieved stable high titer production of vectors. At the research scale, transient transfection remains the preferred method for production, due to the labor-intensive process of selecting high producer cell line clones. The first clinical lentiviral vector was also produced by transient transfection.[14] However, as clinical application of lentiviral vectors progresses, cell lines will ultimately be the primary source for production, both for scalability and for purity. Purity is higher with stable cell lines because transient transfection results in high levels of DNA contamination, which can be reduced by benzonase treatment but is difficult to remove entirely.

Transient Transfection

Vector production by transfection is the most common method for production. Production systems have used two,[15] three,[16] four,[17] or five[18] plasmids for vector manufacture. Increasing the number of plasmids is typically done to improve safety by reducing the chance for recombination. However, the two-plasmid system was used for the first lentiviral vector clinical trials, and the extensive safety engineering ensured safety of the production system.[15] Fewer numbers of plasmids reduces the costs of large-scale manufacture and may result in higher production yields during scale-up.

Notably, transient transfection for retroviral vector production was not successful until it was found that inclusion of the SV40 origin of replication in the expression plasmids, and incorporation of these plasmids into cells expressing the SV40 T antigen (such as 293T cells) greatly enhanced gene expression.[19] When combined with strong constitutive expression by a promoter such as the cytomegalovirus (CMV) promoter, expression levels were high enough to achieve titers useful for research.[20]

Transfection of DNA into mammalian cells by calcium phosphate requires circular DNA, as linear DNA is virtually ineffective.[21] Therefore, the ratio of linear to closed circular DNA is important for transfection efficiency. Closed circular DNA can be isolated preferentially by density gradient using the cesium chloride/ethidium bromide standard molecular technique.[22] This may be suitable for small-scale production, but it is not a scalable process. As the field of gene therapy and gene based vaccines has advanced, the need for development of large-scale plasmid purification has expanded. Purification of DNA by charge using column chromatography has been around since the 1960s.[23,24] Current application of hydroxyapatite columns or anion-exchange chromatography offer the opportunity to produce highly purified plasmid DNA that distinguish between closed circular and linear DNA under certain conditions.[25–27] Recently, plasmid purification by tangential flow filtration has been reported, which is also scalable and is in general a simpler approach to purification.[28] Plasmids produced by any of these methods have been shown to retain their ability to transfect cells efficiently, although a comprehensive side-by-side comparison of efficiency has not been published.

Transfection efficiency is a critical step in optimizing titers. Small-scale transfection by SuperFect (Qiagen) reports high titers with low amounts of DNA.[29] Direct comparison between Fugene (Roche) and calcium phosphate precipitation showed equivalency in vector production.[18] A study comparing three commonly used transfection techniques—Lipofectamine 2000, calcium phosphate precipitation in HEPES-buffered saline, or calcium phosphate precipitation in N,N-bis(2-hydroxyethyl)-2-aminoethanesulfonic acid (BES)—found that calcium phosphate precipitation in BES produced twice as much virus as did the other two methods.[30] Surprisingly, using this method, DNA purified either by the cesium chloride technique or by Qiagen column (which does not distinguish between closed circular and linear DNA) resulted in equivalent titers, suggesting that the far simpler Qiagen purification method may be suitable for small-scale laboratory production of lentiviral vector.

The amount of DNA used in the transfection is directly related to the efficiency of gene transfer, as more DNA results in a coarser precipitate that reduces delivery.[21] A lower pH of the calcium phosphate solution leads to slower formation of this precipitate (the phosphate DNA complex), which seems to improve transfer efficiencies. Higher DNA concentration leading to lower vector titers has been reported by others.[30,31] For optimal vector production, the appropriate stoichiometry of the packaging plasmids must be determined empirically, in part due to the toxicity of packaging genes.[32]

Transfection by calcium phosphate is attractive for scale-up since it is cheaper than commercially available specialty reagents. Scale-up is straightforward using multi-level tissue culture trays or cell factories (Nunc). These are 632-cm^2 tissue culture trays that are offered in single-, double-, four-, 10-, or 40-tray options, and they carry a recommended 200 mL of culture media per tray. To reduce volumes for transfection and concentration of virus produced, volumes of 100 mL per tray can be used.[29] Using this technology, vector production can be linearly scaled up to many liters of vector. Alternative large-scale culture vessels such as roller bottles or a cell cube are not ideal for transient transfection since they do not allow the precipitate to fall on the cells overnight, and therefore are likely to yield lower production efficiency.

It is well known that histone acetylation is associated with areas of high gene transcription.[33] Histone acetylation is also associated with improved expression of plasmid DNA in the cell.[34] Sodium butyrate inhibits deacetylation of histones and can therefore be used to boost gene expression in vitro.[35] Several groups have reported improved vector production after exposure of cells to 10 mM sodium butyrate.[20,31,30] One report did not find an improved titer for VSV-G pseudotyped vector after induction, although production of vectors pseudotyped with other envelopes was improved[31]; however, this is probably a result of a later addition of the butyrate to the culture (16 hours posttransfection instead of just prior to transfection).

Removal of serum from the collection phase of vector production significantly reduces the immunogenicity of the vector produced.[4] Somewhat surprisingly, when using the appropriate serum-free media, production titers generally do not decrease. Culturing cells in the absence of serum but without optimizing the medium to that specialized for serum-free conditions indeed resulted in a drop in titer of about five fold.[4] Removing the serum only at the time of production yielded similar titers but resulted in a shorter collection time due to cell death.[18] This could be a result of the shock to the cells of the late change in serum. Plating and transfection of cells in serum-free media did not result in significant viability issues, and higher vector titers were achieved, possibly as a result of removal of a serum binding factor.[36] The results from these studies are encouraging and indicate that serum can easily be removed from vector production, at least on a small scale.

Collection of vector usually occurs between 24 and 48 hours posttransfection, and sometimes will go as late as 72 hours posttransfection. Around 48 hours, the titers start to decline and cellular debris increases, due to cell toxicity from the transfection and from the *gag* and *VSV-G* genes, which are toxic to the cells.[8,13] Temperature plays a significant role in the stability of retrovirus in culture, and harvest at a lower temperature, such as 32°C, tends to preserve titers at later times.[37,38] Vector is stable if stored appropriately at −80°C, but about 25% of titer is lost during each of the first two freeze–thaws.[37]

Packaging Cell Lines

As mentioned above, packaging cell lines for lentiviral vector production were challenging at first, due to the toxicity of many of the genes expressed in the cell. The toxicity led to low viral titers in the very first cell lines, of no better than 2×10^4 TU/mL.[39,40] To improve titers by reducing cellular toxicity, the packaging genes were placed under the control of the tetracycline response element for inducible expression.[9] This particular cell line used a two-level *tet* off system, where the tTA (the *tet*-controlled transcriptional regulator, described in Gossen and Bujard[41]) controlled the expression of *rev* and HIV *env* by the tetracycline response element (TRE). *Rev*, in turn, drove the expression of the *gag-pol* gene. Although the inducible system worked, titers did not improve.

Replacement of the HIV envelope with the VSV-G envelope in an inducible expression vector greatly improved titers.[42] In this cell line, the envelope was expressed under the control of TRE and on a separate plasmid, all of the HIV proteins minus the envelope were expressed as well under the TRE. This packaging cell yielded titers of over 1×10^6 TU/mL. Expression of the packaging genes declined over time, however, presumably by gene silencing. Addition of sodium butyrate (discussed earlier) helped to recuperate some of the lost gene expression. This was encouraging, but the design of the cell line was very unsafe and could easily lead to an RCL.

As vectors evolved for removal of accessory genes and the requirement for *tat*, the biosafety greatly improved since not enough virus elements were present during packaging to result in a replication-competent recombinant.[17,43,44] A packaging cell line was developed for these highly attenuated vectors.[45] This was again a dual level of regulation, where *VSV-G* and *rev* were under the control of the TRE and *gag–pol* expression was modulated by *rev* availability. High titers of 5×10^6 were achieved in the system, ranging from 1 to 20 TU/cell, with a production period lasting almost one week. This represented the first lentiviral vector packaging line with suitable production and biosafety for regular application, and it (or a similar cell line) is appropriate for use for large-scale clinical production.

A second cell line was developed at Cell Genesys in anticipation of clinical application, in collaboration with Naldini[46] (Cell Genesys later closed down their lentiviral vector R&D department). This cell line was of a similar level of biosafety as the Trono line[45] but utilized only a single level of transcriptional control and expressed *tat* in the system. Farson et al. discovered that the level of vector RNA expression in producer cell is a rate-limiting step for infectious vector production. They also used sodium butyrate, but did not find enhanced overall vector production. Titers reaching above 4×10^6 TU/mL were reported over a 4- to 6- day period.

Ikeda et al. observed that constitutive expression of the *gag/pol* proteins could be achieved if the construct was delivered by a murine retroviral vector.[47] Although the reasons for this are unknown, greater than 1×10^7 TU/mL was reported. If extensive expansion of these packaging cells can be achieved for large-scale production, this represents an important advancement for cell line production. This report also used codon-optimized sequences for maximum expression in mammalian cells. Codon optimization has long been known to improve expression of genes in prokaryotic and eukaryotic cells[48,49] and had recently been shown to improve production of helper proteins for HIV.[50]

Recently, Ni et al. incorporated many of the aspects of prior cell lines to increase titer and the length of the production period for maximum vector collection.[51] This packaging line reduces cellular toxicity by using a three-level regulation cascade intended to reduce leakiness of toxic genes, which can decrease the stability of a cell line.[46] In this cell line, removal of tetracycline induces expression of more tTA and also *rev/tat*, both under the control of the TRE. *Rev* then drove expression of *VSV-G*, and *tat* drove expression of *gag/pol*. tTA amplified expression of the *tat/rev*. In addition, *gag/pol* and *tat/rev* genes were codon optimized for maximum expression, and cells were cultured in the presence of sodium butyrate to improve production. The cell line resulted in prolonged expression of titers over 2×10^7, and an unprecedented production period of over 10 days. Avoidance of gene silencing in this cell line was also achieved partially by simultaneous transfection of cells with all three expression plasmids and a high-throughput method of cell line screening by titer. This allowed time for vector production before the levels of protein expression began to decrease.

Removal of serum from lentivirus vector packaging cell lines has not been reported. Serum is known to reduce vector titers[36] and greatly enhance immunogenicity.[4] The recent concern of transmission of bovine spongiform encephalitis to humans through bovine products has emphasized the importance of removing bovine serum from any vector production process.[52] Serum-free adaptation of cell lines for the purpose of large-scale protein production in suspension has been reported,[53] and successful serum-free suspension culture of 293 cells has also been achieved.[54] Suspension culture will allow production of vector in bioreactors for phase III and beyond levels of vector production.

DOWNSTREAM PROCESSES

In this section on vector purification we focus on VSV-G pseudotyped vectors, since the majority of research and development have used these vectors. VSV-G is a durable cell surface protein that improves vector titers, broadens target cell range, and is sturdy enough to enable retention of titers upon centrifugation or column chromatography.[55] For most laboratory research applications, the simple method of centrifugation is used to concentrate virus titers. However, centrifugation causes cosedimentation of cellular DNA[56] and proteins such as proteoglycans, which are known to inhibit vector infectivity.[57,58] Sucrose gradient ultracentrifugation can help to improve the purity of the virus, but this is not scalable. Accordingly, several methods have been developed for scalable purification based on existing technologies for protein and virus purification. Examples of different purification protocols can be reviewed in Figure 21.1.

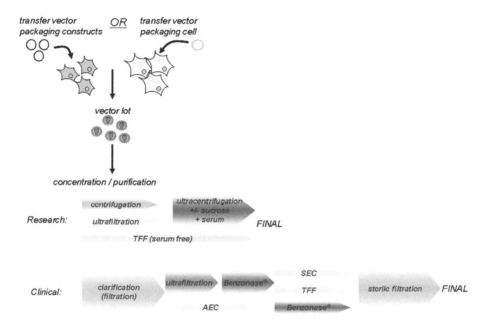

Figure 21.1 Common options for concentration and purification of vector for research or clinical application. Vector can be made by transient transfection or by packaging cell line (top). For research applications, vector is typically centrifuged. Depending on the starting volume, supernatant may first be concentrated by low-speed centrifugation or ultrafiltration. Optimal concentration of titer is achieved by ultracentrifugation. Recovery of vector produced in the absence of serum is poor with ultracentrifugation, so tangential flow filtration (TFF) can be used instead to preserve titers. For clinical applications, vector is first clarified and then concentrated by ultrafiltration and treated with Benzonase to remove residual nucleic acid. Vector is further purified by size using size exclusion chromatography (SEC) or TFF. Alternatively, vector can be concentrated and purified by charge using anion-exchange chromatography (AEC), which obviates the need for an initial concentration step. Vector is then treated with Benzonase. All clinical vector undergoes a final sterile filtration.

Clarification

An optional first step prior to vector concentration or purification is clarification to remove gross cellular debris. For extensive clinical-grade purification of vector, this step is a necessity to avoid disruption of subsequent purification steps. For standard vector applications, filtration is performed using a 0.45-μm filter.[36,59] Filtration through sequentially decreasing pore sizes can improve the clarification process for clinical purification.[14]

Centrifugation and Gradient Purification

Ultracentrifugation (50,000 to 60,000 × g for 1 to 2 hours) is used to concentrate small volumes of virus. This method can concentrate about 300 mL of supernatant (6 × 50 mL) to about 1000-fold of the original titer.[60] This can be followed by subsequent purification on a 20% sucrose gradient.[61] A 20% sucrose cushion is helpful to preserve recovery during concentration of ultracentrifuged vector.[7] For larger culture volumes, lower-speed centrifugation (26,000 × g for about 5 hours) can concentrate about 3 L of supernatant (6 × 300 mL), but to a lesser amount (~800-fold). Low-speed centrifugation can be used for initial concentration, then vector can be resuspended in a smaller volume and subjected to ultracentrifugation for an overall concentration of 8000-fold.[60] Concentration of vector during low-speed centrifugation can be enhanced by vector aggregation induced by poly-l-lysine (PLL) as an alternative to ultracentrifugation, although a direct comparison of fold concentration is not available.[62] The addition of PLL to the vector supernatant was not found to be toxic to cells, but possibly could cause aggregation that would impede sterile filtration.

Vector produced in serum containing media can be recovered significantly better by centrifugation than vector produced in the absence of serum (~70% versus ~10%). Therefore, for vector grown without serum, alternative methods for concentration are needed.

Benzonase Treatment

Purification techniques for vectors based on size, such as cross-flow filtration and size exclusion chromatography, will retain host cell DNA as well, which could impede optimal vector recovery. Inclusion of DNA in the final vector preparation is also a safety issue, in particular if the final preparation step contains packaging genes, which might increase the opportunity for recombination to occur. After concentration but prior to purification based on size, vector can be treated with concentrations of the nuclease Benzonase, ranging from 200 to 500 units/mL without affecting overall recovery of titer[7]. Purification methods not based on size can treat the manufactured vector after purification with Benzonase.[14]

Ultrafiltration

Ultrafiltration is a method of concentration for large biomolecules that allows filtration of small-molecular-weight moieties while retaining the larger-molecular-weight species. Filtration occurs during low-speed centrifugation (2500 to 3500 $\times$ g), and therefore scalability is limited by centrifugation volume and saturation of the filter. Ultrafiltration can be used as a concentration step prior to ultracentrifugation[29,59] or can be used as an alternative to ultracentrifugation to avoid the problems associated with vector aggregation.[36]

Cross-Flow Filtration

Cross-flow filtration, also known as tangential flow filtration (TFF), is similar in concept to ultrafiltration in that it separates out small-molecular-weight molecules while blocking transfer of the larger molecules. However, unlike ultrafiltration, TFF is scalable since the flow of sample is across the filter as opposed to through the filter (see Figure 3 of Lyddiatt and O'Sullivan for a visual explanation[63]). This prevents aggregation of the larger molecules on the filter surface and allows continuous flow of sample, which can be collected at the end of the flow on a final capture filter. This process can purify several liters of vector containing supernatant at a time[5] and is easily scalable. TFF offers a high recovery of vector ($>90\%$)[6] and does not suffer from the loss of recovery in the absence of serum as is seen with centrifugation.[60] For vectors intended for clinical application, additional purification steps will be necessary, in particular treatment of the vector with a nuclease such as benzonase to remove residual cellular and packaging DNA.

Column Purification

Column chromatography has been used extensively in the past for scalable purification of large biomolecules such as proteins and DNA. Purification of viral vectors is also achievable using size exclusion chromatography,[7,14] anion exchange chromatography,[14,64] or hydroxyapatite chromatography.[5] Although the VSV-G envelope protein is quite stable,[55] chromatographic purification based on charge requires a harsh elution buffer (sodium chloride) that can inactivate vector particles, and a 65% recovery for lentiviral vectors has been reported.[14] Charge-based purification columns are more scalable, however, and are attractive since they can be used without an initial concentration step. Overall recovery must be balanced with total vector yield, and the final total titer needed will dictate the choice of column purification. Size exclusion chromatography yields from 70%[7] of input vector to almost 100%, which is comparable to TFF.[14] Since harsh salts are not required for elution of SEC purification, the eluate can be immediately sterile filtered and stored.

RELEASE TESTING

The amount of release testing for a vector lot naturally depends on its intended use. Minimal testing for vector for laboratory research is titer and optionally, RCL testing for biosafety (usually in the context of cell line development). For direct injection into animals, vector should be further purified and evaluated for purity by silver-stained protein gel in addition to titration and RCL testing.[4]

Clincal-grade vector must undergo extensive testing in accordance with the *Code of Federal Regulations* (CFR) 21 for pharmaceutical and bulk chemical GMPs,[65] and the *United States Pharmacopeia* (USP) 1046 for cell and gene therapy products.[66] These regulations require testing for safety, potency, purity, and identity. A review of the quality control (QC) release testing for the first clinical lentiviral vector is presented in Figure 1 of Schonely et al.[67] Testing will vary for each vector but will follow these general principles.

Titration

Titration of research vector is most commonly performed by serial dilution of the vector, transduction of target cells, and then measuring expression of a marker gene by flow cytometry and calculating back the vector titer.[7] Most commonly, HeLa-tat or 293 cells are used for the titration assay. Titration on 293 or HeLa-tat is adequate for QC, and comparisons between laboratories (provided that the titer assays are comparable), but ultimately, titers should be determined in the final target cells since lentiviral vectors demonstrate significant transduction variability in different cell types and can be sensitive to species-specific restrictions.

Titration by marker gene expression is not very accurate, and titration by GFP expression specifically has been found to be a log lower than titration by DNA polymerase chain reaction (PCR) in transduced cells.[68] This is logical since titration by marker gene cannot distinguish between single or multiple integration events. Titration by real-time PCR of the vector stock and comparison to real-time DNA PCR on transduced cells can provide an accurate determination of infectious units for the target cells and provide an indication of the number of defective particles in the preparation.[69] For clinical applications, monitoring of the p24/titer ratio is also helpful in monitoring the amount of defective particles in the vector preparation between lots.[14]

RCL

Testing for recombination or replication-competent lentivirus (RCL) typically involves exposure of cells sensitive to HIV or the vector, and following the culture for about two weeks, monitoring for p24 production by ELISA and for persisting or increasing numbers of packaging DNA measured by PCR.[46,51] Functional assays for detection of tat or helper (by marker rescue assay) have also been used.[42] To date, there is no report of an RCL generation.

Rigorous biological testing for an RCL is a requisite step for release of clinical vector, and the guidelines for testing are based on those provided by the U.S. Food and Drug Administration for detection of replication-competent retrovirus (RCR).[70] Many reports have been made over the past few years regarding optimal RCL assays for clinical vector.[67,71–74] The test article for these assays, in accordance with the FDA guidelines, is 1×10^8, or 1% of the end of production

(EOP) or packaging cell line master cell bank (MCB), whichever is less, *and* 5% or 300 mL of culture supernatant, whichever is less. The working cell bank for the packaging cell line should also be tested, according to the same guidelines.

For detection of an RCL, the most permissive cell line should be used, and this has been reported in two studies to be C8166 cells.[67,74] A positive control that is expected to behave similarly to an anticipated RCL should be used. RCLs are not expected to replicate at high levels,[75] and therefore an attenuated HIV is optimal.[67] Pseudotyping the positive control with VSV-G is perhaps more sensitive.[74,75] The number of passages should be determined by the positive control in the setting of the assay, and is likely to be about two weeks. Previous culture times have varied, due to residual p24 from vector addition and the method of passage. An optional final transfer step of supernatant to indicator cells to distinguish a partial recombinant from an RCL should be performed if residual p24 is detected in the culture at the last passage.

Overlapping detection assays should be used, most commonly p24 detection by ELISA and DNA PCR for helper genes (e.g., *VSV-G* or *gag*). Alternatively, an assay for reverse transcription activity, the product-enhanced reverse transcription (PERT) assay, is useful as a similarly sensitive method for detection of virions in the culture superanant.[72]

DISCUSSION AND PERSPECTIVE

Researchers have a multitude of choices for vector production. Several areas can be modified to improve titers, including DNA purity and titration, transfection conditions, culture conditions, and concentration conditions. Putting the right combination of steps together should ensure successful and fairly reproducible results at the laboratory scale. Careful titration by DNA PCR in HeLa–tat or 293 cells should allow comparability between laboratories.

Cell line production of clinical-grade lentiviral vectors is expected to advance as lentiviral gene therapy trials progress into phase II and beyond.[76] Until then, however, vector will probably be produced by transient transfection due to the flexibility needed in early stage trials and the length of time that it takes to develop a GMP-grade producer cell line.

To date, no single purification method has dominated clinical-grade purification, and the ultimate process will be determined by the need for scale and purity. Anion-exchange chromatography or tangential flow filtration are likely to emerge as a phase III method of purification as a result of its ability to meet these criteria. Notwithstanding this, vector elements other than VSV-G are likely to be used more in the future. Although it has high utility and stability, VSV-G is toxic to cells, highly immunogenic, and is not cell specific. This makes it an unattractive candidate for directly injectable vectors. As more delicate envelopes are incorporated, gentler alternative methods of scalable purification will be used, such as cross-flow filtration.

Release testing of clinical-grade vector to date has been relatively rudimentary, with silver-stained gels and p24/total protein as the primary determinants of purity. As vector production matures, more in-depth description of vector quantification and purity will be required, such as high-performance liquid chromatography and mass spectrophometric monitoring of vector lots.[77]

To date, nine clinical lentiviral vector clinical trials have opened, and laboratory-scale research applying these vectors has exploded. Although good tools exist today for manufacture of vector, it is expected that improved protocols using in part the tools presented in this chapter will continue to emerge and evolve in parallel.

REFERENCES

1. Slepushkin V, Chang N, Cohen R, et al. Large-scale purification of a lentiviral vecor by size exclusion chromatography or mustang Q ion exchange capsule. *Bioprocess J*. 2003;2:89–95.

2. Schonely K, Afable C, Slepushkin V, et al. QC release testing of an HIV-1 based lentiviral vector lot and transduced cellular product. *Bioprocess J*. 2003;2:39–47.

3. Samakoglu S, Lisowski L, Budak-Alpdogan T, et al. A genetic strategy to treat sickle cell anemia by coregulating globin transgene expression and RNA interference. *Nat Biotechnol*. 2006;24:89–94.

4. Baekelandt V, Eggermont K, Michiels M, Nuttin B, Debyser Z. Optimized lentiviral vector production and purification procedure prevents immune response after transduction of mouse brain. *Gene Ther*. 2003;10:1933–1940.

5. Kuiper M, Sanches R, Walford J, Slater N. Purification of a functional gene therapy vector derived from Moloney murine leukaemia virus using membrane filtration and ceramic hydroxyapatite chromatography [abstract]. *Biotechnol Bioeng*. 2002;80:445–453.

6. Kotani H, Newton PB, Zhang SY, et al. Improved methods of retroviral vector transduction and production for gene-therapy. *Hum Gene Ther*. 1994;5:19–28.

7. Transfiguracion J, Jaalouk DE, Ghani K, Galipeau J, Kamen A. Size-exclusion chromatography purification of high-titer vesicular stomatitis virus G glycoprotein-pseudotyped retrovectors for cell and gene therapy applications. *Hum Gene Ther*. 2003;14:1139–1153.

8. Kaplan AH, Swanstrom R. The HIV-1 gag precursor is processed via 2 pathways: implications for cytotoxicity. *Biomed Biochim Acta*. 1991;50:647–653.

9. Yu H, Rabson AB, Kaul M, Ron Y, Dougherty JP. Inducible human immunodeficiency virus type 1 packaging cell lines. *J Virol*. 1996;70:4530–4537.

10. Li CJ, Friedman DJ, Wang CL, Metelev V, Pardee AB. Induction of apoptosis in uninfected lymphocytes by HIV-1 tat protein. *Science*. 1995;268:429–431.

11. Miyazaki Y, Takamatsu T, Nosaka T, et al. The cytotoxicity of human-immunodeficiency-virus type-1 Rev: implications for its interaction with the nucleolar protein B23. *Exp Cell Res*. 1995;219:93–101.

12. Rogel ME, Wu LI, Emerman M. The human-immunodeficiency-virus type-1 Vpr gene prevents cell-proliferation during chronic infection. *J Virol*. 1995;69:882–888.

13. Yang YP, Vanin EF, Whitt MA, et al. Inducible, high-level production of infectious murine leukemia retroviral vector particles pseudotyped with vesicular stomatitis-virus-G envelope protein. *Hum Gene Ther*. 1995;6:1203–1213.

14. Slepushkin V, Chang N, Cohen R, et al. Large-scale purification of a lentiviral vecor by size exclusion chromatography or mustang Q ion exchange capsule. *Bioprocess J*. 2003;2:89–95.

15. Lu X, Humeau L, Slepushkin V, et al. Safe two-plasmid production for the first clinical lentivirus vector that achieves > 99% transduction in primary cells using a one-step protocol. *J Gene Med*. 2004;6:963–973.

16. Naldini L, Blomer U, Gallay P, et al. In vivo gene delivery and stable transduction of nondividing cells by a lentiviral vector. *Science*. 1996;272:263–267.

17. Dull T, Zuffercy R, Kelly M, et al. A third-generation lentivirus vector with a conditional packaging system. *J Virol*. 1998;72:8463–8471.

18. Koldej R, Cmielewski P, Stocker A, Parsons DW, Anson DS. Optimisation of a multipartite human immunodeficiency virus based vector system; control of virus infectivity and large-scale production. *J Gene Med*. 2005;7:1390–1399.

19. Landau NR, Littman DR. Packaging system for rapid production of murine leukemia-virus vectors with variable tropism. *J Virol*. 1992;66:5110–5113.

20. Soneoka Y, Cannon PM, Ramsdale EE, et al. A transient 3-plasmid expression system for the production of high-titer retroviral vectors. *Nucleic Acids Res*. 1995;23:628–633.

21. Chen C, Okayama H. High-efficiency transformation of mammalian cells by plasmid DNA. *Mol Cell Biol*. 1987;7:2745–2752.

22. Garger SJ, Griffith OM, Grill LK. Rapid purification of plasmid DNA by a single centrifugation in a two-step cesium chloride–ethidium bromide gradient. *Biochem Biophys Res Commun*. 1983;117:835–842.

23. Junowicz E, Spencer JH. Rapid separation of nuclcosides and nuclcotides by cation-exchange column chromatography. *J Chromatogr*. 1969;44:342–348.

24. Markov GG, Ivanov IG. Hydroxyapatite column chromatography in procedures for isolation of purified DNA. *Anal Biochem*. 1974;59:555–563.

25. Garon CF, Petersen LL. An improved method for the isolation of supercoiled DNA-molecules using ion-exchange column chromatography. *Gene Anal Tech*. 1987;4:5–8.

26. Giovannini R, Freitag R. Continuous isolation of plasmid DNA by annular chromatography. *Biotechnol Bioeng*. 2002;77:445–454.

27. Prazeres DMF, Schluep T, Cooney C. Preparative purification of supercoiled plasmid DNA using anion-exchange chromatography. *J Chromatogr A*. 1998;806:31–45.

28. Kahn DW, Butler MD, Cohen DL, et al. Purification of plasmid DNA by tangential flow filtration. *Biotechnol Bioeng*. 2000;69:101–106.

29. Coleman JE, Huentelman MJ, Kasparov S, et al. Efficient large-scale production and concentration of HIV-1-based lentiviral vectors for use in vivo. *Physiol Genom*. 2003;12:221–228.

30. Karolewski BA, Watson DJ, Parente MK, Wolfe JH. Comparison of transfection conditions for a lentivirus vector produced in large volumes. *Hum Gene Ther*. 2003;14:1287–1296.

31. Sena-Esteves M, Tebbets JC, Steffens S, Crombleholme T, Flake AW. Optimized large-scale production of high titer lentivirus vector pseudotypes. *J Virol Methods*. 2004;122:131–139.

32. Yap MW, Kingsman SM, Kingsman AJ. Effects of stoichiometry of retroviral components on virus production. *J Gen Virol*. 2000;81:2195–2202.

33. Workman JL, Kingston RE. Alteration of nucleosome structure as a mechanism of transcriptional regulation. *Annu Rev Biochem*. 1998;67:545–579.

34. Thomsen B, Bendixen C, Westergaard O. Histone hyperacetylation is accompanied by changes in DNA topology in vivo. *Eur J Biochem*. 1991;201:107–111.

35. Lea MA, Randolph VM. Induction of reporter gene expression by inhibitors of histone deacetylase. *Anticancer Res*. 1998;18:2717–2721.

36. Reiser J. Production and concentration of pseudotyped HIV-1-based gene transfer vectors. *Gene Ther*. 2000;7:910–913.

37. Kaptein LCM, Greijer AE, Valerio D, van Beusechem VW. Optimized conditions for the production of recombinant amphotropic retroviral vector preparations. *Gene Ther*. 1997;4:172–176.

38. Le Doux JM, Davis HE, Morgan JR, Yarmush ML. Kinetics of retrovirus production and decay. *Biotechnol Bioeng*. 1999;63:654–662.

39. Kaul M, Yu H, Ron Y, Dougherty JP. Regulated lentiviral packaging cell line devoid of most viral cis-acting sequences. *Virology*. 1998;249:167–174.

40. Carroll R, Lin JT, Dacquel EJ, et al. A human-immunodeficiency-virus type-1 (HIV-1)-based retroviral vector system utilizing stable HIV-1 packaging cell-lines. *J Virol*. 1994;68:6047–6051.

41. Gossen M, Bujard H. Tight control of gene expression in mammalian cells by tetracycline-responsive promoters. *Proc Natl Acad Sci U S A*. 1992;89:5547–5551.

42. Kafri T, van Praag H, Ouyang L, Gage FH, Verma IM. A packaging cell line for lentivirus vectors. *J Virol*. 1999;73:576–584.

43. Miyoshi H, Blomer U, Takahashi M, Gage FH, Verma IM. Development of a self-inactivating lentivirus vector. *J Virol*. 1998;72:8150–8157.

44. Zufferey R, Dull T, Mandel RJ, et al. Self-inactivating lentivirus vector for safe and efficient in vivo gene delivery. *J Virol*. 1998;72:9873–9880.

45. Klages N, Zufferey R, Trono D. A stable system for the high-titer production of multiply attenuated lentiviral vectors. *Mol Ther*. 2000;2:170–176.

46. Farson D, Witt R, McGuinness R, et al. A new-generation stable inducible packaging cell line for lentiviral vectors. *Hum Gene Ther*. 2001;12:981–997.

47. Ikeda Y, Takeuchi Y, Martin F, et al. Continuous high-titer HIV-1 vector production. *Nat Biotechnol*. 2003;21:569–572.

48. Makoff AJ, Oxer MD, Romanos MA, Fairweather NF, Ballantine S. Expression of tetanus toxin fragment-C in *Escherichia coli*: high-level expression by removing rare codons. *Nucleic Acids Res*. 1989;17:10191–10202.

49. Holm L. Codon usage and gene-expression. *Nucleic Acids Res*. 1986;14:3075–3087.

50. Fuller M, Anson DS. Helper plasmids for production of HIV-1-derived vectors. *Hum Gene Ther*. 2001;12:2081–2093.

51. Ni YJ, Sun SS, Oparaocha T, et al. Generation of a packaging cell tine for prolonged large-scale production of high-titer HIV-1-based lentiviral vector. *J Gene Med*. 2005;7:818–834.

52. Asher D. Bovine sera used in the manufacture of biologicals: current concerns and policies of the U.S. Food and Drug Administration regarding the transmissible spongiform encephalopathies [abstract]. *Dev Biol Stand*. 1999;99:41–44.

53. Sinacore MS, Drapeau D, Adamson SR. Adaptation of mammalian cells to growth in serum-free media. *Mol Biotechnol*. 2000;15:249–257.

54. Baldi L, Muller N, Picasso S, et al. Transient gene expression in suspension HEK-293 cells: application to large-scale protein production. *Biotechnol Prog*. 2005;21:148–153.

55. Burns JC, Friedmann T, Driever W, Burrascano M, Yee J. Vesicular stomatitis virus G glycoprotein pseudotyped retroviral vectors: concentration to very high titer and efficient gene transfer into mammalian and nonmammalian cells. *Proc Natl Acad Sci U S A*. 1993;90:8033–8037.

56. Chen J, Reeves L, Sanburn N, et al. Packaging cell line DNA contamination of vector supernatants: Implication for laboratory and clinical research. *Virology*. 2001;282:186–197.

57. LeDoux JM, Morgan JR, Snow RG, Yarmush ML. Proteoglycans secreted by packaging cell lines inhibit retrovirus infection. *J Virol*. 1996;70:6468–6473.

58. Le Doux J, Morgan J, Yarmusch M. Removal of proteoglycans increases efficiency of retroviral gene transfer [abstract]. *Biotechnol Bioeng*. 1998;58:23–34.

59. Koldej R, Anson DS. The optimisation of methods for the purification and concentration of human immunodeficiency virus type-1 derived gene transfer vectors. *J Gene Med*. 2005;7:1135–1136.

60. Geraerts M, Michiels M, Baekelandt V, Debyser Z, Gijsbers R. Upscaling of lentiviral vector production by tangential flow filtration. *J Gene Med*. 2005;7:1299–1310.

61. Kootstra NA, Matsumura R, Verma IM. Efficient production of human FVIII in hemophilic mice using lentiviral vectors. *Mol Ther*. 2003;7:623–631.

62. Zhang B, Xia HQ, Cleghorn G, et al. A highly efficient and consistent method for harvesting large volumes of high-titre lentiviral vectors. *Gene Ther*. 2001;8:1745–1751.

63. Lyddiatt A, O'Sullivan DA. Biochemical recovery and purification of gene therapy vectors. *Curr Opin Biotechnol*. 1998;9:177–185.

64. Marino M, Kutner R, Lajmi A, Nocumson S, Reiser J. Development of scalable purification protocols for lentiviral vectors. [abstract]. *Mol Ther*. 2003;7:S178.

65. Pharmaceutical and bulk chemical GMPs. CFR 21:210–211.

66. Cell and gene therapy products. U.S. Pharmacopeia. 1999:1046.

67. Schonely K, Afable C, Slepushkin V et al. QC release testing of an HIV-1 based lentiviral vector lot and transduced cellular product. *Bioprocess J*. 2003;2:39–47.

68. Sastry L, Johnson T, Hobson M, Smucker B, Cornetta K. Titering lentiviral vectors: comparison of DNA, RNA and marker expression methods. *Gene Ther*. 2002;9:1155–1162.

69. Martin-Rendon E, White LJ, Olsen A, Mitrophanous KA, Mazarakis ND. New methods to titrate EIAV-based lentiviral vectors. *Mol Ther*. 2002;5:566–570.

70. U.S. Department of Health and Human Services. Guidance for Industry: Supplemental guidance on testing for replication competent retrovirus in retroviral vector based gene therapy products and during follow-up of patients in clinical trials using retroviral vectors. 2000:1–13.

71. Sastry L, Xu Y, Johnson T, et al. Certification assays for HIV-1-based vectors: Frequent passage of gag sequences without evidence of replication-competent viruses. *Mol Ther*. 2003;8:830–839.

72. Sastry L, Xu Y, Duffy L, et al. Product-enhanced reverse transcriptase assay for replication-competent retrovirus and lentivirus detection. *Hum Gene Ther*. 2005;16:1227–1236.

73. Miskin J, Chipchase D, Rohll J, et al. A replication competent lentivirus (RCL) assay for equine infectious anaemia virus (EIAV)-based lentiviral vectors. *Gene Ther*. 2006;13:196–205.

74. Escarpe P, Zayek N, Chin P, et al. Development of a sensitive assay for detection of replication-competent recombinant lentivirus in large-scale HIV-based vector preparations. *Mol Ther*. 2003;8:332–341.

75. Segall HI, Yoo E, Sutton RE. Characterization and detection of artificial replication-competent lentivirus of altered host range. *Mol Ther*. 2003;8:118–129.

76. Rebello T, Afable C, Callahan S, et al. Phase II clinical trial demonstrates the safety and tolerability of multiple doses of autologous CD4+ T cells transduced with VRX496, a lentiviral vector delivering anti-HIV antisense in patients failing one or more HAART treatments. [abstract]. *Mol Ther*. 2006;13:S292.

77. Transfiguracion J, Coelho H, Kamen A. High-performance liquid chromatographic total particles quantification of retroviral vectors pseudotyped with vesicular stomatitis virus-G glycoprotein. *J Chromatogr B*. 2004;813:167–173.

22 Assays for the Release of Viral Vector Gene Therapy Products for Human Clinical Trials

FLAVIA BORELLINI

Genentech, South San Francisco, California

The development of novel gene delivery systems and the possible applications of gene therapy to the treatment of non-life-threatening conditions have brought new quality and safety issues to the attention of the scientific and regulatory communities. Like other biopharmaceuticals destined for use in humans, viral vectors for gene therapy must meet a variety of well-defined criteria for identity, safety, purity, potency, and stability prior to their use in the clinic. Several regulatory authorities worldwide have developed quality and safety guidelines that specifically address various aspects related to quality assurance of gene therapy products (Table 22.1). In addition, regulatory guidelines generally applicable to biotechnology-derived products may also be relevant to viral gene therapy vectors and should be consulted early in development.

Among the safety tests required for the release of viral gene therapy vectors for human use is a test to detect the presence of wild-type virus in the engineered viral vector stock. Wild-type virus may be present as a contaminant in the vector seed or originate by genetic recombination during the viral vector production process. For replication-competent (oncolytic) adenoviral vectors and replication-defective lentiviral vectors, the detection of wild-type virus or undesired viral recombinants represents a significant hurdle in the transition from the laboratory bench to the clinic. This chapter focuses on approaches to address the unique challenges posed by the detection of replicating recombinants in these unique viral vector systems.

ONCOLYTIC ADENOVIRAL VECTORS

Oncolytic adenoviruses with the ability to replicate preferentially in tumor cells are showing great promise in the treatment of cancer [1–4]. Unlike their replication-defective counterparts, which lack one or more essential viral genes

Concepts in Genetic Medicine, Edited by Boro Dropulic and Barrie Carter
Copyright © 2008 John Wiley & Sons, Inc.

TABLE 22.1   Regulatory Documents Relating to Gene Therapy[a]

- Points to Consider in the Production and Testing of New Drugs and Biologicals Produced by Recombinant DNA Technology, 1985, U.S. FDA (57 FR 33201)
- Regulation of Gene Therapy in Europe: A Current Statement Including References to US Regulation, 1994
- Points to Consider in the Characterization of Cell Lines Used to Produce Biologicals, 1993, U.S. FDA (58 FR 42974)
- Points to Consider in Human Somatic Cell Therapy and Gene Therapy, 1991; update 1996, U.S. FDA
- Guidance for Industry: Guidance for Human Somatic Cell Therapy and Gene Therapy, 1998, U.S. FDA
- Guidance for Industry: Supplemental Guidance on Testing for Replication-Competent Retroviral Vector Based Gene Therapy Products and During Follow-up of Patients in Clinical Trials Using Retroviral Vectors, 2000
- A Proposed Approach to the Regulation of Cellular and Tissue-Based Products, 1997, U.S. FDA (62 FR 9721)
- ICH Draft Guidelines Q5A: Viral Safety Evaluation of Biotechnology Products Derived from Cell Lines of Human or Animal Origin
- ICH Draft Guideline Q5D: Derivation and Characterization of Cell Substrates Used for the Production of Biotechnological/Biotechnology Products
- ICH Draft Guideline Q6B: Specifications, Tests and Procedures for Biotechnological/Biological Products
- ICH Draft Guideline S6: Preclinical Safety Evaluation of Biotechnology-Derived Pharmaceuticals
- Directive 75/318/EEC: Gene Therapy Products—Quality Aspects in the Production of Vectors and Genetically Modified Somatic Cells, 1995, and draft annex, 1998

---

[a]U.S. FDA documents can be obtained via the Internet at http//www.fda.gov.cber/guidelines.htm.

and can replicate only in cells capable of trans-complementation, oncolytic adenoviruses contain all viral genes necessary for replication. Preferential replication in selected target cells is achieved by placing the expression of one or more essential gene(s) (*E1a*, *E1b*) under the control of heterologous tissue- or tumor-specific promoters. In permissive tumor cells, these engineered viruses are capable of multiple cycles of replication, cellular lysis, and reinfection, thereby leading to oncolysis.

Replication-defective adenoviral vectors for gene therapy are commonly tested for the presence of wild-type replication-competent adenovirus (RCA) by amplification of the vector on a cell line that is highly permissive for RCA but does not support replication of the defective vectors. The RCA contaminant is detected and quantified by plaque formation or observation of cytopathic effects in the substrate cells; both endpoints are a specific manifestation of viral replication. Current U.S. Food and Drug Administration (FDA) guidelines indicate that an adenoviral vector preparation for clinical use should contain less than one RCA in 1E10 adenoviral particles.

The detection of RCA in oncolytic virus lots presents a unique dilemma: Although these viruses are engineered to replicate preferentially in the target cells selected, they also exhibit low-level replication in immortalized cell lines and thus cause cytopathic effects. This is not surprising, as the events that lead to cell line immortalization and carcinogenesis produce similar alterations in the control of cell cycle and differentiation. It is also important to keep in mind that in the case of oncolytic viruses, undesirable recombinants are not limited to wild-type virus but include any replication-competent adenoviral variant that may exhibit greater potency, altered tropism, or both, and that has a negative impact on tumor selectivity, potency, and overall safety and efficacy of the oncolytic virus product. The traditional RCA assay is therefore not appropriate for the detection of wild-type adenovirus in oncolytic adenovirus vector lots.

Development of a RCA amplification assay for the testing of oncolytic viruses thus requires (1) the identification of a bioamplification system which is maximally permissive for wild-type virus and minimally permissive for the engineered oncolytic adenovirus, even when the latter is present in large excess; (2) the development of alternative quantitative assay endpoints with absolute specificity for wild-type to replace the nonspecific cytotoxicity endpoints (plaque formation, induction of cytopathic effects); and (3) the development of alternative endpoints that can detect non-wild-type replicating recombinants. Unless the nature of potential recombinants can be predicted, assay development must be conducted using wild-type adenovirus as a model.

The first step in the development of a bioamplification assay is the identification of a cell line that is least permissive for replication of the oncolytic construct while supporting replication of wild-type or nonselective adenovirus. Screening of several tumor and normal cell lines can be conducted by comparing yields of oncolytic virus after a single amplification cycle; cell lines that are least permissive for replication of the oncolytic vector are then screened in a similar fashion to determine if they support replication of wild-type adenovirus. Virus yields for wild-type adenovirus and the engineered vector are then compared; ideally, the yield of wild-type adenovirus in the cell line selected should be at least 3 logs higher than the yield of oncolytic virus over a broad range of MOI (multiplicity of infection) values in order to provide adequate assay sensitivity and specificity. Amplification by serial passaging in nonpermissive cells in vitro mimics the situation in which a tumor-selective oncolytic adenovirus infects a normal, nontumor cell; in addition, the selective pressure associated with passage in nonpermissive cells in vitro provides a sensitive method to monitor genetic stability of an engineered adenovirus. Once a cell line is identified, several assay parameters [virus infection procedures, culture medium composition, MOI, procedures for secondary infection (passage of cells versus supernatant, fixed MOI versus fixed volume of harvest material), number of amplification passages, and assay scale] are optimized to maximize detection of replicating wild-type virus.

Optimization requires the selection of a quantitative assay endpoint with absolute specificity for wild-type. Although direct measurements of viral replication (plaque formation, induction of cytopathic effects) are most relevant to the scope of the bioamplification assay, in the presence of a large excess of oncolytic virus vector these endpoints are neither specific nor quantifiable. In this context, specific quantitative measurement of wild-type virus can only be achieved by a physical method such as quantitative or real-time polymerase chain reaction (qPCR) [5], which can discriminate between wild-type and oncolytic adenovirus on the basis of genomic sequence differences. Quantities of amplified wild-type can be normalized relative to the total number of adenovirus genome copies. Although a qPCR assay per se is incapable of distinguishing between biologically inert or replicating wild-type recombinants, increasing yield of wild-type virus genomes over successive culture passages specifically indicates the presence of replicating wild-type virus in the test material. Non-wild-type recombinants may also be detected by PCR if the structure of the potential recombinant is known or can be predicted a priori.

To increase assay sensitivity, multiple independent replicate cultures may be run for each test sample. When this is done and wild-type virus yield is measured by qPCR after each passage for each replicate culture, the frequency of replicating wild type in the initial oncolytic vector stock can then be estimated using Poisson's distribution:

$$\text{amount in test sample} = -\ln(p_0)$$

where p_0 is the number of negative replicates/total replicates. Therefore, an amount of wild type that can be detected $\sim63\%$ of the time in a test sample (a single replicate) constitutes a detectable "unit":

$$\text{amount in test sample} = -\ln(37/100) = 1$$

The probability of detection for a given amount of wild-type (i.e., the probability that at least one replicate will be positive) increases with the number of replicates N as follows:

$$P = (1 - p_0^N)$$

If the wild-type contaminant is indeed replicating in the bioamplification system, frequency of detection (positive/total replicates) should increase with each successive passage. With careful optimization, a cell-based assay like that described above can achieve a sensitivity of 1 pfu of wild-type virus in 5E8 viral particles with a 98% probability of detection.

Importantly, this semiquantitative assessment of wild-type frequency is based on the assumptions that replicating wild-type contaminants (1) would have a vp/pfu ratio similar to that of the wild-type virus employed for assay development, and (2) would exhibit similar replication kinetics. For any replicating contaminant with replication kinetics significantly different than the wild-type virus lot used as standard, or with a different vp/pfu ratio, assessment of the presence of wild-type must be considered qualitative.

The viral population amplified by multiple passages on nonpermissive cells may be further characterized by comparison of the cytotoxicity (potency) of the viral population produced by bioamplification to the cytotoxicity of the starting (nonamplified) test sample in target and nontarget cells. Altered potency in late-passage virus indicates that there has been a significant change in the viral population, resulting in progressively increasing cytotoxicity on nontarget cells, and subsequent decreasing selectivity with successive amplification passages. The viral population derived from bioamplification can also be characterized by comparing the gross genetic structure of the starting test sample and amplified viral population by restriction digest pattern analysis. Appearance of anomalous fragments may indicate the presence of rearranged, replicating recombinants that may not be detectable by the qPCR assay.

Finally, when interpreting the results of a bioamplification assay, it is also important to keep in mind that recombinants detected after prolonged culture may not represent contaminants present in the original viral stock but may in fact be "adaptive" variants of the engineered virus that emerge upon repeated passaging on poorly permissive cells during the bioamplification assay. One therefore needs to balance the need for high sensitivity (and therefore prolonged amplification in culture) with the risk of forcing the emergence of adaptive variants by selective pressure.

LENTIVIRAL VECTORS

Replication-defective lentiviral vectors combine the advantages of transduction of nondividing cells, efficient integration, and stable long-term expression of the transgene in vivo and are well suited for long-term delivery of therapeutic genes. Regardless of the specific clinical application, very stringent safety standards must be applied to the manufacturing and testing of lentiviral vectors for human use, due to the pathogenicity of the parental virus. A critical safety issue is the detection of replication-competent lentivirus recombinants (RCLs) that may arise by genetic recombination during the vector production process. Recombination may also generate "partial recombinants" which lack the capacity to replicate autonomously but are potential precursors to replicating recombinants.

The development of sensitive and specific RCL assays presents unique challenges; (1) it is difficult to predict with any accuracy the structure of a recombinant that would be replication competent and therefore to design specific detection assays; and (2) most vector production systems employ transient transfection procedures, which often result in detectable levels of residual input plasmid DNA and its derivative RNA and proteins in the lentiviral vector product. For this reason, RCL assays that rely on physical detection of viral components cannot be directly applied lentiviral product testing. Therefore, bioamplification of RCL by culture on a permissive cell line, combined with a variety of physical and biological endpoints, currently provides the best system for achieving sensitive and specific detection of RCL.

The first step in the development of a bioamplification assay for detection of RCL is the identification of a positive control lentivirus that adequately represents the replication characteristics of the RCL predicted to arise from the particular lentivirus vector production system (e.g., deletion of accessory viral genes in the vector construct should be mirrored in the positive control). Ideally, the positive control virus should carry the same envelope as that used in the vector particles in order to reflect the same in vitro cell entry properties. When the introduction of the envelope into the positive control viral genome may result in a virus with expanded tropism and pose an undesirable biosafety risk, an alternative approach is to use a phenotypic pseudotype (i.e., a phenotypically mixed viral particle bearing both envelope proteins) as a positive control [6,7]; the engineered vector envelope glycoproteins mediate the first round of infection, while subsequent amplification depends on the native envelope of the lentivirus.

To achieve good RCL detection sensitivity, a cell line that permits efficient replication of the relevant positive control RCL must be identified. The cell line need not be a human cell line. In one recent survey of human cell lines, C8166-45, a human T-cell line, was identified as a sensitive substrate for amplification of HIV-1-derived, attenuated RCL [6,7]. Selection of an endpoint is also of critical importance. Given the difficulty in predicting the nature of a potential RCL, more than one endpoint should be considered that targets both structural (viral RNA, proviral DNA, proteins) and biological features (reverse transcriptase activity). The analyses based on the detection of structural features of a RCL should be designed based on the most likely identity and structure of the RCL predicted. If the vector is pseudotyped, it may be useful to target additional components of the vector production system, such as the pseudotyping envelope protein or its coding sequence. In any case, to avoid background problems, these analyses should be conducted when the components from the input test material are no longer detectable. For example, input p24 capsid protein can be detected by ELISA for at least 20 days in culture, although at declining concentrations [6,7]. Nevertheless, any assay that relies on detection of a specific sequence or protein ultimately relies on the accuracy of the RCL predicted. Therefore, it is also important to consider using less specific methods that do not rely on a requisite knowledge of the genetic structure of the RCL, such as an assay for reverse transcriptase activity. An alternative approach to RCL detection is to employ a marker-rescue assay [8,9].

Since RCL generation is expected to be a very rare event, the detection assays should be as sensitive as technically feasible. The assay sensitivity should be evaluated in the presence of vector particles, at concentrations comparable to final lentiviral product preparation, and verified by spike-recovery experiments. The minimal duration of the culture period required to ensure detection of limiting amounts of RCL should be determined using the relevant positive control RCL.

Other assay optimization parameters include determination of the optimal MOI and test volume.

Ideally, a release assay for lentiviral vectors intended for clinical use should demonstrate that there is no RCL in a patient dose. Considering that the RCL distribution in a vector sample obeys a Poisson distribution, a statistical rationale based on the Poisson distribution with a high confidence interval (95%) can be applied to determine the amount of vector that should be tested to detect an RCL infectious dose [10]. However, at the current scales of lentiviral vector production this ideal approach may not be feasible. An alternative approach is to estimate what would constitute an infectious dose of RCL based on the infectivity of the parental virus compared to the estimated infectivity of the RCL positive control, taking into consideration effects on replication that would either reduce infectivity (such as deletions of accessory genes) or increase infectivity or cell tropism (such as the use of VSV-G envelope). Although these estimates may be extremely difficult to make, they may provide a rough approximation of the minimal RCL infectious dose.

In the CBER Guidance for Industry for RCR testing (see Table 22.1), the end of production (EOP) cells are tested directly for the presence of an RCR. Currently, the majority of lentivirus vectors are made using a transient transfection process, in which considerable cell toxicity may result from overexpression of helper functions. In these cases, testing of the EOP may not be useful.

CONCLUSIONS

Establishment of a comprehensive quality assurance and safety testing program is critical to the development of safe and effective gene delivery systems. Ultimately, the development of characterization and release assays should be science driven, use the best available science and technology, and must consider the unique nature of these products.

REFERENCES

1. Lichtenstein DL, Wold WS. *Cancer Gene Ther*. 2004;11(12):819–829.
2. Chu RL, et al. *Clin Cancer Res*. 2004;10(16):5299–5312.
3. Oosterhoff D, van Beusechem VW. *J Exp Ther Oncol*. 2004;4(1):37–57.
4. Dobbelstein M. *Curr Top Microbiol Immunol*. 2004;273:291–334.
5. Bernt RM, et al. *J Virol*. 2002;76:10994–11002.
6. Escarpe P, et al. *Mol Ther*. 2003;8(2):332–341.
7. Sastry L, et al. *Mol Ther*. 2003;8(5):830–839.
8. Segall HI, Yoo E, Sutton RE. *Mol Ther*. 2003;8(1):118–129.
9. Segall H, Sutton RE. *Methods Mol Biol*. 2003;229:87–94.
10. Guidance to Industry: Supplemental Guidance on Testing for Replication Competent Retroviral Vector Based Gene Therapy Products and During Follow-up of Patients in Clinical Trials Using Retroviral Vectors. 2000.

23 Safety of Retroviral Vectors: Regulatory and Technical Considerations

KENNETH CORNETTA
Department of Medical and Molecular Genetics, Indiana University
School of Medicine, Indianapolis, Indiana

CAROLYN A. WILSON
Division of Cellular and Gene Therapies, Center for Biologics
Evaluation and Research, Bethesda, Maryland

Gamma retroviral vectors based on Moloney murine leukemia virus (MoMLV) have been in clinical use for over a decade. While retroviral vectors are designed to be replication defective, recombination events during vector production have led to the generation of replication-competent retroviruses (RCRs). The known pathogenicity of RCR dictates strict monitoring of gene therapy products intended for clinical use. Guidelines for assays to detect RCRs have been set forth by the U.S. Food and Drug Administration (FDA), and detection methods for RCRs pseudotyped with the GALV, RD114, and ecotropic viral envelopes have been described. More recent events in clinical trials have underscored that even in the absence of RCR, the replication-defective retroviral vector poses more than a theoretical risk through insertional mutagenesis, as evidenced by children developing leukemia in a gene therapy clinical trial in France as a direct result of the insertion of the retroviral vector DNA. Therefore, additional regulatory issues have arisen relative to these observations, focused primarily on accurate and clear informed consent of subjects who participate in clinical trials using retroviral vectors, risk/benefit justifications of using retroviral vectors in the proposed clinical indication, and additional subject monitoring for evidence of oligoclonal or monoclonal patterns of retroviral vector integration in transduced cell populations. In this chapter we review both the regulatory and technical issues relevant to reducing the risk of using retroviral vectors in clinical trials.

Gammaretrovirus-based retroviral vectors (herein referred to as *retroviral vectors*) have been used since the early 1990s in a variety of clinical indications

Concepts in Genetic Medicine, Edited by Boro Dropulic and Barrie Carter
Copyright © 2008 John Wiley & Sons, Inc.

(cancer, HIV, monogenic disorders, and others) in part, because the ability to integrate their genetic material into the host cell genome allows for long-term expression of the desired transgene. Unfortunately, this advantage of using retroviral vectors is also associated with a risk of malignant transformation.

Gammaretroviruses have long been known to participate in oncogenesis. This may occur in those instances where genomic integration causes dysregulation of endogenous cellular gene expression, a process often termed *insertional mutagenesis*. There are three known mechanisms by which gammaretroviruses induce this biological effect (shown in Figure 23.1; reviewed by Rosenberg and Joelicoer, 1997): (1) the genomic site of integration of the retroviral DNA interrupts key regulatory elements of a genetic locus; (2) the enhancer element, located in U3 within the 3′ long terminal repeat (LTR), causes transcriptional read-through of a downstream gene; and (3) the U3 enhancer in either the 5′ or 3′ LTR may induce gene transcription at distal sites, up to 300 kb away from the site of insertion via enhancer activation. Although not all integration events will necessarily induce gene-dysregulation, nor will all gene dysregulating events cause tumors, in rare instances the integration will contribute to malignant transformation of the cell.

As retroviral vectors entered clinical trials, the risk of insertional mutagenesis was thought to be associated primarily with the potential for inadvertent exposure of clinical trial subjects to replication-competent retrovirus (RCR). Previously, the data available indicated that the risk of insertional mutagenesis associated with replication-defective retroviral vectors would be very low, but not zero (Cornetta, 1992; Li et al., 2002) and that the risk of insertional mutagenesis would be greatest when RCR was present, due to the potential for a much greater number of integration events, one of which may be oncogenic. The theoretical risk of RCR-mediated oncogenesis was translated into a true risk when three out of 10

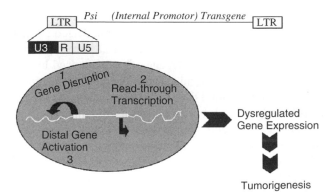

Figure 23.1 Gamma retroviral–mediated endogenous gene activation. The double-stranded DNA proviral configuration of a retroviral vector is shown, containing the long terminal repeats (LTRs) at either end of the provirus genome. Upon integration in the host cell genome, the U3 element within the LTR may act to cause dysregulated gene expression by one of three mechanisms, as shown. In some cases, altered gene expression may lead to tumor formation.

nonhuman primates undergoing autologous transplantation of vector-transduced hematopoietic progenitor cells developed lymphoma (Donahue et al., 1992). The monkeys were exposed to high doses of RCR which contaminated the retroviral vector product, thereby infecting the vector-transduced cells subsequently infused into these animals. This led to an increased regulatory emphasis on performing rigorous testing for RCR contamination in the retroviral vector and in clinical trial subjects (reviewed in more detail below). Indeed, until 2002, the rationale for using RCR-free vectors for clinical trials was borne out by the safety record of gene therapy clinical trials using retroviral vectors.

Unfortunately, in 2002, both preclinical and clinical data emerged that indicated that even an RCR-free (hence, replication-defective) retroviral vector may cause insertional mutagenesis. First, results from a preclinical study in mice demonstrated a strong correlation between the integration of the retroviral vector into a known murine oncogene, Evi-1, and the development of myeloid leukemia (Li et al., 2002). Later that year, initial reports were presented at meetings of various advisory bodies indicating that integration of the retroviral vector caused development of leukemias in subjects participating in a gene therapy trial for X-linked severe combined immunodeficiency (SCID) (Cavazzana-Calvo et al., 2000; Hacein-Bey-Abina et al., 2002,2003a,b). In at least two of the cases, the integration caused activated gene expression of a known human onco-gene, LMO-2, normally transcriptionally silent in mature T cells (Cavazzana-Calvo et al., 2000; Hacein-Bey-Abina et al., 2002,2003a,b). The reasons that these children developed leukemia is complex, but preliminary evidence suggests the possibility that the transgene in this study (the common gamma-chain cytokine receptor) may act cooperatively with vector-induced gene dysregulation (i.e., a second "hit") (Berns, 2004; Dave et al., 2004). This hypothesis is also partly supported by preclinical studies suggesting a collaborative role between gamma-c and LMO-2 in the development of certain murine leukemias (Dave et al., 2004). The adverse events with replication-defective retroviral vectors have led to a new set of regulatory recommendations relevant to the clinical use of retroviral vectors.

REGULATORY CONSIDERATIONS

The most relevant regulatory recommendations from the FDA regarding the clinical use of retroviral vectors, including recommendations on subject monitoring, are found in two guidance documents: (1) *Supplemental Guidance on Testing for Replication Competent Retrovirus in Retroviral Vectors Based Gene Therapy Products During Follow-up of Patients in Clinical Trials Using Retroviral Vectors* (herein referred to as *RCR Guidance*); and (2) *Guidance for Industry: Gene Therapy Clinical Trials — Observing Participants for Delayed Adverse Events* (herein referred to as *Follow-up Guidance*). These recommendations provide specific guidance on what and how much of vector manufacturing materials should be tested for RCR, as well as information on how often and what type of follow-up should be performed on subjects who participate in retroviral vector-based gene therapy clinical trials.

During retroviral vector manufacture, the RCR guidance recommends that testing for RCR should be performed throughout the process, in recognition that the recombination events that give rise to RCR are stochastic and may occur at any point during the retroviral vector production process. Therefore, RCR testing needs to be performed on the master cell bank of the vector producer cells, the working cell bank, the production lot (including the end of production cells), and the ex vivo transduced cells (when cultured longer than four days past exposure to the retroviral vector). The guidance also provides information on how to use a statistical approach to determine how much material should be tested; however, in the absence of an available titered reference for RCR testing, the default for vector supernatant is to use 5% of the volume and for cell banks or postproduction cells to use 1% or 10^8 cells (whichever is smaller).

The guidance also describes when and what type of subject monitoring should be performed. In addition to a pretreatment sample, relevant clinical samples of subjects should be obtained at 3, 6, and 12 months after exposure to a retroviral vector-based product and should be assayed for evidence of RCR infection. The test method may be chosen by the sponsor, with consideration for the clinical indication. Typical assays include detection of RCR-specific antibodies (Martineau et al., 1997; Long et al., 1998) or analysis of patient PBMC by polymerase chain reaction (PCR) for RCR-specific sequences (Morgan et al., 1990; Martineau et al., 1997; Long et al., 1998). The test method chosen should consider both the mode of exposure to a retroviral vector (and potential RCR) and the immune status of the patient. In either case, a positive result should be confirmed by attempting to culture infectious virus from the subject. If the analyses of these initial samples are all negative, the guidance recommends archiving of yearly samples, as well as annual clinical follow-up of subjects, where attention is paid to development of new hematologic, neurologic, or malignant conditions. The guidance also recommends that an autopsy should be requested upon the death of the subject. In the event that any subject samples test positive for RCR, the sponsor should contact CBER for further guidance and report the test results as an adverse experience in an IND safety report (according to Title 21, *Code of Federal Regulations,* part 312.32).

Since January 2003, and recently published in the *Follow-up Guidance*, the FDA has recommended that the informed consent documents accurately reflect the risk of tumorigenesis from retroviral vector gene therapy and provide clear language about the results in the clinical trial in France using retroviral vectors for X-SCID (described above). Additional information has been requested from sponsors who propose performing gene therapy clinical trials using retroviral vectors to transduce hematopoietic stem cells or other cell types with similar properties of high replicative capacity and long life span. Sponsors must provide a clear risk/benefit justification for using retroviral vectors for the proposed clinical indication, taking into account alternative therapies available for the clinical condition. FDA has also requested additional laboratory monitoring for evidence of trends toward oligoclonality or monoclonality of vector integration sites in the transduced cell population, when vector-positive cells are detectable and if it is feasible to obtain a surrogate clinical sample (e.g., PBMC as a surrogate for transduced hematopoietic stem cells). These most current recommendations have been published in the *Follow-up Guidance*, in addition to previous FDA presentations and discussions at advisory committee meetings of both the FDA and the NIH (see transcripts of the October 10, 2002, February 28, 2003, and March 4, 2005 meetings of the Cells, Tissues, and Gene Therapies Advisory Committee, formerly the Biologics Response Modifiers Advisory Committee, available at http://www.fda.gov/cber/advisory/ctgt/ctgtmain.htm; and transcripts of the Fifth National NIH Safety Symposium: Current Perspectives on Gene Transfer for X-SCID, March 15, 2005, available at http://www4.od.nih.gov/oba/rac/SSMar05/index.htm).

TECHNICAL CONSIDERATIONS

Most retroviral vectors are based on the MoMLV and take advantage of the unique reproductive cycle of the retrovirus, which allows for the deletion of the viral protein coding sequences (*gag*, *pol*, and *env*) and substitution of this region with an exogenous gene(s) of interest. Deletion of the viral protein coding sequences renders the vectors replication defective. Vector particles must be generated by coexpressing the vector sequences along with the viral genes. This can be done using plasmids expressing the vector and viral genes, either by transient transfection methods or by the use of stable packaging cell lines (Mann et al., 1983; Watanabe and Temin, 1983) (see Miller, 1990 for a review). In retroviral vector products, the most likely source of RCR is recombination between the vector and viral genes used in vector packaging. RCR was frequently detected in early versions of vector packaging cell lines in which all the viral genes (*gag/pol/env*) were expressed from a single plasmid (Bodine et al., 1990; Muenchau et al., 1990; Scarpa et al., 1991; Otto et al., 1994). By minimizing homology between vector and packaging cell sequences and segregating *gag–pol* and *env* genes onto separate plasmids, the rate of RCR development can be substantially decreased but not eliminated (Bosselman et al., 1987; Danos and Mulligan, 1988; Markowitz et al., 1988a, 1988b; Miller and Rosman, 1989; Miller et al., 1991). As the recombination frequency of production plasmids decreased, a variety of novel RCRs have been detected in which cellular sequences contribute to the RCR. For example, Chong et al. reported a RCR in which the 5′ LTR, *gag*, and most of the *pol* genes in the RCR were derived from ecotropic endogenous retroviral sequences contained in the packaging cell (Chong et al., 1998). Garrett et al. identified an RCR arising in an amphotropic producer cell line that contained the ecotropic envelope and endogenous sequences carried over from an ecotropic packaging cell line used in generating the amphotropic producer cell line (Garrett et al., 2000). As murine cells contain a large number of endogenous retroviral sequences, the recent move to utilize human cells for vector packaging may decrease the incidence of RCR (Patience et al., 2001), although possible recombination with human endogenous retroviral sequences must be considered. Finally, although recombination is the most likely source of a RCR, other explanations should be considered. As an example, Miller and colleagues identified a novel retrovirus, the *Mus dunni* endogenous virus (MDEV), which was present in the *Mus dunni* cell line used in a marker rescue assay. The virus was activated by hydrocortisone in the medium being tested for RCR (Miller et al., 1996; Bonham et al., 1997). Therefore, cell lines used for amplification and assay must be considered as a possible source of RCR unrelated to the vector product.

Screening vector products for RCR has generally utilized biological assays, as molecular tests such as PCR are less sensitive and are prone to false positives. If using PCR, care must be taken in the samples selected for testing by the PCR method, since cells tested shortly after transduction may be contaminated with plasmids carried over from transient production methods or from producer cell line DNA that can yield a false positive result (Chen et al., 2001b). Therefore, screening products have relied on biological assays that aim to detect viral replication as the determinant of a true RCR. The biological assays most commonly used to qualify clinical-grade material include the extended S+/L− assay and the marker rescue assay (see Figure 23.2) (Cornetta et al., 1993; Printz et al., 1995; Forestell et al., 1996; Miller et al., 1996). In these assays test material is placed on a permissive cell line and the cells are passaged for a minimum of three weeks to amplify virus (amplification phase). In the marker rescue assay, the permissive cell line has been engineered to contain a retroviral vector genome with an easily identifiable transgene (e.g., a "marker" gene such as the neomycin phosphotransferase gene). After three weeks, the cell media from the amplification phase is collected. If RCR is present, it will package both the RCR genomes and also "rescue" the marker vector. Cell-free media from the amplification phase cells is then used to transduce a naive cell line, which is then subjected to drug selection. Demonstration of drug resistance in the transduced cell population is indicative of RCR.

In the extended S+/L− assay, virus is amplified in an identical manner to marker rescue except that the amplification cells do not contain vector. Instead, virus is detected using indicator cell lines, such as the cat cell line PG-4 (Bassin et al., 1982). The PG-4 cell line is referred to as a S+/L− cell line, as it contains the murine sarcoma virus genome (S+) but lacks the murine leukemia virus genome (L−). Cells that express the murine sarcoma virus induce a transformed phenotype but only in cells coexpressing a murine leukemia virus. Therefore, if media collected from the amplification phase cells contain RCR, the PG-4 cells will be transformed and can be detected as foci within the PG-4 cell culture. The S+/L− assay can also be performed without the amplification phase (a direct S+/L− assay). While a direct S+/L− assay allows a quantitative determination of viral infectious particles, when performed with limiting dilutions of the test material it is less sensitive than when the amplification phase precedes the direct assay.

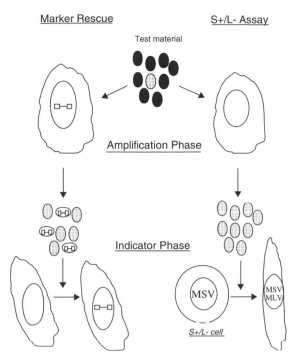

Marker Rescue   S+/L- Assay

Test material

Amplification Phase

Indicator Phase

MSV

MSV
MLV

S+/L- cell

Figure 23.2 Detection of replication-competent retrovirus using biological assays: amplification phase. Test material depicts retroviral vector supernatant in which a small portion of the replication-defective vector material (solid ovals) is contaminated with RCR (stippled ovals). Biological assays often utilize a three-week amplification phase in which a permissive cell line is used to increase the titer of any RCR present in the test material. In the marker rescue assay the cell lines used in the amplification phase contain an integrated retroviral vector that expresses a marker gene (such as a drug resistance gene). If RCR is present, it will "rescue" the marker vector and the cell supernatant will contain RCR along with virions capable of conferring drug resistance to naive cells in the indicator phase. The S+/L− assay also has an amplification step, but in this case the indicator cell line detects RCR directly. The indicator cell is termed an S+/L− cell since it contains the murine sarcoma virus (MSV), which will transform the cell phenotype but only in the presence of a murine leukemia virus (MSV) RCR.

The selection of the amplification phase cell line and the indicator cell assay will depend in part on the vector pseudotype. *Pseudotype* refers to the viral envelope selected for expression on the surface of the vector particle. The MoMLV from which many vectors are derived normally expressed the ecotropic envelope. As the ecotropic receptor is limited to rodent cells, vectors for human cell transduction were initially pseudotyped with the envelope from the amphotropic 4070A virus, whose receptor is present on most mammalian cells. Methods detecting RCR pseudotyped with the 4070A envelope were developed and the *Mus dunni* cell line is commonly used in the amplification phase due to the suscepti-bility to and amplification of a wide variety of murine leukemia viruses (Lander and Chattopadhyay, 1984; Wilson et al., 1997). Although *Mus dunni* propagates many RCRs, viruses enveloped with the ecotropic MoMLV glycoprotein are a notable exception and alternative cell lines must be used for their detection (Reeves et al., 2002). Also, the recent use of nonmurine retroviral envelopes to pseudotype retroviral vectors has complicated the screening for RCRs. One that has now been used in a variety of clinical applications is the envelope derived from the gibbon ape leukemia virus (GALV) (Wilson et al., 1989; Miller et al., 1991). The GALV envelope has demonstrated improved transduction efficiency in a number of target cells, in part, due to the increased expression of the GALV receptor on many target cells (Bayle et al., 1993; von Kalle et al., 1994; Bauer et al., 1995; Bunnell et al., 1995). While GALV acts as a xenotropic virus in that it infects primate and other mammalian cells, it cannot infect murine cells (Miller et al., 1991). Therefore, *Mus dunni* cells are not suitable for GALV amplifica-tion. To address this, 293 cells have been substituted for *Mus dunni* during the amplification phase of the extended S+/L− assay with similar levels of virus detection (Chen et al., 2001a). Another retroviral envelope being developed for clinical trial use was cloned from the RD114 virus, which also displays proper-ties of xenotropic viruses (Cosset et al., 1995; Kelly et al., 2000; Goerner et al., 2001). The 293 cell line is also useful for amplifying RD114 pseudotyped RCR in an extended S+/L− assay (Duffy et al., 2003).

Given the importance of generating material free of RCR, the methods used to detect RCR should be continually reviewed and improved upon when appropriate. For example, the amount of material to be tested and whether the supernatant or postproduction cells are the optimal test material require continued evaluations. It has been the experience of the National Gene Vector Laboratory at Indiana University that when RCR is present it is generally detected in both supernatant and postproduction cells. When only one test has been positive, it is usually the postproduction cells, but there have been rare incidences when only the super-natant was positive (unpublished data). As production using transient transfection methods is developed, the relative sensitivity of postproduction screening will require further evaluation, as the cells are generally less viable at the time of vector harvest. Additional modifications to retroviral vector production, such as use of the vesicular stomatitis virus G protein to pseudotype the vector parti-cles, may preclude testing of postproduction cells due to toxicity from G protein expression. These issues will need to be evaluated experimentally.

For subject monitoring for evidence of RCR infection, most investigators have chosen PCR and serologic assays. The obvious advantage of using PCR or sero-logic methods is the rapid, high-throughput nature of the assay; however, this may be offset by the potential for false positives. Also, one must consider that complex recombinations have led to the RCR, so that the target sequence may not be present. Clinical suspicion of RCR with a negative PCR or serologic result should prompt further testing for other target sequences (e.g., *gag* sequences in cases where *env* PCR was negative) as well as analysis for RCR using bio-logic assays. Further refinements of the existing biological assays to decrease the labor-intensive nature of these assays are warranted if sensitivity can be maintained.

The finding that no documented RCR exposure has occurred using products tested with current screening methods is encouraging, but the known risk of insertional mutagenesis mandates continued vigilance in testing for RCR in the product, combined with appropriate clinical and laboratory follow-up of clinical trial subjects.

REFERENCES

Bassin RH, Ruscetti S, Ali I, Haapala D, Rein A (1982). Normal DBA/2 mouse cells synthesize a glycoprotein which interferes with MCF virus infection. *Virology*. 123: 139–151.

Bauer Jr. TR, Miller AD, Hickstein DD (1995). Improved transfer of the leukocyte integrin CD18 subunit into hematopoietic cell lines by using retroviral vectors having a gibbon ape leukemia virus envelope. *Blood*. 86:2379–2387.

Bayle JY, Johnson LG, St. George JA, Boucher RC, Olsen JC (1993). High-efficiency gene transfer to primary monkey airway epithelial cells with retrovirus vectors using the gibbon ape leukemia virus receptor. *Hum Gene Ther*. 4:161–170.

Berns A (2004). Good news for gene therapy. *New Engl J Med*. 350:1679–1680.

Bodine DM, McDonagh KT, Brandt SJ, et al. (1990). Development of a high-titer retro-virus producer cell line capable of gene transfer into rhesus monkey hematopoietic stem cells. *Proc the Nat Acad Sci U S A*. 87:3738–3742.

Bonham L, Wolgamot G, Miller AD (1997). Molecular cloning of *Mus dunni* endogenous virus: an unusual retrovirus in a new murine viral interference group with a wide host range. *J Virol*. 71:4663–4670.

Bosselman RA, Hsu R-Y, Bruszewski J, Hu S, Martin F, Nicolson M (1987). Replication-defective chimeric helper proviruses and factors affecting generation of competent virus: expression of Moloney leukemia virus structural genes via the metallothionein promoter. *Mol Cell Biol*. 7:1797–1806.

Bunnell BA, Muul LM, Donahue RE, Blaese RM, Morgan RA (1995). High-efficiency retroviral-mediated gene transfer into human and non-human primate peripheral blood lymphocytes. *Proc Nat Acad Sci, U S A*. 92:7739–7743.

Cavazzana-Calvo M, Hacein-Bey S, de Saint Basile G, et al. (2000). Gene therapy of human severe combined immunodeficiency (SCID)-X1 disease. *Science* 288:669–672.

Chen J, Reeves L, Cornetta K (2001a). Safety testing for replication-competent retrovirus (RCR) associated with gibbon ape leukemia virus pseudotyped retroviral vectors. *Hum Gene Ther*. 12:61–70.

Chen J, Reeves L, Sanburn N, Croop J, Williams DA, Cornetta K (2001b). Packaging cell line DNA contamination of vector supernatants: implication for laboratory and clinical research. *Virology*. 282:186–197.

Chong H, Starkey W, Vile RG (1998). A replication-competent retrovirus arising from a split-function packaging cell line was generated by recombination events between the vector, one of the packaging constructs, and endogenous retroviral sequences. *J Virol*. 72:2663–2670.

Cornetta K (1992). Safety aspects of human gene therapy. *Br J Haematol*. 80:421–426.

Cornetta K, Nguyen N, Morgan RA, Muenchau DD, Hartley J, Anderson WF (1993). Infection of human cells with murine amphotropic replication-competent retroviruses. *Hum Gene Ther*. 4:579–588.

Cosset F, Takeuchi Y, Battini J, Weiss RA, Collins MKL (1995). High-titer packaging cells producing recombinant retroviruses resistant to human serum. *J Virol*. 69:7430–7436.

Danos O, Mulligan RC (1988). Safe and efficient generation of recombinant retroviruses with amphotroic and ecotropic host ranges. *Proc Nat Acad Sci, U S A*. 85:6460–6464.

Dave UP, Jenkins NA, Copeland NG (2004). Gene therapy insertional mutagenesis insights. *Science*. 303:333.

Donahue RE, Kessler SW, Bodine D, et al. (1992). Helper virus induction T cell lymphoma in nonhuman primates after retroviral mediated gene transfer. *J Exp Med*. 176:1125–1135.

Duffy L, Koop S, Fyffe J, Cornetta K (2003). Extended S+/L− assay for detecting replication competent retroviruses (RCR) pseudotyped with the RD114 viral envelope. *Preclinica*. May–June:53–59.

Forestell SP, Dando JS, Bohnlein E, Rigg RJ (1996). Improved detection of replication-competent retrovirus. *J Virol Methods*. 60:171–178.

Garrett E, Miller AR-M, Goldman J, Apperley JF, Melo JV (2000). Characterization of recombinant events leading to the production of an ecotropic replication-competent retrovirus in a GP+ *env* AM12-derived producer cell line. *Virology*. 266:170–179.

Goerner M, Horn PA, Peterson L, et al. (2001). Sustained multilineage gene persistence and expression in dogs transplanted with CD34(+) marrow cells transduced by RD114-pseudotyped oncoretrovirus vectors. *Blood*. 98:2065–2070.

Hacein-Bey-Abina S, Le Deist F, Carlier F, et al. (2002). Sustained correction of X-linked severe combined immunodeficiency by ex vivo gene therapy. *New Engl J Med*. 346:1185–1193.

Hacein-Bey-Abina S, von Kalle C, Schmidt M, et al. (2003a). A serious adverse event after successful gene therapy for X-linked severe combined immunodeficiency. *New Engl J Med*. 348:255–256.

Hacein-Bey-Abina S, von Kalle C, Schmidt M, et al. (2003b). LMO2-associated clonal T cell proliferation in two patients after gene therapy for SCID-X1. *Science*. 302:415–419 [erratum appears in *Science*. 2003;302;568].

Kelly PF, Vandergriff J, Nathwani A, Nienhuis AW, Vanin EF (2000). Highly efficient gene transfer into cord blood nonobese diabetic/severe combined immunodeficiency repopulating cells by oncoretroviral vector particles pseudotyped with the feline endogenous retrovirus (RD114) envelope protein. *Blood*. 96:1206–1214.

Lander MR, Chattopadhyay SK (1984). A *Mus dunni* cell line that lacks sequences closely related to endogenous murine leukemia viruses and can be infected by ecotropic, amphotropic, xenotropic and mink cell focus-forming viruses. *J Virol*. 52:695–696.

Li Z, Dullman J, Schiedlmeier B, et al. (2002). Murine leukemia induced by retroviral gene marking. *Science*. 296:497.

Long Z, Li L-P, Grooms T, et al. (1998). Biosafety monitoring of patients receiving intracerebral injections of murine retroviral vector producer cells. *Hum Gene Ther*. 9:1165–1172.

Mann R, Mulligan RC, Baltimore D (1983). Construction of a retrovirus packaging mutant and its use to produce helper-free defective retrovirus. *Cell*. 33:153–159.

Markowitz D, Goff S, Bank A (1988a). Construction and use of a safe and efficient amphotropic packaging line. *Virology*. 167:400–406.

Markowitz D, Goff S, Bank A (1988b). A safe packaging line for gene transfer: seperating viral genes on two different plasmids. *J Virol*. 62:1120–1124.

Martineau D, Klump WM, McCormack JE, et al. (1997). Evaluation of PCR and ELISA assays for screening clinical trial subjects for recplication competent retrovirus. *Hum Gene Ther*. 8:1231–1241.

Miller AD (1990). Retrovirus packaging cells. *Hum Gene Ther*. 1:5–14.

Miller AD, Rosman GJ (1989). Improved retroviral vectors for gene transfer and expression. *BioTechniques*. 7:980–990.

Miller AD, Garcia JV, Von Suhr N, Lynch CM, Wilson C, Eiden MV (1991). Construction and properties of retrovirus packaging cells based on gibbon ape leukemia virus. *J Virol*. 65:2220–2224.

Miller AD, Bonham L, Alfano J, Kiem HP, Reynolds T, Wolgamot G (1996). A novel murine retrovirus identified during testing for helper virus in human gene transfer trials. *J Virol*. 70:1804–1809.

Morgan RA, Cornetta K, Anderson WF (1990). Application of polymerase chain reaction in retroviral mediated gene transfer and the analysis of gene-marked human TIL cells. *Hum Gene Ther*. 1:136–149.

Muenchau DD, Freeman SM, Cornetta K, Zwiebel JA, Anderson WF (1990). Analysis of retroviral packaging lines for generation of replication-competent virus. *Virology* 176:262–265.

Otto E, Jones-Trower A, Vanin EF, et al. (1994). Characterization of a replication-competent retrovirus resulting from recombination of packaging and vector sequences. *Hum Gene Ther*. 5:567–575.

Paticncc C, Takeuch Y, Cosset FL, Weiss RA (2001). MuLV packaging systems as models for estimating/measuring retrovirus recombination frequency. *Dev Biol*. 106:169–179.

Printz M, Reynolds J, Mento SJ, Jolly D, Kowal K, Sajjadi N (1995). Recombinant retroviral vector interferes with the detection of amphotropic replication competent retrovirus in standard culture assays. *Gene Ther*. 2:143–150.

Reeves L, Duffy L, Koop S, Fyffe J, Cornetta K (2002). Detection of ecotropic replication-competent retroviruses: Comparison of S+/L− and marker rescue assays. *Hum Gene Ther*. 13:1783–1790.

Rosenberg N, Joelicoer P (1997). Retroviral pathogenesis. In: Coffin JM, Hughes SH, Varmus HE, eds. *Retroviruses*. Cold Spring Harbor, NY: Cold Spring Harbor Laboratory Press: 475–586.

Scarpa M, Cournoyer D, Muzny DM, Moore KA, Belmont JW, Caskey CT (1991). Characterization of recombinant helper retroviruses from Moloney-based vectors in ecotropic and amphotropic packaging cell lines. *Virology*. 180:849–852.

von Kalle C, Kiem HP, Goehle S, et al. (1994). Increased gene transfer into human hematopoietic progenitor cells by extended in vitro exposure to a pseudotyped retroviral vector. *Blood*. 84(9):2890–2897.

Watanabe S, Temin HM (1983). Construction of a helper cell line for avian reticuloendotheliosis virus cloning vectors. *Mol Cell Biol*. 3:2241–2249.

Wilson C, Reitz MS, Okayama H, Eiden MV (1989). Formation of infectious hybrid virions with gibbon ape leukemia virus and human T-cell leukemia virus retroviral envelope glycoproteins and the *gag* and *pol* proteins of Moloney murine leukemia virus. *J Virol*. 63:2374–2378.

Wilson CA, Ng T, Miller AE (1997). Evaluation of recommendations for replication-competent retrovirus testing associated with use of retroviral vectors. *Hum Gene Ther*. 8:869–874.

24 Assays for the Quality Control of Lentiviral Vectors

JAMES E. MISKIN, SUSAN M. KINGSMAN,
and KYRIACOS A. MITROPHANOUS
Oxford BioMedica, Oxford, UK

To advance lentiviral vectors from a promising research tool into a vector that can be used in human clinical trials, it is necessary to be able to test a range of parameters for each vector preparation. Through performing these tests, the manufacturer is able to demonstrate equivalence between manufactured batches of vector and to ensure that each batch meets certain preset conditions that have been agreed with the regulatory authorities [e.g., the Food and Drug Administration (FDA) in the United States or the Medicines and Healthcare Products Regulatory Agency in the UK]. These criteria are based on comparison with vectors that have been shown to be safe and efficacious in appropriate preclinical studies. There are a number of differences between the various lentiviral vector systems, whether derived from primate (e.g., HIV-1) or nonprimate [e.g., equine infections anemia virus (EIAV)] lentiviruses, but the concepts of the assays are broadly applicable to all systems. Although regulatory guidelines for quality control (QC) testing are quite prescriptive in terms of what information must be made available (e.g., particle number, titer, host cell DNA contamination), there is limited guidance on the choice of method that should be used to determine the information required. The QC assays we describe here have been developed specifically to check batches of lentiviral vectors based on EIAV although the approaches taken could be adapted relatively simply for any lentiviral vector system. The assays described in this chapter do not constitute an exhaustive list of the QC requirements for release of a batch of vector destined for the clinic, but some of the key assays pertinent to lentiviruses are described.

We have developed assays for the detection of replication-competent viruses and discuss methods that we have established for determining the titer of therapeutic vectors lacking marker genes, measuring their potency, demonstrating the identity, and determining the particle number within vector preparations. A schematic diagram of some of the QC assays tailor made for testing batches

Concepts in Genetic Medicine, Edited by Boro Dropulic and Barrie Carter
Copyright © 2008 John Wiley & Sons, Inc.

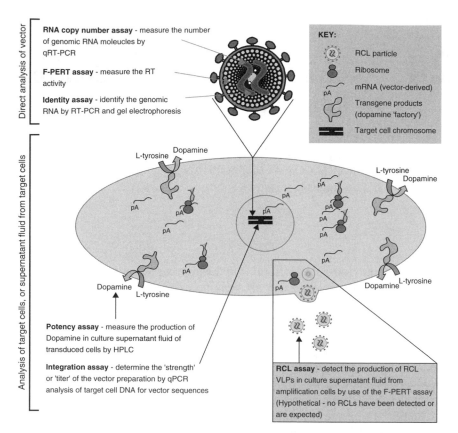

Figure 24.1 Key QC assays developed for testing batches of ProSavin® an EIAV vector designed to treat Parkinson's disease. As indicated, assays are either conducted directly on vector material or on target cells or supernatant fluid following treatment of cells with ProSavin in culture.

of ProSavin® vector, our gene therapy treatment for Parkinson's disease [1,2], is shown in Figure 24.1. In addition to these vector-specific assays, more general assays have been adopted or have been adapted to be applicable for testing lentiviral vector preparations. The general assays (e.g., total DNA, total protein, pH, osmolarity, sterility, mycoplasma) are not described here.

REPLICATION-COMPETENT LENTIVIRUS ASSAY

One key assay is a test for the presence of replication-competent lentiviruses (RCLs) within a vector preparation, as the presence of such entities within a batch could have serious implications if administered to patients. Each vector system is typically tailored to minimize the potential for generating RCLs, but despite our best efforts, biology is sometimes unpredictable, so it is impossible to be certain that no RCL could arise during production. The EIAV vector system we have developed is completely minimal, meaning that the only gene from the parental virus expressed during production is codon-optimized *Gag-Pol*, which is required to form the vector particles and enzymes required for gene delivery (reverse transcriptase, integrase). The use of codon-optimized *Gag-Pol* meant that the Rev/RRE (rev response element) system was not required for particle production but was required initially for efficient packaging of full-length genomic RNA within particles. The final step toward a completely minimal system, dispensing with the Rev/RRE system, was achieved by including a short open reading frame immediately downstream of the packaging signal (Ψ), such as the neomycin-resistance gene (*Neo*) [3]. The envelope used to pseudotype these vectors is often the glycoprotein from vesicular stomatitis virus (VSV-G). To develop an RCL assay for minimal EIAV vectors, there were four key questions that we needed to address: (1) to determine an appropriate positive control replication-competent virus, (2) to choose a suitable amplification cell line, (3) to establish culture conditions for the amplification of RCL, and (4) to pick a suitable assay for the detection of amplified RCL and positive control. Layered on top of these questions was the consideration that the assay needed to be relatively simple to perform robustly in a regulatory-compliant setting. The scientific rationale underpinning the choice of RCL assay conditions as well as the details of the assay have been described [4].

Assays for replication-competent retrovirus (RCR) can act as a guide for the development of an RCL assay. Traditionally, RCR assays have consisted of passaging the test article on a permissive cell line to amplify any RCR present. The supernatant from these cultures is then assayed for the presence of RCR by virological methods such as focus-forming assays. The positive control used is usually the parental retrovirus. As the minimal lentiviral vectors are produced from human cells and destined for human use, the amplification cell line chosen was a human cell line (HEK293). HEK293 cells have been shown to be permissive for infection/transduction by a wide range of vector systems/viruses. As wild-type EIAV cannot enter or replicate in human cells, it cannot act as a positive control. We therefore sought to use a wild-type virus that would have the same replication dynamics in human cells as putative RCL derived from EIAV. We showed that in equine dermal (ED) cells, EIAV and MLV replicated with almost identical kinetics. As expected, EIAV did not replicate at all in human cells, as it is blocked by two independent mechanisms: the lack of the EIAV receptor, which has been identified recently [5], and the fact that human Cyclin-T1 (hCT1) is unable to interact with the Tat–TAR complex to allow efficient transcription from the EIAV long terminal repeat (LTR) in human cells [6]. From these data we demonstrated that under conditions where EIAV and murine leukemia virus (MLV) could be compared, their replication rates were the same, but a human cell comparison was not possible. Engineering human cells to express equine Cyclin-T1 (eCT1) was not sufficient to "rescue" EIAV replication. At this point there were two clear choices to us: either to generate a novel human cell replication-competent entity derived from EIAV, or to test whether a surrogate control virus could be used instead. Ethical and safety considerations made the former choice one that was far from ideal, as highlighted in a recent draft guideline issued by the European Medicines Agency (EMEA) [7]. Therefore, we chose to pursue the latter option by modeling the replication kinetics of viruses using a series of replication-deficient vectors that were increasingly disabled but had structural similarities to the most likely RCL that one could predict from the vector system components. The EIAV vectors were called the EMOB (EIAV mobilizable) series, and all contained the components necessary for packaging, reverse transcription, and integration as well as the codon-optimized *Gag–Pol* cassette. A total of eight vectors were tested containing variations in the LTR sequences and the presence or absence of the EIAV accessory gene region (encoding Tat, Rev, and S2). The rate of particle production from the EMOB vectors was examined in equine cells (EDs) as well as in unmodified human cells (HEK293) and in human cells expressing eCT1 (HEK293eCT1). The results of these studies indicated that particle production by EMOB vectors was completely dependent on the presence of all of the following features: (1) a functional LTR sequence such as the full-length EIAV LTR, or an EIAV-MLV hybrid LTR where the EIAV U3 sequence was replaced with the U3 from MLV; (2) the presence of eCT1 (in either ED or HEK293eCT1 cells); and (3) the presence of the EIAV accessory gene region. These experiments allowed us to make two critical observations. The first observation was that the particle production kinetics of MLV and EMOB-2, which was effectively an *Env*-deleted surrogate of EIAV as it contained the EIAV accessory gene region and the full-length EIAV LTR, were almost identical in ED and HEK293eCT1 cells. This observation meant that if EIAV was to overcome the blocks to productive infection in human cells, it would presumably replicate with kinetics similar to MLV. The second observation was that particle production from EMOB vectors absolutely required three features that were entirely absent from the vector production system. The minimal vector system has a self-inactivating (SIN) LTR, contains none of the accessory gene region, and there is no expression of eCT1 in the production cells. Taken together, these observations made a very strong argument for the adoption of MLV 4070A and human cells as the RCL assay positive control, and also made a convincing argument that the use of EIAV and equine cells would be inappropriate to test the minimal EIAV vectors for the presence of RCL. MLV 4070A is a reference standard for RCR assays that can easily be obtained from the ATCC.

We reasoned that a unifying feature of all RCLs would be the presence of reverse transcriptase (RT) within the particles. The use of RT as an indicator of the presence of retroviral or lentiviral particles meant that a generic assay could be chosen and also that prior knowledge of the structure and identity of a putative RCL was not needed. Recently, a number of similar quantitative PCR-based assays have been developed to detect RT activity, notably the fluorescent product–enhanced reverse transcriptase (F-PERT) assay [8,9]. Finally, the choices of MLV 4070A as the positive control, HEK293 cells for amplification, and F-PERT as a sensitive endpoint assay for RCL led us to devise a suitable passage and amplification regime for putative EIAV-derived RCLs. The passaging process takes approximately four to five weeks and includes nine or 10 passages, to ensure that the vector-associated RT activity has been diluted out and that a minimal dose of the positive control virus has been amplified effectively [4]. This extended period was required, as EIAV vector particles and RT activity were demonstrated to be very stable in culture; RT activity in culture supernatant fluid was stable for at least seven days at 37 °C. This was notably different from other vector systems, where RT activity was not stable in culture. To match RCR regulatory guidelines [10] that suggest testing 5% of a vector product and 10^8 postproduction cells, two RCL assays were devised. The vector (clinical lot) RCL assay was designed to be scalable to allow testing of 5% of a vector from a wide range of manufacturing scales, whereas the postproduction cell (co-cult) RCL assay was designed at a single scale. The RCL assays have now been validated at the 20-L manufacturing scale, during which no RCL was detected. The assay is also theoretically applicable to any retroviral or lentiviral vector and pseudotype combination, provided that a suitable approach is used to demonstrate that the choice of positive control, cell line, and passage regime are all appropriate.

DETERMINATION OF VECTOR TITER

An assay that is suitable to determine the biological activity (also referred to as *strength* or *titer*) of a lentiviral vector is an absolute requirement for clinical development. It is important to be able to benchmark a given vector preparation to other preparations that have been shown to possess the accepted characteristics of a vector that was efficacious and safe in the appropriate preclinical models. To be considered *functional*, a lentiviral vector must be able to enter a target cell through envelope glycoprotein–cell interactions, and must contain packaged vector genomic RNA, and must be able to reverse transcribe this RNA into a DNA entity that, together with integrase, forms the preintegration complex, which ultimately becomes integrated within the DNA genome of the target cell. An assay that directly measures the vector particles for a physical characteristic (such as RNA content or RT activity) would be, by definition, incapable of demonstrating whether any of the criteria to be considered functional have been met. The chosen assay must therefore be able to measure the functional integration efficiency of the vector, as through doing this information is gained that demonstrates that the appropriate proportion of particles are active. The majority of vectors destined for the clinic will have been pared down to minimize the amount of exogenous protein and DNA that are transferred to target cells. Therefore, most clinical vectors will not possess a generic marker gene, and as a consequence, a generic assay of gene expression would be impossible to devise.

However, one feature that is retained in all vectors is their ability to package genomic RNA, which is subsequently converted into DNA and integrated.

By definition, the genetic payload of each vector will differ, depending on the intended therapeutic area, but one aspect of the vector genome that is always preserved is the packaging signal (Ψ). Through bringing together all these requirements for the assay and commonality between different vectors, we have devised an assay that tests the integration performance of a vector in tissue culture cells (HEK293T) by the use of quantitative real-time PCR. This assay can be thought of in three distinct phases. The first phase involves transduction and passage of the HEK293T cells in tissue culture; the transduction and passage regimes have been determined empirically to ensure that any DNA sequences detected at the end of the assay (10-days posttransduction) are due to integrated vector sequences, to which nonintegrated entities such as LTR circles and plasmid DNA do not contribute. To achieve this we have demonstrated that cells should undergo at least eight population doublings, with the effect being that nonintegrated sequences are theoretically diluted out by a factor of 2^8 (256-fold). The second phase of the assay involves the isolation of genomic DNA from the target cells and quantification, which is achieved by the use of a high-throughput DNA extraction instrument (MagNA Pure LC, Roche) and a spectrophotometer. The final stage of the assay uses TaqMan quantitative PCR technology to analyze a known amount of DNA (150 ng), which is equivalent to approximately 22,000 human cells' worth of DNA, alongside DNA extracted from a HEK293T standard that has been shown to contain a single copy of an EIAV vector genome. However, it is not sufficient to validate such an assay using a generic vector and assume that the results are valid for any genetic payload. It is critical that each vector genome be tested in this assay over an extended period in culture. This is to determine whether the vector can be reverse transcribed and integrated and to ensure that the particular vector genome does not result in reduced or enhanced growth kinetics of the target cells because of expression of the transgene. If this is the case, any titer value obtained from this in vitro assay would not reliably predict the biological activity of the vector preparation. If expression of the transgene is problematic in the integration assay, it may be possible, or even advantageous, to prevent expression of the transgene except within the intended target tissue in vivo (such as use of a tissue-specific promoter). The titer obtained using the integration assay should be used to compare vector preparations containing the same transgene, and the relationship between this value and efficacy should be established in an appropriate model. Diverse vector genomes may perform differently in this assay for reasons such as altered pseudotype, efficiency of reverse transcription, and packaging efficiency. However, the performance of different batches of the same vector should be predictable within the limits of the assay. It is important to note that any in vitro titer assay will be biased by the actual conditions used (e.g., volume of vector, number of target cells, addition of polycations, culture medium), so the integration titer value that is determined by the assay does not necessarily reflect the entire active population of particles within a vector prep; rather, it is a "snapshot" of the integrative potential of the preparation.

POTENCY AND IDENTITY

The majority of the QC assays required for the testing of lentiviral vectors can be generic, at least at the level of the vector system (i.e., suitable for QC testing of any EIAV-based vector). However, the nature of the potency and identity assays means that it is not possible to devise single assays to test all the potential vector transgene combinations for treatment of different diseases by gene therapy. As an overview, the potency assay must be devised to measure the function of the vector. It is not considered sufficient merely to devise an assay that tests for expression of the transgene, but instead, one that tests an effect of gene expression. For example, the potency assay we have devised to measure the potency of ProSavin measures the amount of dopamine produced per integrated copy in the supernatant fluid of target cells. ProSavin expresses three transgenes that together produce dopamine, which is then measured in cell culture medium using high-performance liquid chromatography.

The identity assay must be designed to be able to identify the presence of the specific vector transgene combination within the vial from which vector will ultimately be administered to patients. Each lentiviral vector will have a large number of structural components in common with all other vectors from the same system, but a unique feature will be the structure of the vector genomic RNA packaged within particles. Therefore, the identity assays we have devised for each of the EIAV-based vectors rely on the isolation, reverse transcription, amplification, and identification of the RNA through its unique banding pattern following gel electrophoresis. The region amplified encompasses the transgenes, at least in part, and positive and negative controls are included to ensure that the amplification was from RNA and not contaminating DNA species.

RNA COPY NUMBER AND F-PERT

Various approaches can be thought of to determine or estimate the number of particles, functional or inactive, within vector preparations. Physical methods, such as electron microscopy, are useful but are not very quantitative and do not lend themselves well to being routine QC release tests. Two characteristics of retroviruses and lentiviruses can simply be exploited using quantitative real time PCR (qRT-PCR)-based assays to measure particle number, resulting in either relative or absolute numbers. The first of these uses the F-PERT assay discussed previously [8,9] to measure the amount of RT activity within vector prepartions. It is known that retroviruses contain between 10 and 100 molecules of RT enzyme per particle [11–14]. Through qRT-PCR, the number of molecules of cDNA generated by the RT activity released from a known amount of a vector, using an excess of an unrelated RNA as template, can be converted into a relative particle number. Cross-comparison of these results with other assays can allow estimations to be made of the true particle number. The second of the two assays relies on the quantification of the number of genomic RNA molecules within a given vector preparation. As retroviral particles typically package two RNA molecules per particle as a dimer, the number of RNA molecules can be converted into a vector particle number. The F-PERT assay has the advantage that it will measure all viruslike particles (VLPs), irrespective of whether the particle is functional (i.e., envelope and RNA are not required), but has the disadvantage that it is a more complex process to determine a particle number from such an assay. The qRT-PCR RNA copy number assay has the advantage that it lends itself to absolute quantification, but the disadvantage is that empty VLPs will not be measured. Therefore, we have used a pragmatic approach by using both of these assays as part of the QC process, and through a comparison with results from other assays, an accurate measure of the purity, strength, and equivalence of a preparation can be obtained.

THE FUTURE

The culmination of years of development of lentiviral vectors to make them increasingly minimal, improvements to production and purification strategies, and the development of an appropriate array of QC tests together will allow the progression of these vectors into the clinic. The long-held promise of gene therapy for the successful treatment of a variety of diseases is hopefully just around the corner.

REFERENCES

1. Azzouz M, et al. Multicistronic lentiviral vector-mediated striatal gene transfer of aromatic L-amino acid decarboxylase, tyrosine hydroxylase, and GTP cyclohydrolase I induces sustained transgene expression, dopamine production, and functional improvement in a rat model of Parkinson's disease. *J Neurosci*. 2002; 22(23):10302–10312.

2. Azzouz M, Kingsman SM, Mazarakis ND. Lentiviral vectors for treating and modeling human CNS disorders. *J Gene Med*. 2004;6(9):951–962.

3. Wilkes FJ, In preparation, 2005.

4. Miskin J, Chipchase D, Rohll J, et al. A replication competent lentivirus (RCL) assay for equine infectious anaemia virus (EIAV)–based lentiviral vectors. *Gene Ther*. 2006; 13(3):196–205.

5. Zhang B, et al. A tumor necrosis factor receptor family protein serves as a cellular receptor for the macrophage-tropic equine lentivirus. *Proc Natl Acad Sci U S A*. 2005; 102(28):9918–9923.

6. Bieniasz PD, et al. Highly divergent lentiviral Tat proteins activate viral gene expression by a common mechanism. *Mol Cell Biol*. 1999;19(7):4592–4599.

7. EMEA Guideline on development and manufacture of lentiviral vectors. European Medicines Agency, Evaluation of Medicines for Human Use, Committee for medicinal products for human use (CHMP). 2005;CHMP/BWP/2458/03:1–8.

8. Arnold BA, Hepler RW, Keller PM. One-step fluorescent probe product-enhanced reverse transcriptase assay. *BioTechniques*. 1998;25(1):98–106.

9. Lovatt A, et al. High throughput detection of retrovirus-associated reverse transcriptase using an improved fluorescent product enhanced reverse transcriptase assay and its comparison to conventional detection methods. *J Virol Methods*. 1999; 82(2):185–200.

10. CBER et al. *Guidance for Industry*: Supplemental guidance on testing for replication competent retrovirus in retroviral vector based gene therapy products and during follow-up of patients in clinical trials using retroviral vectors. CBER document. 2000; N/A(N/A):1–12.

11. Stromberg K, et al. Structural studies of avian myeloblastosis virus: comparison of polypeptides in virion and core component by dodecyl sulfate–polyacrylamide gel electrophoresis. *J Virol*. 1974;13(2):513–528.

12. Panet A, Baltimore D, Hanafusa T. Quantitation of avian RNA tumor virus reverse transcriptase by radioimmunoassay. *J Virol*. 1975;16(1):146–152.

13. Krakower JM, Barbacid M, Aaronson SA. Radioimmunoassay for mammalian type C viral reverse transcriptase. *J Virol*. 1977;22(2):331–339.

14. Layne SP, et al. Factors underlying spontaneous inactivation and susceptibility to neutralization of human immunodeficiency virus. *Virology*. 1992;189(2):695–714.

25 Assays for Nonviral Vectors

RALPH W. PAUL

Targeted Genetics Corporation, Seattle, Washington

Plasmid DNA purified from *Escherichia coli* can be the complete vector and gene expression system to be delivered in an in vivo setting to direct protein expression for a genetic vaccine or therapeutic gene therapy application, or it can function as the core building block of any number of nonviral gene delivery systems. High-quality plasmid DNA may also be a key constituent of production processes used to generate viral vectors for gene therapy applications. At present, the method of DNA generation from bacteria still represents the most viable, scalable, cost-effective (but not cheap) means of producing sufficient quantities of multi-kilobase-sized double-stranded DNA for clinical trials. Laboratory-scale purification of quantities of plasmid DNA with sufficient quality for in vitro and small in vivo studies is readily possible. It is in the transition from small laboratory-scale purification to the scale required to generate sufficient quantities for larger-scale animal efficacy and toxicology studies, followed by the hoped-for clinical studies and commercialization, that a number of issues may arise in the generation of appropriate quantities of high-quality plasmid DNA. To ensure the quality, purity, stability, biological potency, and equivalency of DNA lots to be used in clinical applications, a number of assays have typically been developed and utilized. These assays are meant to answer or address any product issues or questions raised by regulatory agencies and to prevent spurious biological results that may come about due to inconsistencies in any of these parameters. Despite the use of plasmid DNA in many clinical trials to date, this is still an evolving and dynamic field. New methods of evaluating DNA are constantly being developed in an effort to bring our understanding of the physical parameters of this biological molecule to that of pharmaceutical products generated by defined organic syntheses.

PRODUCTION AND ANALYSIS OF PLASMID DNA

Production of plasmid DNA using bacterial fermentation is clearly an eminently scalable process based on years of experience in pharmaceutical manufacturing.

Concepts in Genetic Medicine, Edited by Boro Dropulic and Barrie Carter
Copyright © 2008 John Wiley & Sons, Inc.

In contrast to most production processes for biologics, however, the purification strategy for this product is directed toward recovery of DNA as opposed to protein. Upon embarking on a plan that will ideally lead to the initiation of a clinical trial, a critical evaluation of the guidance documents and points to consider such as those which have been generated by the FDA[1,2] may be useful in providing insight. The elements identified in these documents as being crucial for such a plan can aid in determining which assays and their measured parameters are acceptable for success in an investigational new drug (IND) filing. Through 2004, roughly 23% of gene therapy trials worldwide have utilized naked DNA or DNA-based formulations.[3] As a result of this interest, a number of commercial contractors can now provide quantities of GMP (good manufacturing practice)–compliant plasmid DNA for clinical use and have a number of production and validated assay systems in place. However, each plasmid/product may have specific characteristics and require the development of unique assays (often those with biological readouts). A good understanding of the type of assays applicable to a DNA plasmid-based system (common or unique) by those pursuing the use of such a system may have a significant impact on the timeliness and success of the program. Typically, it is recommended that an initial analysis is performed to determine the best combination of *Escherichia coli* host to use together with the plasmid of interest by evaluating yield, ease of lysis, and separation of cellular debris, as well as the general state of the DNA generated (supercoiled, linear, full length, etc.) after purification. Ideally, the purification process used in this evaluation would closely mimic that to be used at a larger scale. It is also recommended that unless using a suppressor tRNA system for plasmid-positive bacterial selection, the resistance gene used should not be a β-lactam (e.g., ampicillin) since they are commonly used and more likely to induce levels of allergic reactions up to anaphylaxis. To address this issue, a commonly used resistance marker is kanamycin or neomycin.[1,2] In contrast to β-lactams, these aminoglyoside antibiotics are not commonly used in clinical practice. Once a plasmid–host cell combination is chosen, the generation of a master cell bank (MCB) and working cell bank (WCB) derived from the MCB is essential.[4] Production runs are then made from the WCB with multiple purity and characterization assays being applied both in process (during purification) and at the bulk or final product stages.

Following bacterial fermentation and harvest, the first step in purification of plasmid DNA is the lysis of the cells. Most processes still rely on a variation of the Birnboim and Doly alkaline lysis protocol. Alternative approaches are being explored, such as heat lysis protocols[5,6] which introduce fewer reagents into the process (consequently, obviating the need to be assayed for after downstream clearance) and may yield purified DNA with fewer intermediate steps. The bacterial cell lysate is subsequently clarified and plasmid DNA isolated away from contaminants, purified, and characterized. Downstream processes typically rely on a series of column chromatography steps using any of a number of ion-exchange

TABLE 25.1   Typical Assays Used to Measure Parameters of Plasmid DNA Preparations Used in Preclinical and Clinical Studies

Parameter Measured	Assay(s) Used[a]	Typical Acceptance Criteria
Bioburden	Agar plating	0 cfu/mL of product
Endotoxin	Chromogenic, kinetic LAL	1–10 EU/mg DNA
Total protein	Micro BCA	<1%
Host cell protein	*E. coli*–specific ELISA	<100 ng/mg DNA
Host cell DNA	Real-time PCR	<1%
RNA	Electrophoresis, HPLC, PCR, fluorescent dye binding	Undetectable–5%
Residual chemicals/ reagents	GC, HPLC	Limits dependent on specific chemical or reagent; guidelines for most in *U.S. Pharmacopeia*
Plasmid concentration	A_{260}, fluorescent dye binding, electrophoresis	For A_{260}-specified concentration when O.D. 260/280=1.7 to 2.0
Percent supercoiled plasmid	Electrophoresis, HPLC	>70%
Plasmid size	Electrophoresis ± restriction digests, MALDI-TOF	Identity with known standards
Plasmid identity	Electrophoresis ± restriction digests, sequencing, DNA array hybridization	Identity with known standards and sequence composition predicted
Appearance	Visual observation, dynamic light scattering	Clear solution with specified particle size range and distribution
Potency	Biological readout based on expression from functional plasmid	Dependent on indication, expression level required for biological effect, and acceptability of surrogate readouts/endpoints

[a]LAL, *Limulus* amebocyte lysate; BCA, bicinhoninic acid; ELISA, enzyme linked immunosorbent assay; PCR, polymerase chain reaction; HPLC, high performance liquid chromatography; GC, gas chromatography; A_{260}, adsorbance at light wavelength of 260 nm; MALDI-TOF, matrix assisted laser desorption/ionization time-of-flight mass spectrometry.

or hydrophobic interaction resins for purification and final product polishing. Often, these matrices are also chosen based on their potential scalability and history of use in pharmaceutical production.

A summary of typical assays applied to plasmid DNA which is to be used in preclinical toxicology/efficacy studies and/or clinical trials is given in Table 25.1. The focus of these assays is typically to demonstrate either the clearance of possible contaminating materials or the presence of pure, high-quality, plasmid DNA, ensuring the safety and enhancing efficacy of the DNA product.

PURITY AND SAFETY ASSAYS

Bioburden plating assays are designed to demonstrate the presence of viable bacterial cells which have passed successfully through the purification process or, more likely, been introduced as a contaminant. Minimizing the level of and assaying for the lipopolysaccharide–protein complexes or endotoxins derived from the outer bacterial cell wall of gram-negative bacteria is of significant importance. These represent a process impurity that must be removed and are typically measured using variants of the *Limulus* amebocyte lysate (LAL) assay. These variations may measure the turbidity increases characteristic of the assay by following this reaction kinetically, or they may have a terminal chromophore step for a colorimetric readout. Some assays can measure a combination of kinetic and colorimetric outputs. These negatively charged endotoxins can cause pronounced immunological effects over a range of concentrations in vivo.[7] Also problematic is that these are charged molecules that can interfere with the charge balancing and interaction between DNA and other constituents, such as lipids or polymers, that make up a nonviral formulation. Total protein can be measured by a number of standard protein assay techniques, but host-cell-specific protein is now typically measured by an *E. coli*–specific ELISA. Host cell DNA is commonly quantified by real-time polymerase chain reaction (RT-PCR) assays. RNA may be measured by gel electrophoresis and staining, but RT-PCR coupled with subsequent quantitative PCR, high-performance liquid chromatography (HPLC), and fluorescent dye–based assays have all been described[8] for this purpose. As for the plasmid DNA itself, these same approaches are meant to generate assays that are more sensitive, quantitative over a wider dynamic range, less subject to interfering contaminants, and capable of being validated. The assays for determinations of residual reagents (e.g., alcohols, organic solvents) or chemicals (e.g., kanamycin, detergents) will depend on the exact process used for DNA purification. Many of these materials are measured using gas chromatography (GC) or HPLC. It should be noted that purification processes that require certain organic reagents will need to be performed in facilities built to accommodate the flammability or explosive potential of such reagents.

DNA QUALITY AND QUANTITY

In determinations that involve the assay of final plasmid DNA product for both physical and biological parameters, it is crucial that thought be given to preparation of DNA standards that remain stable over time (most commonly achieved through low-temperature storage) and can act as internal assay controls for the DNA product being assessed. Ideally, these control samples will have been prepared using processes similar, if not identical, to those used to generate the new plasmid preparation. Plasmid concentration is typically determined using the absorption reading at 260 nm. This simple measurement is useful for DNA solutions with concentrations in excess of 500 ng/mL and if additional assays have been performed to verify a low level of contaminants such as RNA and proteins, whose presence can affect this absorption value. Typically, the concentration determined in this manner is taken in the context of acceptance criteria value whereby the DNA preparation must have an O.D. 260/280 ratio being 1.8 or higher, indicative of a clean preparation of DNA. Other methods used to determine DNA concentration include fluorescence-based assays using PicoGreen staining, which can be very facile and sensitive, and assays that rely on electrophoretic separation followed by staining. The latter assays can have higher sensitivity but are more time consuming and instrumentation intensive. Plasmid size and identity are typically measured by electrophoresis of both uncut and restriction-digested material. Sizes are compared to known standards for confirmation of identity. To generate more accurate size and identification data, efforts have been directed toward the use of laser desorption time-of-flight analysis (MALDI-TOF) of restriction fragments to yield significantly higher resolution and accuracy in measurement of these parameters.[9] Size and identity analyses are closely coupled with actual DNA sequencing of the entire plasmid, which is required in the characterization of the MCB and of an initial purified plasmid bulk preparation.

The detection of mutations in a fraction of the final plasmid product, most importantly in the transgene to be expressed, is a potential issue that currently isn't actively assessed, but ongoing preclinical and clinical outcomes and analyses, along with new technology, may make it feasible to incorporate this as an acceptance criterion in the future. Chemical cleavage of mismatched base pairs and RNase cleavage assays[9] have been developed to address the issue of contaminating mutations in a plasmid population, but long term the approach will likely be to use DNA chip hybridization to screen point mutations, insertions, and deletions rapidly and accurately.[10] A logical extension of the use of DNA arrays would be for rapid confirmatory sequencing of all purified plasmid preparations generated for a specific product. This approach is of particular appeal at commercial-scale production, where ongoing production runs coupled with rapid confirmatory sequencing would be desirable. As a single parameter of plasmid quality and stability, the percentage supercoiling in preparations is closely monitored. The percentage of supercoiling can be assessed electrophoretically followed by scanning but is now measured more commonly using HPLC-based assays.[11] Since a single break in the DNA phosphodiester backbone can convert supercoiled plasmid to an open circular form and further to linear forms, the monitoring of the total supercoiled content is an indicator of physical stability, possibly correlated with biological effectiveness. There is some debate about the absolute correlation between biological potency of plasmid preparations and the amount of supercoiled plasmid versus other forms, as long as the nonsupercoiled forms have not had substantial degradation of the actual transgene coding sequence.[12,13] In synthetic systems where the plasmid is a component of a formulation, the percentage of supercoiled plasmid may play a role in determining the physical and biological characteristics of the final formulation. Long-term stability studies of DNA products as a requirement for clinical trials invariably measure percentage supercoiled plasmid as a stability indicator, and the incorporation of stability-enhancing agents such as chelating and/or reducing agents to minimize oxidation effects may be considered.[9] Plasmid appearance is generally a simple visual inspection of the preparation to ascertain that there are no large aggregates or undesired particulates that have been introduced by the purification or final vialing process. This measurement also has the potential of being refined and quantitated through the application of dynamic light-scattering (DLS) techniques. DLS can be used to determine the size and representational percentages of the particulate population(s) in solution, allowing for an acceptance standard to be developed. One of the more difficult parameters to develop an assay for is the biological potency of the plasmid preparation. This assay will clearly be unique for each plasmid product and dependent on the nature of the transgene being expressed. The ultimate nature of any individual assay may be dependent on discussion with regulatory agencies. A simple in vitro expression experiment through transfection of a target cell line and measurement of the expression level of the transgene may be acceptable for early-stage trials or for comparison to a standard, but such an assay may not be completely predictive of a biological readout. In such areas as DNA vaccines, the development of an immunological readout may take many weeks or months and may need to be repeated for each new plasmid preparation. Such an assay may be extremely onerous, and the pursuit of suitable surrogate endpoints with a more rapid turnaround time is highly desirable.

Despite the numerous parameters of DNA that can now be assessed through both simple and sophisticated characterization assays, more direct relationships still need to be drawn between the physical parameters that can be measured for one of the most predictable and structurally coherent of biological molecules and its biological effects. Work described recently[14, 15] compared the biological activity of an unformulated or "naked" muIL12 expressing plasmid, prepared by three different purification processes, intratumorally injected into intradermally implanted CT-26 melanoma cells. Each of the three processes yielded DNA preparations with comparable characteristics in each of the 10 assays applied to them, yet yielded from 2- to 40-fold differences in biological activity as measured by tumor reduction 21 days postinjection. The preparation found to be most stable in an accelerated stability study (60 °C) also appeared to have the highest biological activity. Additional differences were observed between the preparations when assessed by differential scanning calorimetry (DSC), measuring thermodynamic stability as determined by DNA structural motifs, and Fourier transform analysis (FTIR), measuring base and backbone interactions. How these physical characteristics directly relate to the biological outcomes is currently under evaluation.

Clearly, the physical and biological evaluation of DNA for its use either alone or as a component of a more complex nonviral gene delivery system has been sufficient to satisfy the requirements of regulatory agencies for clinical trials in humans as well as commercial licensure for vaccines in animal health applications (West Nile virus for horses[16] and infectious haematopoietic necrosis virus

(IHNV) for commercially raised salmon[17]). However, there is still a desire and demand for additional analytical techniques to address questions that remain unanswered. These questions revolve around the interplay between purification processes, sequence, structure, stability, and biological outcome.

REFERENCES

1. Draft Guidance for Industry: Considerations for plasmid DNA vaccines for infectious disease indications. Rockville, MD: CBER; February 2005.
2. Guidance for Industry: Guidance for human somatic cell therapy and gene therapy. Rockville, MD: CBER; March 1998.
3. Edelstein ML, Abedi MR, Wixon J, Edelstein RM. Gene therapy clinical trials worldwide 1989–2004: an overview. *J Gene Med*. 2004;6:597–602.
4. Robertson JS, Griffiths E. Assuring the quality, safety, and efficacy of DNA vaccines. *Mol Biotechnol*. 2001;17:143–149.
5. O'Mahony K, Freitag R, Hilbrig F, Müller P, Schumacher I. Proposal for a better integration of bacterial lysis into the production of plasmid DNA at large scale. *J Biotechnol*. 2005;119:118–132.
6. Zhu K, Jin H, Zma Y, et al. A continuous thermal lysis procedure for the large-scale preparation of plasmid DNA. *J Biotechnol*. 2005;118:257–264.
7. Burrell R. Human responses to bacterial endotoxin. *Circ Shock*. 1994;43:137–153.
8. Murphy JC, Winters MA, Watson MP, Konz JO, Sagar S. Monitoring of RNA clearance in a novel plasmid DNA purification process. *Biotechnol Prog*. 2005;21:1213–1219.
9. Middaugh CR, Evens RK, Montgomery DL, Casimiro DR. Analysis of plasmid DNA from a pharmaceutical perspective. *J Pharm Sci*. 1998;87:130–146.
10. Karaman MW, Groshen S, Lee CC, Pike BL, Hacia JG. Comparisons of substitution, insertion and deletion probes for resequencing and mutational analysis using oligonucleotide microarrays. *Nucleic Acids Res*. 2005;33:e33.
11. Molloy MJ, Hall VS, Bailey SI, Friffin KJ, Faulkner J, Uden M. Effective and robust plasmid topology analysis and the subsequent characterization of the plasmid isoforms thereby observed. *Nucleic Acids Res*. 2004;32:129.
12. Bergan D, Galbraith T, Sloane DL. Gene transfer in vitro and in vivo by cationic lipids is not significantly affected by levels of supercoiling of a reporter plasmid. *Pharm Res*. 2000;17:967–973.
13. Cupillard L, Juillard V, Latour S, et al. Impact of plasmid supercoiling on the efficacy of a rabies DNA vaccine to protect cats. *Vaccine* 2005;23:1910–1916.
14. Green AP, Tumanova I, Burzynski J, et al. In vivo evaluation of supercoiled plasmids. *Mol Ther*. 2005;11:S222.
15. Green AP, Tumanova I, Burzynski J, et al. Analytical characterization of supercoiled plasmids. *Mol Ther*. 2005;11:S216.
16. Powell K. DNA vaccines: back in the saddle again? *Nat. Biotechnol*. 2004;22:799–801.
17. Crabtree P. DNA vaccines approved for animals. *San Diego Union-Tribune*. July 20, 2005.

26 Assays for the Release of Cellular Gene Therapy Products

PHILIP J. CROSS
Harvard Gene Therapy Initiative, Boston, Massachusetts, and
Philip J. Cross & Associates, Inc., Wilmington, Delaware

BRUCE L. LEVINE
Clinical Cell and Vaccine Production Facility and
Department of Pathology and Laboratory Medicine,
University of Pennsylvania, Philadelphia, Pennsylvania

In this chapter we first define basic aspects of quality related to cellular gene therapy products. We then discuss release-testing considerations when submitting clinical protocols for review by regulatory agencies, specific tests, and testing strategies. Somatic cellular gene therapy refers to autologous, allogeneic, or xenogeneic cells that have been manipulated ex vivo to constitutively or inducibly express a marker or potentially therapeutic gene and then are reintroduced into the body. Conceivably, these products could also be used as part of a medical device which is implanted or through which body fluids are perfused. The scope of this chapter does not include directly administered gene vectors to whole organs or tissues for transplant, or germ-line cells such as sperm and oocytes.

Release testing for cellular gene therapy products is both more laborious and more convenient than release testing for most other cellular therapy products. On the one hand, testing related to the vector transduction efficiency and residuals of the vector production process and replication-competent virus must be performed in addition to the tests performed on a cellular therapy product. On the other hand, due to the length of time required to perform replication-competent virus testing, most gene therapy products are cryopreserved. Thus, cellular gene therapy product testing can be performed and repeated as necessary without compromising the potency of the final product.

Concepts in Genetic Medicine, Edited by Boro Dropulic and Barrie Carter
Copyright © 2008 John Wiley & Sons, Inc.

REGULATORY CONTEXT FOR RELEASE TESTING
OF CELLULAR GENE THERAPY PRODUCTS

All gene-modified cellular therapy products are regulated by the Food and Drug Administration (FDA)'s Center for Biologics Evaluation and Research (CBER) in the United States, by the European Medicines Agency (EMEA) in the European Union, or by equivalent agencies in other countries. Release testing as discussed in this chapter will highlight the U.S. regulatory environment and the International Conference on Harmonisation (ICH). Cells intended for use in humans (either investigational or licensed) must be manufactured using current good manufacturing practice (cGMP). cGMP is the current set of principles as defined by 21CFR210, 211, 600, 610, and 820 (U.S. *Code of Federal Regulations*). Use of the word *current* in cGMP indicates that the regulations and methods used to implement them change over time and stress the need for manufacturing establishments to constantly review and modify the way they implement these practices.

The terms *quality assurance* (QA) and *quality control* (QC) have often been used synonymously but in fact describe very different functions. The QC unit was originally defined in the drug GMP regulations (21CFR211.22) as the group with the responsibility for approval and rejection of all materials used in manufacture and the final product itself. This group also had responsibility for performing release testing and assuring that the final product met all specifications. This definition has changed over the years. The QC unit is now generally responsible for testing raw materials, in-process materials, and final products. The QA unit is responsible for compliance oversight and review of manufacturing and testing of the final product. Generally, it is current practice for the QA and QC groups to have separate reporting structures within the organization. QA should be independent of both QC and manufacturing. A good recent description of a "quality program" is provided in the good tissue practice regulations (see 21 CFR1271.160). Elements of the quality program include establishing and maintaining procedures, ensuring that appropriate corrective actions are taken and documented, establishing a system for the maintenance of records, investigating and documenting deviations, conducting audits and evaluations, and ensuring compliance with the regulations.

Release testing on cellular gene therapy products is performed in the context of the quality program as described above to meet regulatory requirements on characterizing the final product. Quality control testing must ensure the *safety, sterility, purity, potency*, and *identity* of the final product (see 21CFR600.3). The types of individual tests that may be used for cellular gene therapy products are described in more detail below. In a general sense, the word *safety* means the relative freedom from harmful effects to persons affected directly or indirectly by a product when prudently administered, taking into consideration the character of the product in relation to the condition of the recipient at the time. Safety testing may include preclinical experiments to document removal of reagents used in the manufacturing process or animal toxicity studies. The word *sterility* is interpreted to mean freedom from viable contaminating microorganisms. *Purity* means relative freedom from extraneous matter in the finished product, whether or not harmful to the recipient or deleterious to the product. *Purity* includes but is not limited to relative freedom from sensitizing and pyrogenic substances. The word *potency* is interpreted to mean the therapeutic capacity of the final product to function as anticipated or for relevant products synthesized by the final product to function as anticipated. In early-phase trials, potency may not be completely characterized. Testing and labeling controls must also be in place to ensure final product *identity*, which may be established either through the physical or chemical characteristics of the product, inspection by macroscopic or microscopic methods, specific cultural tests, or in vitro or in vivo immunological tests.

PRECLINICAL DEVELOPMENT OF RELEASE TEST ASSAYS

Preclinical studies must be conducted in preparation for submission of a chemistry, manufacturing, and controls (CMC) section of an investigational new drug (IND) application to the FDA and should be seen as an investment that will save time, money, and regulatory headaches later. These studies may include refining methods for isolation or differentiation of cells to be gene modified, refining the method of transduction or transfection, and toxicology studies in animals conducted according to good laboratory practice. A new look must be taken at procedures that were developed in the research lab to translate these techniques to clinically compatible reagents and materials and to delineate the plan for release testing of a clinical product.

These studies should be designed to validate novel release tests or to validate established release tests on novel products or processes. For example, the purity of gene-modified cells following a newly established method of isolation, activation, or transduction must be established in preclinical development. Preclinical studies should also be designed to characterize the biological effects or potency of the gene-modified cell product. Full-scale validation runs serve as a "dress rehearsal" for the standard operating procedures for processing and release testing. Critical to establish during validation runs are the volumes and cell numbers required for each release test, whether a sample is taken in process or from the final product, and the timing of release test performance and the availability of test results.

An additional component of the CMC section is a description of the facilities in which the gene-modified cells will be manufactured. The laboratory must be segregated from all research activities and have controlled access. To comply with new regulations on good tissue practice, procedures should be in place for environmental monitoring of nonviable and viable particles, decontamination, and changeover. Changeover procedures should detail what cleaning should take place in between manufacture of different vectors or cell products. Equipment used in the laboratory should be monitored and calibrated regularly. Detailed records of equipment calibration, environmental monitoring, and processing should be maintained during preclinical development and validation and especially during clinical processing. Space limitations preclude a detailed description here of the regulatory and quality considerations for facilities for the production of gene-modified cellular products. More detailed reviews (Burger, 2000,2003; Gee, 2003; Smith and Lowdell, 2003) and relevant regulations and guidances listed in the Appendix should be consulted.

ASSAYS FOR MASTER CELL BANKS AND RAW MATERIALS

Concurrent with preclinical development is the preparation, validation, and testing of the upstream components of the final gene-modified cellular therapy product. Screening of individual components allows for the detection of problems before significant additional time and resources are invested in the final product. A product developed from an autologous source is exempt from many tests for infectious agents but is still required to pass testing for possible contamination by microorganisms during processing, as described in the section below. A product prepared from primary cells (other than reproductive cells) obtained from a directed allogeneic source, usually a tissue-type-matched related or unrelated donor, must undergo testing for the following infectious agents: HIV-1, HIV-2, hepatitis B, hepatitis C, and *Treponema pallidum*. Viable leukocyte-rich cells and tissues must also be tested for cytomegalovirus, human T-lymphotrophic virus (HTLV)-I, and HTLV-II. Other infectious agents, depending on certain environmental risk factors, may be required. In most cases, screening of the donor takes place in advance of the collection of cells for processing. The most recent regulations on donor screening should be consulted (for U.S. regulations, see the *Code of Federal Regulations*, 21CFR 1271.85 and 1217.90).

Cell banks are used for vector production or the production of gene-modified cells made repeatedly from the same source material. Master cell banks undergo extensive testing, while working cell banks, if used, should undergo limited testing for phenotypic or genotypic markers and testing for microbiological contamination. In choosing a cell line to develop, consideration of the origin and history of the cells should be taken into account. The identity of the cells should be confirmed by a combination of isoenzyme analysis, phenotypic markers, and genotypic markers. Cell lines that have been cultured or processed in media or components derived from animals require more extensive testing. Bovine serum or animal-derived enzymes present a risk of contamination with adventitious organisms. In addition, bovine- or ovine-derived components should be avoided if at all possible, as the lack of an adequate test for prion contamination (the causative agent in transmissible spongiform encephalopathies) presents a particular problem. Cell lines that have been or are cultured in media with antibiotics added should be tested for mycoplasma and other microbiological contaminants and adventitious viral contaminants following culture for at least two weeks in an antibiotic-free medium. For cell lines that will be used to produce viral vectors, a preliminary screen for the presence of replication-competent viruses should be performed. For allogeneic cell lines or preparations to be directly infused or injected, tumorigenicity studies or validation of irradiation may be needed. The cell harvest from a master cell bank or working bank used for vector production should be tested for sterility, mycoplasma, adventitious viral contaminants, and replication-competent virus. Final testing on the vector will also include vector sequence and restriction maps, pH, and residual host cell DNA and proteins.

The raw materials to be used in vector production, transduction, or transfection and cellular processing provide an opportunity to build quality into the production of a gene-modified cell product. Reagents should be clinically approved, USP or infusion grade, whenever possible. Other media, solution, or buffer components or columns should be the highest grade available and may require additional testing. Reagents derived from animals should be avoided, as additional testing for a panel of adventitious agents may be required. Reagents derived from humans should be tested as described above for allogeneic cells and tissues. Certificates of analysis should be obtained for all lots, and raw material specification sheets should be prepared recording the values from the certificate of analysis and any additional testing, such as sterility testing, performed for each reagent lot prior to release from quarantine.

ASSAYS FOR GENE-MODIFIED CELLULAR PRODUCTS

The use of cellular products in phase I clinical trials is generally based on the safety of the cells and on assuring the identification, purity, and strength or potency of the preparation (see Table 1). Assays used to characterize the cells should be developed and validated throughout the transition from phase I to phase III. The test methodology and acceptance criteria may change during development. The full characterization and final specifications for the product are usually not needed until phase III trials. In vitro and in vivo tests conducted on investigational agents to determine their safety should be performed in compliance with good laboratory practice [GLP; see 21CFR58.3(d)]. Tests of an exploratory nature or tests that are used to determine the physical or chemical characteristics of the product do not need to be performed under GLP. Once a license is granted to market the cells, all release tests are governed by cGMP regulations. Most release tests for gene-modified cellular products should be performed on the final product. In-process samples may be taken for the following assays: (1) the mycoplasma assay, which should be performed on the preharvest cells plus media prior to initiation of washing or harvest; (2) assays for replication-competent viruses, where preharvest supernatant and cells should be tested; (3) assays for minimal residual tumor cells in cancer study subjects to track the decline or absence of contaminating tumor cells; and (4) assays for HIV p24/viral load in HIV study subjects to track the decline in HIV viral load during transduction and ex vivo processing.

Safety testing of cellular gene therapy products encompasses tests to ensure that the product is free of microbial contamination and tests to ensure that the transduced or transfected cells are free of detectable replication-competent viruses. Cell therapy products that are not gene transduced or transfected are often infused or injected immediately after processing and require rapid release,

TABLE 26.1 Assays for the Release of Cellular Therapy Products for Human Use

Group	Test[a]	Master cell Bank	Working Cell Bank	Gene Modified Cellular Product
Identity	Cell surface markers (FACS)	X	X	X
	Cellular morphology	X	X	
	Growth characteristics	X		
	Isoenzyme analysis to confirm species	X	X	
	Plasmid number (transfected cells)	X	X	
	Biochemical markers	X	X	X[d]
Dose (Strength)	Cell number	X	X	X
	Viability	X	X	X
Potency	Expression of proteins (e.g., GM-CSF) and/or transgene	X	X	X
	Bioassays for function of expressed protein	X	X	X
Purity	Removal of ancillary products (e.g., beads, media components)	X		X
	Packaging cell residuals			X
	Enumeration of contaminating cell types			X
Safety	Sterility	X	X	
	Endotoxin or pyrogens	X	X	
	Mycoplasma	X	X	X[c]
	In vivo adventitious virus	X		
	In vitro adventitious virus	X	X	
	Specific pathogens (HIV, HTLV, HBV, HCV, etc.)	X		X[d]
	Contaminants from media components (e.g., bovine, porcine)[b]	X		
	Replication-competent viruses (transfected cells)	X		X
	Cell growth after irradiation (cancer cells)	X		X
	Tumorigenicity (soft agar or nude mice injections for nontransformed lines)	X		

[a] Not all tests in this table may be needed for different cell types. The types of tests should be determined on a case by case basis.
[b] Not needed if media components of animal origin have been tested for adventitious agents.
[c] Should be performed on cells plus culture media prior to washing and harvest.
[d] Mandatory for allogeneic products, recommended for autologous products.

thus affecting the choice of microbial contamination detection assays. For most cellular gene therapy products, because they must also be tested for replication-competent viruses using assays that can take from four to eight weeks, cryopreservation of the final product is the only option. Although there is usually a loss of cell yield and perhaps potency in cryopreserved and thawed gene therapy products compared to fresh products, from a quality assurance perspective the time provided by cryopreservation is a delay that allows time for more vigorous microbial contamination testing. The *Code of Federal Regulations* specifies sterility testing in 21CFR610.12 or an equivalent method, such as described in USP <71>. These methods, developed over 30 years ago, although sensitive to the most common cell culture contaminants, are cumbersome and expensive if sent to a contract laboratory. More recently developed and commercially available methods for detection of blood and body fluid contamination such as the Bactec (Becton Dickinson) and the BacT/Alert (bioMerieux) are in use in the majority of hospital and clinical laboratories. A recent study comparing these automated culture systems with the 21CFR610.12 method and the USP method found that both the Bactec and the BacT/Alert were superior for overall detection and time to detection (Khuu et al., 2004). Although these newer methods are not currently encoded in regulations, agencies such as the FDA should take this study and others into consideration when reviewing cellular gene therapy IND applications.

Processing laboratories may also supplement the CFR/USP method or the automated methods with testing for bacterial endotoxin. An observation by Bang (1956) that gram-negative infections of the horseshoe crab, *Limulus polyphemus*, resulted in fatal intravascular coagulation resulted in the development of a gel clot method for the detection of gram-negative bacteria. ELISA-based endotoxin kits are available from several manufacturers, in either an endpoint assay or a kinetic assay where readings are taken at several time points. Both types of ELISA-based assays should be run with standard-spiked samples to test for inhibition or enhancement of the test article. The ELISA-based assays have two advantages over the gel clot assay. First, multiple samples can be run more easily in the ELISA 96-well plate format. Second, ELISA-based assays are more objective in that readings are taken on a spectrophotometer rather than relying on visual inspection of a clot. However, the endpoint ELISA assays are generally less sensitive than the gel clot assay, and regulatory agencies may ask laboratories for comparability data for ELISA-based endotoxin assays to the gel clot assay. The current FDA limit for somatic cell and gene therapy products is 5 EU/kg body weight per dose for parenteral administration or 0.2 EU/kg body weight per dose for intrathecal administration.

Mycoplasma is a common contaminant of cell lines cultured for extended periods of time, most commonly from media additives such as serum. Although rare in cell preparations processed for short periods of time, regulatory agencies still require mycoplasma testing on cellular-based gene therapy products. The FDA-preferred method of mycoplasma testing is specified in 21CFR610.30 and must be performed by both the agar and broth media procedure (with subculture) and the indicator cell culture procedure of at least 28 days in duration or by a procedure demonstrated to be comparable. As with the sterility testing described in 21CFR610.12, the FDA-preferred method is cumbersome or expensive if sent to a contracting laboratory. Alternatives are PCR- or enzyme-based mycoplasma detection kits. The PCR-based kits are sensitive and specific, but care must be taken in the correct dilution of cell lysate or supernatant tested. The enzyme-based bioluminescence detection kit is quick and relatively simple to perform, but without the specificity of the PCR methods. However, regulatory agencies may well require additional data from laboratories performing these alternative methods of mycoplasma testing compared to the extended culture method of mycoplasma testing.

Safety testing specific to gene therapy includes testing for replication-competent viruses and is based on the potential lack of predictable or manageable pathogenesis when viruses are administered in a route different than natural infection and when viruses are engineered with a pseudotyped envelope. Testing for replication-competent retroviruses (RCRs) should be performed at multiple stages of production, starting with the master cell bank used for vector production and the individual vector lots. For lot testing of ex vivo transduced cells that are cultured four days or more after transduction, the FDA guidance is to test 1% of the pooled transduced cells or 10^8 cells, whichever is fewer, and to test separately 5% of the supernatant of the transduced cells. There is an alternative to testing 5% of the supernatant volume for RCR (see the FDA Guidance of October 2000 for details). The test for RCRs involves culture with a permissive cell line for amplification, such as *Mus dunni* for amphotrophic Moloney murine leukemia virus, for a minimum of five passages (Lander and Chattopadhyay, 1984; Wilson et al., 1997). An assay for vectors pseudotyped with gibbon ape leukemia virus has been reported using human 293 cells for amplification (Chen et al., 2001). The amplified supernatant is then incubated, along with positive and negative controls on an indicator cell line, such as PG-4. Hybrid Moloney/amphotropic murine leukemia virus available from the American Type Culture Collection may be used as an RCR-positive control. A novel PCR-based RCR detection assay was recently reported to detect RCR with more sensitivity and much more rapidly than the culture amplification method (Uchida et al., 2004). The assay developed for replication-competent lentivirus uses the permissive cell line C8166 for amplification, with detection of RCL by measuring p24 in the supernatant by ELISA (Escarpe et al., 2003; Schonely et al., 2003). The first lentiviral clinical trial used a VSV-G pseudotyped vector and presented unique issues due to the unacceptable consequence of developing a true RCL-positive control with the wide tropism of VSV-G. The RCL assay for this trial was developed in consultations with the FDA (Schonely et al., 2003). For replication-competent adenoviruses (RCAs), a minimum of 3×10^{10} virus particles should be tested. Virus is tested on a cell line permissive for the growth of wild-type virus only, such as A549 cells. After inoculation using several dilutions, the cells (and appropriate controls) are incubated for 28 days with two subcultures. Evidence of any cytopathic effect in the cell line is indicative of RCAs (Dion et al., 1996; Hehir et al., 1996). A sensitive and rapid PCR test for the *E1a* region of adenovirus has also been developed (Ishii-Watabe et al., 2003). Study subjects who receive gene-modified cells must be monitored for replication-competent viruses after administration (see the FDA Guidance of October 2000). As an alternative to the cell line amplification and detection culture assay described above, investigators may consider a PCR- or ELISA-based assay, which should demonstrate comparability for the particular vector used (Martineau et al., 1997). For vectors other than retroviruses, adenoviruses, or lentiviruses or for lipofection or electroporated-modified cells, investigators should consult the FDA or relevant regulatory agency far in advance to develop and agree on a testing strategy.

Other required release testing includes tests performed to assure the identity and/or phenotype of the gene-modified cell product. These can include flow cytometry, cellular morphology and growth characteristics, isoenzyme analysis, or the presence of plasmids in transfected cells. The type of test will depend on the particular cell product. Purity tests include tests for the removal of ancillary products, such as assays for residual peptides, proteins, DNA, RNA, solvents, and reagents used during vector production and purification, cell separation or culture media components, and beads or other additives used in cell processing. In a clinical trial using gene-modified dendritic cells or artificial antigen-presenting cells as an ancillary reagent to generate activated T cells, the absence of the gene-modified ancillary reagent may need to be demonstrated. Enumeration and limits of contaminating cell types in mixed populations of cells (T cells/NK cells, dendritic cells/monocytes, etc.) may also be required. The dose or strength of the cell product should include the quantitation of the number of cells using manual or automated methods. For complex cell types or final products with low cell numbers, manual cell counts may be needed. A determination of the viability of the cells should be performed using trypan blue or fluorescent methods. A minimum of 70% viable cells is usually required for administration. Potency is a measure of the pharmacological effect of the cell product and is usually the determination of expression and/or function of the cells or transgene in genetically modified cells. Transgene expression is usually measured by PCR or flow cytometry when a surface marker is encoded. Potency assays may also include bioassays demonstrating transgene function. Correlating expression and function with desired pharmacologic effect may be difficult, and a validated potency assay is needed prior to phase III clinical trials. Often, the initial tests are qualitative but are developed into quantitative tests by phase III.

In addition to tests used for release of cellular products, stability assays must be performed (see 21CFR211.166). The stability program is used to ensure that the product maintains its strength, potency, purity, identity, and safety throughout its use in the clinic and is generally used for cellular products that are cryopreserved or not used immediately. Tests used to establish the stability of a cell product generally include cell number and viability, potency (expression or function), integrity of transgene structure, and determination of morphology or phenotype. A periodic test for sterility to assure storage container integrity is also performed. Time periods for testing depend on the expected storage period of the product. Testing at 0, 6, and 12 months and annually thereafter is often used. If the cells are cultured rather than cryopreserved, stability should include time points over the normal culture period.

As the "c" in cGMP implies, current good manufacturing practices are a constantly moving target. Testing and reporting requirements, study subject monitoring requirements, and other recommendations may be updated. Investigators should frequently consult with regulatory authorities well in advance of initiating cellular gene therapy clinical trials, and after trial completion.

APPENDIX: REGULATIONS, GUIDANCE DOCUMENTS, AND REGULATORY RESOURCES

U.S. Code of Federal Regulations Resources   These documents are available http://www.access.gpo.gov/nara/cfr/cfr-table-search.html.

- 21CFR610.1: Regulation for Release of Licensed Biological Products
- 21CFR211.165: Release Requirements for Drugs
- 21CFR312.23 (7): Testing, Reporting, and Release of Investigational Drugs
- 21CFR820.80: Receiving, In-Process, and Finished Device Acceptance
- 21CFR1271: Human Cells, Tissues, and Cellular and Tissue-Based Products

Guidance Documents

- EMEA Points to Consider on the Manufacture and Quality Control of Human Somatic Cell Therapy Medicinal Products (May 2001)
- EMEA Concept Paper on the Development of Good Manufacturing Practices Guidance for Gene Therapy and Somatic Cell Therapy Medicinal Products (December 2003)
- FDA Guideline on Validation of the Limulus Amebocyte Lysate Test as an End-Product Endotoxin Test for Human and Animal Parenteral Drugs, Biological Products and Medical Devices (1987)
- FDA Points to Consider in the Characterization of Cell Lines Used to Produce Biologicals (1993)
- FDA Guidance for Human Somatic Cell Therapy and Gene Therapy (March 1998)
- FDA Guidance for Industry: Supplemental Guidance on Testing for Replication Competent Retovirus in Retroviral Vector Based Gene Therapy Products and During Follow-up of Patients in Clinical Trials Using Retroviral Vectors (October 2000)
- FDA Draft Guidance: Instructions and Template for Chemistry, Manufacturing, and Control (CMC) Reviewers of Human Somatic Cell Therapy Investigational New Drug Applications (INDs) (August 2003)
- FDA Draft Guidance: Eligibility Determination for Donors of Human Cells, Tissues, and Cellular and Tissue-Based Products (HCT/Ps) (May 2004)

- International Conference on Harmonisation (ICH) Q5A: Guidance on Viral Safety Evaluation of Biotechnology Products Derived from Cell Lines of Human or Animal Origin (September 1998)
- ICH Q5D: Guidance on Quality of Biotechnological/Biological Products: Derivation and Characterization of Cell Substrates Used for Production of Biotechnological/Biological Products (September 1998) (this is for cell banks used to produce biologicals and not specifically for somatic cell therapy)
- *United States Pharmacopeia* (USP) <71>: Sterility tests
- *United States Pharmacopeia* (USP) <1046>: Cell and gene therapy products

Other Quality and Regulatory Resources

- American Society for Gene Therapy, http://www.asgt.org/
- Australian Therapeutic Goods Administration, http://www.tga.gov.au/
- Canada's Health Products and Food Branch: Biologics and Genetic Therapies, http://www.hc-sc.gc.ca/dhp-mps/brgtherap/index_e.html
- European Legislation Portal (Eur-Lex), http://europa.eu.int/eur-lex/en/index.html
- European Medicines Agency (EMEA), http://www.emea.eu.int/home.htm
- Food and Drug Administration Center for Biologics Evaluation and Research, http://www.fda.gov/cber/index.html
- FDA/CBER Office of Cellular and Gene Therapy, http://www.fda.gov/cber/gene.htm
- Foundation for the Accreditation of Cellular Therapy, http://www.unmc.edu/Community/fahct/Default.htm
- International Conference on Harmonisation of Technical Requirements for Registration of Pharmaceuticals for Human Use (ICH), http://www.ich.org/
- International Society for Cellular Therapy, http://www.celltherapy.org/
- Japan Pharmaceuticals and Medical Devices Evaluation Center, http://www.nihs.go.jp/pmdec/outline.htm
- United Kingdom Medicines and Healthcare Products Regulatory Agency, http://www.medical-devices.gov.uk/mda/mdawebsitev2.nsf?Open
- United States Pharmacopeial Convention, http://www.usp.org/index.html

REFERENCES

Bang FB (1956). A bacterial disease of *Limulus polyphemus*. *Bull Johns Hopkins Hosp*. 98(5):325–351.

Burger SR (2000). Design and operation of a current good manufacturing practices cell-engineering laboratory. *Cytotherapy*. 2(2):111–122.

Burger SR (2003). Current regulatory issues in cell and tissue therapy. *Cytotherapy*. 5(4):289–298.

Chen J, Reeves L, Cornetta K (2001). Safety testing for replication-competent retrovirus associated with gibbon ape leukemia virus–pseudotyped retroviral vectors. *Hum Gene Ther*. 12(1):61–70.

Dion LD, Fang J, Garver RI Jr (1996). Supernatant rescue assay vs. polymerase chain reaction for detection of wild type adenovirus-contaminating recombinant adenovirus stocks. *J Virol Methods*. 56(1):99–107.

Escarpe P, Zayek N, Chin P, et al. (2003). Development of a sensitive assay for detection of replication-competent recombinant lentivirus in large-scale HIV-based vector preparations. *Mol Ther*. 8(2):332–341.

Gee AP (2003). Regulatory issues in cellular therapies. *Expert Opin Biol Ther*. 3(4): 537–540.

Hehir KM, Armentano D, Cardoza LM, et al. (1996). Molecular characterization of replication-competent variants of adenovirus vectors and genome modifications to prevent their occurrence. *J Virol*. 70(12):8459–8467.

Ishii-Watabe A, Uchida E, Iwata A, et al. (2003). Detection of replication-competent adenoviruses spiked into recombinant adenovirus vector products by infectivity PCR. *Mol Ther*. 8(6):1009–1016.

Khuu HM, Stock F, McGann M, et al. (2004). Comparison of automated culture systems with a CFR/USP-compliant method for sterility testing of cell-therapy products. *Cytotherapy*. 6(3):183–195.

Lander MR, Chattopadhyay SK (1984). A Mus dunni cell line that lacks sequences closely related to endogenous murine leukemia viruses and can be infected by ectropic, amphotropic, xenotropic, and mink cell focus-forming viruses. *J Virol*. 52(2):695–698.

Martineau D, Klump WM, McCormack JE, et al. (1997). Evaluation of PCR and ELISA assays for screening clinical trial subjects for replication-competent retrovirus. *Hum Gene Ther*. 8(10):1231–1241.

Schonely K, Afable C, Slepushkin V, et al. (2003). QC release testing of an HIV-1 based lentiviral vector lot and transduced cellular product. *BioProcessing J*. 2(4):39–47.

Smith L, Lowdell MW (2003). Quality issues in stem cell and immunotherapy laboratories. *Transfus Med*. 13(6):417–423.

Uchida E, Sato K, Iwata A, et al. (2004). An improved method for detection of replication-competent retrovirus in retrovirus vector products. *Biologicals*. 32(3):139–146.

Wilson CA, Ng TH, Miller AE (1997). Evaluation of recommendations for replication-competent retrovirus testing associated with use of retroviral vectors. *Hum Gene Ther*. 8(7):869–874.

27 Toxicology for Gene Therapy Products: Concepts and Challenges

RUSSETTE M. LYONS

Novartis Vaccines and Diagnostics, Cambridge, Massachusetts

The application of traditional toxicological concepts to the evaluation of gene therapy products often presents unique challenges. The complex biological properties, species and tissue specificity, broad spectrum of gene delivery platforms, diverse clinical approaches, and numerous therapeutic indications often associated with gene therapy products preclude the development of standard, universal toxicity study designs. In most cases, product-specific toxicology plans and toxicity study designs will be necessary. However, it is also essential that the objectives of identifying and characterizing potential risks are achieved, which requires a clear understanding of toxicological principles and concepts. Thus, this chapter provides an overview of the fundamental toxicological concepts, their relevance to the assessment of gene therapy products, and their application to developing meaningful toxicity study designs. It would be both impossible and inappropriate to present specific study designs given that individual toxicity studies must be developed within the context of the product's intended clinical use. Therefore, product-specific toxicology studies that integrate traditional toxicological principles will provide the best opportunity for meaningful assessment of the potential risks for gene therapy products.

FUNDAMENTAL TOXICOLOGICAL CONCEPTS

Toxicology studies are conducted to identify and characterize any adverse effects that may result from exposure to the product; they are not conducted to demonstrate safety. This is an important distinction that is vital to the design of meaningful toxicology studies. Furthermore, interpretations of adverse effects identified in toxicology studies must be made within a larger context that includes information gained from mechanistic, biodistribution, and pharmacology studies as

Concepts in Genetic Medicine, Edited by Boro Dropulic and Barrie Carter
Copyright © 2008 John Wiley & Sons, Inc.

well as within the context of the intended clinical use. As part of a comprehensive preclinical package, a toxicology plan is likely to include several individual toxicity studies that identify potential target organs of toxicity under extreme conditions as well as the risk of these findings under more relevant conditions that approximate their intended clinical use. Following is a brief review of important concepts that provide the rationale for toxicity study designs as well as an explanation of general toxicology study objectives. Toxicology reference books should be consulted for a more comprehensive review of traditional toxicology concepts, principles, and methods (Hayes, 2001).

DOSE RELATIONSHIP

Perhaps the most basic concept in toxicology is that of a direct relationship between the dose of a substance administered and the incidence and/or severity of adverse effects. One of the earliest statements of this relationship was by Paracelsus (1493–1541) in his assertion that "all substances are poisons. It is the dose that differentiates a cure from a poison." Because all products, including gene therapy products, can be assumed to have adverse effects if given at high enough doses, the most appropriate interpretation of the absence of adverse effects in a toxicology study is that the dose was not sufficient. Practical limitations, such as product concentration and/or dose volume, may affect the maximum achievable dose for gene therapy products.

The absence of adverse effects at the highest achievable dose cannot be interpreted as an absence of risk; rather, the risks remain unknown. It might be tempting to conclude that toxicity will not occur in patients unless very high doses are administered. However, this conclusion should be made with caution, for several reasons. First, species differences in sensitivity are well known, with humans often being more sensitive than any other species (Eaton and Klaassen, 2001). This is the basis for recommending a starting dose in clinical investigation that is several times lower than doses that produced adverse effects in test animals. In the absence of a toxic dose in test animals, there is a high degree of uncertainty about the shape of the toxicity curve, further complicating selection and justification of a starting clinical dose. From a toxicological point of view, clinical investigation should proceed cautiously, since there is no information about what or when to monitor patients for potential toxicities.

Second, doses administered to test animals may have been calculated using average measurements, such as body weight, rather than individual animal measurements. This results in increased variability in the actual dose that individual animals receive and contributes to overall study variability, making interpretation more difficult. Thus, it is standard practice to dose animals in toxicity studies on an individual basis relative to an appropriate parameter such as body weight or body surface area. This facilitates the comparison of findings at a particular dose (i.e., 10^{10} vp/kg) between multiple species (i.e., mouse, monkey, human).

EXPOSURE

The route and site of administration as well as the frequency and duration of administration will affect exposure levels. Administration of high doses of a product using a route that results in limited or minimal exposure will not provide adequate opportunity to identify potential target organs of toxicity or adverse effects. An example from small-molecule toxicology plans helps to illustrate the value of maximizing exposure using a route of administration that may not be intended for clinical use. Many small-molecule drugs are developed for oral administration; however, low bioavailability by the oral route often limits exposure of test animals. To maximize exposure, the first toxicity studies performed with small molecules intended for oral administration are often single-dose intravenous administration studies. Subsequent toxicity studies are done using the oral route with the knowledge of target organs of toxicity gained from the intravenous studies. The oral administration studies may incorporate additional in-life measurements and more extensive microscopic evaluations of target organs of toxicity identified from the intravenous administration studies to determine if similar, though perhaps less frequent and/or severe findings are present. The application of these concepts to gene therapy products will depend on results obtained from biodistribution investigations to determine the route that provides maximum exposure.

Exposure is also affected by the frequency and duration of administration. The biological properties of gene therapy products introduces additional challenges when considering this aspect of exposure. Unlike small-molecule drugs that in general have relatively rapid elimination kinetics, gene therapy products are intended to express encoded gene products for weeks, months, and perhaps years. Thus, a single administration of a gene therapy vector may result in sustained exposure to the encoded gene product, while administration of the identical recombinant protein at a high dose would result in much lower exposure due to rapid elimination. In this example, the total exposure expressed as the area under the curve (AUC) may be significantly higher for the gene therapy product than the recombinant protein. This type of pharmacokinetic data can be used to guide the duration of toxicity studies.

TYPES OF ADVERSE EFFECTS

There are several distinct categories of adverse effects that may be observed including (1) local versus systemic effects, (2) immediate or acute versus delayed or chronic effects, and (3) reversible versus irreversible effects. The biological properties of the product, such as tissue distribution and pharmacokinetic profile, will contribute to the types of adverse effects that may be observed. For example, a product that has limited tissue distribution may be anticipated to produce few microscopic findings in distal tissues. However, if the toxicology study is not designed to examine distal tissues, the potential for systemic effects cannot be evaluated. The absence of information, in this example "no microscopic examination" of distal tissues, is not equivalent to negative data, or "no microscopic findings" in distal tissues that were examined. Therefore, microscopic examination of distal tissues even though distribution is expected to be limited would enable detection of unanticipated adverse effects and should be considered in at least one key toxicology study.

Similarly, delayed or chronic effects might not be expected with transient gene transfer systems. However, chronic and progressive toxicological responses can be initiated as a result of an acute injury. A toxicology plan that includes assessment of chronic effects which may appear months after initial exposure, as well as the reversibility of acute effects, should be considered regardless of the intended duration of the therapeutic effect. Selection of a final time point is one of the more challenging aspects of designing toxicology studies for gene therapy products that persist for prolonged periods. Other factors, including the clinical indication and patient population, should be considered. For example, a lifetime study may be considered for a retroviral vector product if it were being considered to treat pediatric patients with a serious but non-life-threatening disease. In contrast, a study of much shorter duration might be considered if a retroviral vector was being developed to treat adult patients with a limited life expectancy due to their life-threatening disease. Thus, designing toxicology studies that are informative and feasible requires an understanding of both the biology of the product and the clinical plan.

TOXICOLOGY STUDY OBJECTIVES

The objectives of individual toxicology studies are an important factor in determining the final study design. Clear, specific, and focused study objectives will result in toxicology studies that yield interpretable, biologically meaningful, and clinically relevant results. It is important to note that toxicology studies can only address the objectives that have been prospectively stated; retrospective objectives will generally be limited and incomplete and should be avoided.

For general toxicology studies, the following set of conventional objectives is broadly applicable to most, if not all, gene therapy products:

1. *Identification of target organs of toxicity.* Comprehensive tissue collection and microscopic evaluation by a board-certified veterinary pathologist is needed to satisfy this objective. Information obtained from this analysis will enable decisions regarding the toxicological significance of the findings, the relationship between the safe, effective, and toxic doses to estimate a safety margin and therapeutic index, and the identification of patient populations potentially at risk.

2. *Recommendation of a clinical starting dose.* To address this objective, the study must be conducted with more than one dose, and preferably three doses. A correctly designed study will allow one to determine a maximum

tolerated dose (MTD) and a no observable adverse effect level (NOAEL). This information, together with the knowledge that humans are often more sensitive to the adverse effects of products than other species, will be used to justify a clinical starting dose.

3. *Recommendation of a dose escalation scheme.* The toxicity profile is used to recommend a clinical dose escalation scheme. A toxicity curve having a steep slope would warrant a very conservative dose escalation scheme, since small changes in dose may result in significant toxicity.

4. *Patient monitoring recommendations.* To address this objective, the standard biological samples that should be collected and analyzed are blood, serum, plasma, and urine. Other biological samples, such as saliva, cerebral spinal fluid, feces, or others, may be considered, depending on the biol ogy of the product and feasibility of sample collection. The collection and analysis of in-life biological samples at multiple time points can be used to identify easily accessible markers of toxicity and optimal time points to monitor.

5. *Determination of potential cumulative toxicities.* This objective is relevant for the assessment of products that are intended for repeated administrations or multiple treatment cycles. The number of treatments and the treatment schedule used in the toxicology study should approximate the clinical trial design. It is possible to abbreviate the number of treatments and compress the treatment schedule with appropriate scientific justification.

6. *Determination of the reversibility of findings.* This objective is generally addressed by examination of animals after a recovery period. This period can easily be defined for small-molecule drugs based on the pharmacokinetic profile. However, a recovery period may be difficult to define for gene therapy products that are designed to persist, possibly for life. Long-term studies that include periodic comprehensive examination of treated animals may be considered in these cases. The overall duration of such studies will be based on the specific product, intended clinical use, and scientific judgment.

In addition to general toxicology studies, there are special toxicity studies, such as reproductive toxicology, carcinogenicity, immunotoxicology, and safety pharmacology studies that may be included in a comprehensive toxicology plan. Special toxicology studies focus on specific organ systems and physiological processes. Study designs and objectives for special toxicology studies are well established for small-molecule drugs. While gene therapy products are expected to address these issues as well, the application of special toxicology study designs to gene therapy products is not straightforward. In some cases, the results from a general toxicology study may prompt further investigation. For example, if a statistically significant increase in spleen weights was observed in a general toxicity study, a more in-depth investigation of immunological changes, such as in vivo and in vitro analyses of immune cell subsets, can be included in a subsequent study fairly easily. In contrast, the investigation of potential reproductive toxicities, such as effects on fertility or development, may be required regardless of the results of general toxicology studies. Reproductive toxicity cannot be assessed by incorporating additional analyses in a general toxicology study. Separate studies, designed to ensure adequate exposure of animals during specified stages of reproduction, will be required. It is also important to distinguish reproductive toxicity from the concern of germ line gene transfer. Germ line gene transfer is a concern unique to gene therapy products; it may be considered part of the reproductive toxicity plan but will not address all reproductive toxicity concerns.

TOXICOLOGY CHALLENGES FOR GENE THERAPY PRODUCTS

The preceding review of fundamental toxicological concepts and study objectives was intended to emphasize the relevance of these concepts and objectives for gene therapy products. Due to the biological specificity of gene therapy products, the use of alternative models and novel study designs to address toxicological concerns has been both acknowledged and encouraged (Frederickson et al., 2003). However, it is the application of traditional toxicological concepts to nontraditional models that often presents significant challenges, such as (1) limited experience and lack of historical databases for nontraditional models; (2) model effects may obscure real product-related findings (i.e., false negative); (3) model effects may be misinterpreted as product-related effects (i.e., false positive); and (4) limited availability of animals can delay study initiation or compromise the statistical power and overall value of the study if inadequate numbers of animals are used. Gaining as much information as possible about an alternative model and its limitations before conducting a definitive toxicology study is advisable. In many cases, multiple models, each addressing specific objectives, may be necessary when no single model can adequately address all objectives or concerns.

The issues discussed below represent some of the more significant challenges for gene therapy toxicology studies. This list is not comprehensive; rather, it is intended to highlight the issues that are most common and provide insights as to how these issues might be addressed.

Species Selection

The selection of species for toxicology studies should consider the intended use of the product as well as the biology of the product. A species lacking specific viral receptors would not be appropriate for evaluation of a vector based on that virus. Similarly, if a product is being developed to treat a particular tissue and will be administered directly to that site, a species with anatomical features similar to those of humans may be considered.

Rodents, in particular mice, are a commonly used species for gene therapy research and toxicology investigations. Research studies may use in-bred normal, immunodeficient, or transgenic strains of mice with specific biological properties to demonstrate a therapeutic response. Frequently, the mouse strain used in research investigations will be used in subsequent toxicology studies. However, these strains are not the typical mouse toxicology model. Although these mouse strains may be very well described with regard to the specific genetic attributes, there is considerably less knowledge and experience with these strains in respect to the variability of toxicological parameters. Furthermore, in-bred mouse strains can differ significantly in their response to viral vectors, from minimal to severe toxicity, at identical vector doses. In-bred strains of rats also differ in response to drugs (Kacew and Festing, 1996). These differences provide an opportunity to investigate mechanisms of toxicity and the potential relevance to humans. In the absence of such information, however, a conservative recommendation for a starting clinical dose would be advised.

It has been suggested that nonhuman primates, which are closely related to humans phylogenetically, are the most relevant species for evaluation of a biological product. However, nonhuman primates are an extremely valuable resource, and careful consideration of the need and value added should be done before conducting studies in these animals. In addition, the choice of the specific nonhuman primate species should be considered carefully. The most common nonhuman primate species used in toxicology studies are macaques, either rhesus (*Macaca mulatta*) or cynomologus (*Macaca fascicularis*). Other nonhuman primate species are less commonly used for toxicological investigations. A significant issue to consider with the selection of any nonhuman primate for toxicity studies is the source of animals. The commonly used species are generally purpose bred, while less common species may be wild-caught. In either case, exposure to animal and human pathogens is common and has the potential to affect toxicity studies negatively. Finally, the number of animals needed for a statistically meaningful study in nonhuman primates is not trivial. A study conducted using inadequate numbers of animals is both noninformative and an inappropriate use of this valuable resource.

Other species, such as cotton rats, rabbits, goats, dogs, and others, may also be considered for toxicological investigation. The selection of a nontraditional species for toxicity studies should be scientifically justified. For example, research studies have demonstrated that human adenoviruses replicated, to a limited degree, in lung tissue of cotton rats (Prince et. al. 1993; Mittal et al. 1995). This suggests that cotton rats may be an appropriate species for the evaluation of adenoviral products intended for pulmonary delivery or exposure, but not necessarily for all adenoviral products. The disadvantages of using cotton rats, which include availability and difficulty in handling, among others, should be weighed against potential advantages on a product-by-product basis. Similar assessments of the pros and cons associated with alternative species will be needed to justify their use. Finally, regardless of the species used, adequate numbers of animals must be used for meaningful interpretation of findings. Pilot or exploratory studies using a small number of animals can be quite informative in planning subsequent toxicology studies; however, it is unlikely that they can replace comprehensive, definitive studies.

Disease Models

Some gene therapy products may be inactive in normal animals. A disease model may be necessary to provide the molecular signals for product activation. In these cases, it is important to identify specific toxicities as a result of biological activity of the product as well as general toxicities. Disease models may include transgenic animals, immune-deficient tumor models, chemical, physical, or dietary induction of disease states, and others. In general, disease models will be complemented with toxicology studies performed in normal animals.

Studies performed in disease models are particularly challenging since the health of the animal is already compromised; thus, product-related effects may be obscured. In addition, disease models often have greater variability in the standard pathology parameters used to assess general health, such as hematology and clinical chemistry. This increased variability may require that group sizes be increased so that significant differences between treated and untreated animals can be detected if they occur. Another complication of using disease models for toxicology investigations is that disease progression in untreated control animals may require early termination of these animals. In addition, animals treated at low, nonefficacious doses may also require early termination. The comparison of findings between control and treated animals may only be possible at early time points in these situations. Interim terminations should be scheduled at a time point at which most or all control animals are expected to have survived.

Study Design

Many features of traditional toxicology studies, such as the number of animals per group, clinical pathology parameters, and list of tissues collected for microscopic evaluation, can and should be applied to gene therapy studies that are conducted in common toxicological models. Studies conducted in nontraditional models may require larger group sizes if there is relatively little experience with that model from a toxicological perspective.

Study design features that will be product specific include the route of administration, time points for sample collection, and study duration. The route of administration should include or approximate the intended clinical route of administration. As discussed previously, when the intended clinical route results in limited exposure, a second route of administration that maximizes exposure should be considered. The time points selected for in-life or interim analyses should be based on relevant pharmacokinetic parameters, such as peak vector content in target tissues and peak transgene expression levels. The overall duration of the study should take into consideration persistence of the vector in target tissues as well as the potential for chronic effects even in the absence of detectable vector. For gene therapy products with the potential for lifetime persistence, such as integrating vectors, the duration of toxicology studies will require clinical input, scientific judgment, and discussion with appropriate reviewers.

Regulatory recommendations and guidelines for gene therapy products emphasize the use of relevant models and product-specific toxicology plans. Although a regulatory guidance document has not been issued for gene therapy products, the guideline for other biotechnology-derived pharmaceuticals (ICH S6, 1997) is a relevant resource, and many concepts are likely to be applied to gene therapy products. The product-specific nature of toxicology studies for gene therapy studies places significant responsibility on investigators to have a thorough understanding of both the product and the model being proposed such that a clear, scientifically compelling justification can be made.

In conclusion, fundamental toxicology concepts can and should be applied to the evaluation of gene therapy products. A thorough understanding of traditional toxicology is necessary such that decisions can be made regarding the relevance, or lack of relevance, of a particular study design or model. With this knowledge, product-specific studies can be designed appropriately and alternative models justified that meet regulatory expectations for identification, characterization, and communication of potential risks.

REFERENCES

Eaton DL, Klaassen CD (2001). Principles of toxicology. In: Klaassen CD, ed. *Casarett and Doull's Basic Toxicology: The Science of Poisons*. 6th ed. New York: McGraw-Hill; 11–34.

Frederickson RM, Carter BJ, Pilaro AM (2003). Nonclinical toxicology in support of licensure of gene therapies. *Mol Ther*. 8: 8–10.

Hayes AW (2001). *Principles in Toxicology*. 4th ed. Philadelphia, PA: Taylor & Francis.

ICH (International Conference on Harmonisation of Technical Requirements for Registration of Pharmaceuticals for Human Use) (1997). *Guidance for Industry*: Preclinical safety evaluation of biotechnology-derived pharmaceuticals. http://www.fda.gov/cder/guidance/1859fnl.pdf

Kacew S, Festing MF (1996). Role of rat strain in the differential sensitivity to pharmaceutical agents and naturally occurring substances. *J Toxicol Environ Health*. 47: 1–30.

Mittal SK, Middleton DM, Tikoo SK, Babiuk, LA (1995). Pathogenesis and immunogenicity of bovine adenovirus type 3 in cotton rats (*Sigmodon hispidus*). *Virology*. 213: 131–139.

Prince GA, Porter DD, Jenson AB, Horswood RL, Chanock RM, Ginsberg, HS, (1993). Pathogenesis of adenovirus type 5 pneumonia in cotton rats (*Sigmodon hispidus*). *J Virol*. 67: 101–111.

28 Regulatory Aspects of Gene Therapy Medicinal Products in the European Union

MATTHIAS SCHWEIZER, CHRISTIAN J. BUCHHOLZ, and KLAUS CICHUTEK

Division of Medical Biotechnology, Paul-Ehrlich-Institut, Langen, Germany

Although gene therapy is a novel way of treatment for a variety of diseases by transferring specific, functional genetic material into somatic target cells, the class of gene therapy products has been clearly defined in European Union (EU) legislation. Directive 2003/63/EC,[1] amending Directive 2001/83/EC,[2] lists gene therapy products and cell therapy products under the term *advanced therapy products* in Part IV of Annex I. A new proposal of the European Commission[3] has recently been published to establish *tissue engineering products* as an additional class of advanced therapy products. It is recognized that advanced therapy products will most likely be developed primarily by small and medium-sized enterprises and academic research groups for which procedural help and financial facilitations handled mostly by the European Medicines Agency (EMEA) have been established. It has also been proposed to define good manufacturing and good clinical practices specifically for these products. A number of clinical trial applications have been received by EU member state competent authorities; examples are listed in Table 28.1.

The definition of *gene therapy products* according to Part IV[4] of Annex I to Directive 2001/83/EC as amended by Directive 2003/63/EC is as follows:

Gene Therapy Medicinal Products (Human and Xenogeneic)

For the purposes of this Annex, gene therapy medicinal product shall mean a product obtained through a set of manufacturing processes aimed at the transfer, to be performed either in vivo or ex vivo, of a prophylactic, diagnostic or therapeutic gene (i.e. a piece of nucleic acid), to human/animal cells and its subsequent expression in vivo. The gene transfer involves an expression system contained in a delivery

Concepts in Genetic Medicine, Edited by Boro Dropulic and Barrie Carter
Copyright © 2008 John Wiley & Sons, Inc.

TABLE 28.1   Advanced Therapy Clinical Trial Applications in the EU from 2004 to August 2005[a]

Clinical Use	Number
Somatic cell therapy medicinal products	25/13 generic products
Cardiovascular	4
Cancer immunotherapy	3
Skin/liver/diabetes/bone TE	5
Neurological	1
Gene therapy/transfer medicinal products	19/9 generic products
Cancer	4
Cardiovascular	2
Neuronal	1
HIV vaccine	2
Biologicals	184

[a]The list highlights the number and target disease of gene therapy and somatic cell therapy applications in the EU since the transformation of Directive 2001/20/EC.

system known as a vector, which can be of viral, as well as non-viral origin. The vector can also be included in a human or animal cell.

As an explanation, a variety of more specific products are then named as follows.

Diversity of Gene Therapy Medicinal Products

   a. Gene therapy medicinal products based on allogeneic or xenogeneic cells
- The vector is ready-prepared and stored before its transfer into the host cells.
- The cells have been obtained previously and may be processed as a cell bank (bank collection or bank established from procurement of primary cells) with a limited viability.
- The cells genetically modified by the vector represent an active substance. Additional steps may be carried out in order to obtain the finished product. By essence, such a medicinal product is intended to be administered to a certain number of patients.

   b. Gene therapy medicinal products using autologous human cells
- The active substance is a batch of ready-prepared vector stored before its transfer into the autologous cells.
- Additional steps may be carried out in order to obtain the finished medicinal product.
- Those products are prepared from cells obtained from an individual patient. The cells are then genetically modified using a ready-prepared vector containing the appropriate gene that has been prepared in advance and that constitutes the active substance. The preparation is re-injected into

the patient and is by definition intended to a single patient. The whole manufacturing process from the collection of the cells from the patient up to the re-injection to the patient shall be considered as one intervention.

c. Administration of ready-prepared vectors with inserted (prophylactic, diagnostic or therapeutic) genetic material

- The active substance is a batch of ready-prepared vector.
- Additional steps may be carried out in order to obtain the finished medicinal product. This type of medicinal product is intended to be administered to several patients.
- Transfer of genetic material may be carried out by direct injection of the ready-prepared vector to the recipients.

These explanations clarify that genetically modified cells, be they autologous, allogeneic, or xenogeneic, are classified as gene therapy products. Furthermore, viral and nonviral vectors as well as nucleic acids used in vivo are gene therapy products if used with the intention to transfer a gene or to physically modify a preexisting gene in human cells.

Products containing or consisting of cells genetically modified with a gene that is not intended to serve a therapeutic, preventive, or marker purpose are classified as somatic cell therapy products according to the cell therapy product definition given in Annex I[5] to Directive 2001/83/EC as amended by Directive 2003/63/EC. The somatic cell therapy product definition generally excludes products containing genetically modified cells. There is one exception, however. Cells to be used in humans which have been genetically modified by adding a gene that has no purpose for the relevant indication will fall under the definition of somatic cell therapy products.

There is some discussion of cases that may or may not be classified as gene therapy products. For example, oncolytic and conditionally replication-competent viruses carrying no additional therapeutic gene are often classified as gene therapy products. This classification is in line with the gene therapy product definition given above when thinking of the viral genome (which is intended to mediate the therapeutic effect, i.e., lysis of the infected tumor cells) as the therapeutic gene. Another example may be recombinant replicating microorganisms or viruses intended for the prevention of the disease they cause. Such replication-competent attenuated viruses will probably be treated as live virus vaccines, for which a number of guidance documents exist.

Generally, gene therapy products can be differentiated from other products of molecular medicine if it is kept in mind that gene therapy products none either deliver a gene to human cells in vivo or contain genetically modified (i.e., delivered gene-containing) cells to be used in vivo. For example, siRNA is not a gene therapy product (because RNA is not a gene), whereas siRNA genes are. Despite their name, gene therapy products, can be used for therapeutic or preventive or in vivo diagnostic purposes. Recombinant poxvirus vectors are used as preventive vaccines in clinical trials; blood stem cells modified by a marker gene have been used in clinical trials for in vivo diagnostic purposes, here the analysis of their differentiation properties in vivo. Also, gene therapy products are being used in healthy volunteers: for example, preventive vaccines in patients suffering from non-life-threatening disease (such as rheumatoid arthritis) or patients in a severe life-threatening condition with an expected life span of a few weeks or months (such as certain tumor patients). This makes us understand that the purposes of gene therapy applications can be very different and that the risk–benefit evaluation has to take into account a number of factors. Gene therapy products are also being used in clinical trials for cancer, cardiovascular disease, monogeneic disease, and infectious disease. Gene therapy products are therefore much more than medicinal products for life-threatening orphan diseases.

The main replication-incompetent vector classes currently being investigated[6] in clinical trials are naked plasmid DNA, nonviral vectors (plasmid DNA delivered in a mixture with transfection reagent), gamma retroviral vectors, adenoviral vectors, adeno-associated viral (AAV) vectors, pox viral vectors, and herpes viral vectors. A wide variety of oncolytic viruses are currently being tested,[7] such as attenuated measles virus, herpesvirus, adenovirus, or New Castle disease virus. Classifying a product as a gene therapy product has relevance for licensing (centralized procedure for gene therapy products), the time lines for clinical trial authorization (60 to 180 days maximum), the necessity to obtain contained use and/or deliberate release authorization, and other issues, some of which are explained below.

EU LICENSING OF GENE THERAPY PRODUCTS

Licensing of gene therapy products, both ready prepared and individually prepared products (if produced industrially), is mandatory in the EU.[8] Marketing authorization is obtained via the EMEA by the European Commission. All gene therapy products follow under the centralized licensing procedure, which means that a single application is filed with the EMEA and, if approved, results in a marketing authorization in all EU members states within 270 days, excluding clock stops. Before filing a marketing authorization application, many applicants use the "scientific advice" procedure to get information about critical issues with respect to data showing quality, safety, efficacy, or the environmental risk of their product. This is helpful to avoid unnecessary issues during the licensing procedure.

The decision on a marketing authorization application is proposed to the European Commission by the Committee for Human Medicinal Products (CHMP) at the EMEA. CHMP members are scientific and/or medical experts for medicinal product evaluation, usually educated at and employed by regulatory members state authorities. There is generally one member from the competent regulatory authority of a given EU member state and an alternate member. In addition, five coopted members are selected as members for their special expertise: for example, in blood products, statistics, or other fields.

Filing a marketing authorization is preceded by prefiling meetings with EMEA staff scientists six months or more earlier which provide important procedural information. For a given application the CHMP choses from its members a rapporteur and a co-rapporteur, supported by additional experts, in most cases chosen from the competent authority or member state of the respective (co-) rapporteur, to assess the licensing application file. There is a clearly defined licensing procedure which is finalized by a decision of the CHMP on a request to the European Commission for marketing authorization. This illustrates that what is often perceived outside Europe as the EMEA is really a network of European regulatory authorities coordinated by the EMEA. EMEA staff members play an important role in harmonizing not only procedural but also scientific standards and views within Europe. Concerning medicinal product regulation and evaluation, this system assures harmonized standards, decisions and a pooling of expertise available in the EU while assuring the necessary local regulations and ethics relevant for some medicinal products issues. The EMEA is therefore not a European counterpart of the U.S. Food and Drug Administration. Involvement in the EMEA in clinical trial issues is limited, but important improvements to pave the way from clinical trials to marketing authorization have been made (see below).

CLINICAL TRIAL AUTHORIZATION IN THE EU

Since the transformation of the *clinical trial directive* (Directive 2001/20/EC[9]) in 2004, the procedure and time lines preceding a clinical trial in EU member states have been harmonized. A clinical trial in an EU member state may proceed after obtaining both a clinical trial authorization by the competent member state authority and positive approval by the competent ethics committee of the member state. Thus, a harmonized legal procedure is now established in all EU member states. In Germany, the Paul-Ehrlich-Institut provides gene therapy clinical trial and deliberate release authorization[10, 11] (Figure 28.1). A list is available of the data to be submitted in a clinical trial application. A *national scientific advice* document from the respective member state authority can be obtained prior to or during the clinical trial. There is no mutual recognition of clinical trial authorization between member states, however. For multicenter trials, authorization and approval have to be obtained in each member state in which the trial is to be carried out.

Clinical trial material has to be produced according to good manufacturing practice (GMP),[12] pharmacological-toxicological tests have to be carried out under good laboratory practice (GLP),[13, 14] and clinical trials have to be carried out under good clinical practice (GCP).[9] Prior to applying for a clinical trial, a manufacturing authorization by the competent authority is usually obtained. If a medicinal product intended to be tested in a clinical trial is imported from a non-EU member state, an import license from the EU member state into which the medicinal product is intended to be imported has to be obtained. The relevant member's state authority may choose to inspect the GMP facility outside the EU, a procedure readily followed for medicinal products imported from the United States. The manufacturing authorization of a given EU member's state is mutually recognized by other EU member states.

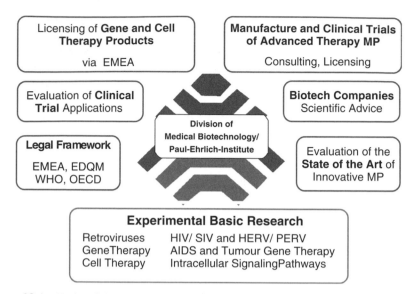

Figure 28.1   Tasks of the Division of Medical Biotechnology of the Paul-Ehrlich-Institut, federal agency for sera and vaccines, in Germany. A list of some of the regulatory tasks related to gene therapy product development is provided. Also illustrated is the combination of experimental scientific research and regulatory work.

The data necessary for the initiation of a given clinical trial are evaluated by the competent authority. During the assessment, naturally standards for clinical trial approval are adopted, although a case-by-case decision is made. There may be a difference, however, between data necessary to obtain clinical trial approval and data necessary for a clinical trial that are pivotal later for obtaining marketing authorization. This difference may not be clarified in the clinical trial authorization in all cases. Within general time limits as defined in Directive 2001/20/EC,[10] there is also a difference between the time lines from application to obtaining clinical trial authorization between member states. There is also a difference between the depth of assessment of the clinical trial application and protocol submitted, which may be relevant for the usefulness of the data to be obtained during a clinical trial for future licensing application. So although the clinical trial procedure has been harmonized in the EU, subtle differences between member state procedures still exist.

Harmonization of views of member state experts from the regulatory authorities providing clinical trial authorization on data and issues critical for clinical trials is enhanced through scientific discussions in CHMP working parties at the EMEA. CHMP working party members are usually medical and/or scientific experts from member state regulatory authorities. Proposals from working parties are endorsed by the CHMP, thus ensuring communication between experts involved in regulatory assessments and decisions at the EMEA and/or member state competent authorities.

CHMP GENE THERAPY WORKING PARTY

The CHMP is supported by a number of CHMP working parties (Figure 28.2). The CHMP Gene Therapy Working Party (GTWP) has been formed to support the CHMP on all relevant issues in gene therapy and clinical gene transfer. It is particularly in charge of updating the current European "Note for Guidance on the Quality, Preclinical and Clinical Aspects of Gene Transfer Medicinal Products" (CPMP/BWP/3088/99).[15] In addition, a number of guidance documents have been proposed by the GTWP to be drafted, including guidance on data necessary for addressing the environmental risk of a gene therapy product, guidance on assessing the risk of inadvertent germ line transmission, a points-to-consider document on issues related to the risk of insertional oncogenesis currently connected with murine leukemia virus (MLV) vectors used to genetically modify stem cells, and other documents. European guidance documents are not legally binding per se, but they define the legally relevant state of the art in a given field and therefore have importance for licensing applications and, in some cases, clinical trials. General technical requirements for data to be submitted for a licensing application of advanced therapy products have been laid down in Directive 2001/83/EC,[1] amended by Directive 2003/63/EC.[2]

The GTWP also encourages interaction of the developing industry and academic groups with the GTWP. There is limited regulatory experience available in the EU on critical issues during licensing of gene therapy products, as only one licensing application of a gene therapy product has been filed so far (the decision on the application is pending). A wealth of regulatory experience is available in those member states where gene therapy trials have been or are being carried out. Sharing scientific principles relevant for the quality, safety, efficacy, and environmental risk of gene therapy products leads to a pooling of expertise in gene therapy in the EU. It may also have a side effect in harmonizing views between member state regulatory experts in the EU.

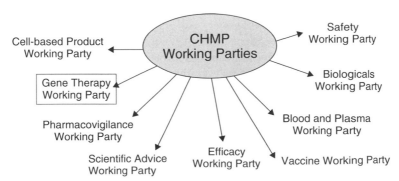

Figure 28.2 Committee of Human Medicinal Products (CHMP) and working parties with expertise relevant for gene therapy product development. The list of working parties is not final; it simply exemplifies support for CHMP with relevance for biological product development and regulation.

The GTWP also provides an EU position on issues for the International Conference on Harmonisation Gene Therapy Discussion Group (ICH-GTDG).[16] Here, gene therapy experts from the United States, Canada, Japan, and the EU regularly meet to harmonize views on critical issues. This group also provides white papers defining common views, such as views, on biodistribution and germ line transmission testing. The ICH-GTDG has also organized regulatory meetings in the ICH realm, (e.g., on oncolytic viruses[7]), as a forum for stakeholders to share their views. As about 60% of all gene therapy clinical trials are carried out in the United States, 35% in the EU, and most of the other gene therapy trials in Japan and Canada, the ICH-GTDG provides an important forum for regulatory exchange between these regions. As gene therapy development is international, the regulatory environment also has to be international.

CRITICAL ISSUES IN GENE THERAPY PRODUCT DEVELOPMENT

Gene therapies are expected to provide beneficial treatment in monogeneic diseases such as severe combined immunodeficiency (SCID), they may lead to improvement in survival rates and quality of life of certain cancer patients, and they may have beneficial effects in cardiovascular diseases. Infectious disease treatment or prevention is another field of expectations. Phase II/III or phase III clinical trials will show whether adequate clinical endpoints can be attained. Licensing applications following the first one filed to the EMEA in 2005[17,18] are expected within the next few years.

A number of adverse reactions are now being recognized as linked causally to particular gene therapy approaches. If used systemically in doses above 10^{13} particles,[19,20] toxicity of adenoviral vectors is an issue as well as the induction of leukemia following infusion of murine leukemia virus (MLV) vector-modified blood stem cells in children less than 1 year of age,[21-24] when a strong selective advantage is conferred upon the modified cells. These are practical risks that have so far been detected in one and three patients, respectively, treated in two gene therapy clinical trials. Fortunately, several hundred other trials, involving thousands of volunteers or patients, have shown a very limited number of suspected serious adverse reactions, meaning serious adverse events possibly related to the gene therapy medicinal product administered. However, effectively, working drugs sometimes have drastic side effects, which are accepted because of the benefit the drugs provide. It is therefore a matter of speculation if clinical use of gene therapy products will be accompanied by additional serious side effects, once gene therapy strategies have been improved sufficiently to allow more efficacious treatment. Gene therapy is still conceptually the most natural way of delivering a drug: In most cases, gene therapy uses human somatic cells to produce a natural physiological protein to provide therapeutic benefit. Iterative clinical trials followed by improvement of the given gene therapy strategy and re-start of trials will therefore lead to effective gene therapy medicinal products in a variety of disease settings. Thus, gene therapy medicinal products are just like other biological products, except for the variety of diseases that can potentially be targeted and for the variety of approaches, genes, vectors, and cells that can potentially be applied. Gene therapy needs time but will be successful in orphan and common diseases. It will not, however, substitute for a large number of other medicinal products but it will offer a new way of advancing molecular medicine.

The currently general issues in gene therapy product development discussed most include (1) absence of vector-derived replication-competent virus (2) risk of insertional oncogenesis due to insertional mutagensis by chromosomally integrating vector genes, (3) limited persistence of therapeutic gene expression (e.g., due to insufficient transcription or immune reactions against vector gene-expressing cells or against the viral vector particle used for delivery), (4) adverse systemic effects induced by therapeutic proteins released from or expressed by the genetically modified vector-harboring cells in vivo and (5) biodistribution of the vector gene to nontarget cells or tissues, particularly germ line cells, modification of which is legally prohibited in the EU.

Practical issues with a view to licensing applications will be (1) the comparability of the expression vector used in early versus late clinical trials, (2) the validation of assays used during nonclinical pharmacological–toxicological and pharmacodynamic–pharmacokinetic testing, (3) providing relevant toxicological observations in animal models relevant for the target disease and the intended mode of action, and (4) obtaining objective evidence of clinical efficacy and/or improved performance compared to a conventional medicinal product on the market.

The issues listed above are solved easily if one keeps in mind that once a gene therapy product has shown the first signs of possible clinical efficacy, all other requirements for obtaining a marketing authorization (known from other biological medicinal products) also have to be followed. It would be great if gene therapy products would be developed that show such clear evidence for efficacy that exceptional circumstances could be considered for releasing some of the not-so-critical data requirements for licensing applications.

REFERENCES

1. European Communities. *Off J Eur Union*. June 27, 2003; L159:46–94. http://pharmacos.eudra.org/F2/eudralex/vol-1/DIR_2003_63/DIR_2003_63_EN.pdf.

2. European Communities. *Off J Eur Commun*. November 28, 2001;L311:67–128. http://pharmacos.eudra.org/F2/eudralex/vol-1/DIR_2001_83/DIR_2001_83_EN.pdf.

3. Commission of the European Communities. Proposal for a Regulation of the European Parliament and of the Council on Advanced Therapy Medicinal Products and Amending. Directive 2001/83/EC and Regulation (EC) 726/2004. COM(2005) 567 final, 2005/0227 (COD). http://pharmacos.eudra.org/F2/advtherapies/docs/COM_2005_567_EN.pdf.

4. European Communities. *Off J Eur Union*. June 27, 2003;L159:88–94. http://pharmacos.eudra.org/F2/eudralex/vol1/DIR_2003_63/DIR_2003_63_EN.pdf.

5. European Communities. *Off J Eur Union*. June 27, 2003;L159:49–94. http://pharmacos.eudra.org/F2/eudralex/vol1/DIR_2003_63/DIR_2003_63_EN.pdf.

6. Cichutek K. Development and regulation of gene therapy drugs in Germany. In: Meager A, ed. *Gene Therapy Technologies, Applications and Regulations: From Laboratory to Clinic*. Chichester, England: Wiley; 1999: 347–355.

7. ICH (International Conference on Harmonisation of Technical Requirements for Registration of Pharmaceuticals for Human Use). Report presented at the ICH Workshop on Oncolytic Viruses. November 7. Chicago: ICH; 2005. http://www.ich.org/LOB/media/MEDIA2695.pdf.

8. European Communities. *Off J Eur Union*. April 30, 2004;L136:1–33. http://pharmacos.eudra.org/F2/eudralex/vol-1/REG_2004_726/REG_2004_726_EN.pdf.

9. European Communities. *Off J Eur Commun*. May 1, 2001;L121:34–44. http://pharmacos.eudra.org/F2/eudralex/vol-1/DIR_2001_20/DIR_2001_20_EN.pdf.

10. German Medicinal Products Act (Arzneimittelgesetz, AMG). *Federal Law Gazette (Bundesgesetzblatt)*. 2005; Pt I(73): 3394–3469.

11. Ordinance on the implementation of good clinical practice in the conduct of clinical trials on medicinal products for human use (GCP-Ordinance–GCP-O) (*GCP-Verordnung–GCP-V*). *Federal Law Gazette (Bundesgesetzblatt)*. 2004;Pt I(42): 2081–2091.

12. European Communities. *Off J Eur Union*. October 14, 2003;L262:22–26. http://pharmacos.eudra.org/F2/eudralex/vol-1/DIR_2003_94/DIR_2003_94_EN.pdf.

13. European Communities. *Off J Eur Union*. February 20, 2004;L50:28–43. http://europa.eu.int/eur-lex/pri/en/oj/dat/2004/l_050/l_05020040220en00280043.pdf.

14. European Communities. *Off J Eur Union*. February 20, 2004;L50:44–49. http://europa.eu.int/eur-lex/pri/en/oj/dat/2004/l_050/l_05020040220en00440059.pdf.

15. EMEA. *Note for Guidance*. London: EMEA; 2001. http://www.emea.eu.int/pdfs/human/bwp/308899en.pdf.

16. International Conference on Harmonisation of Technical Requirements for Registration of Pharmaceuticals for Human Use—Gene Therapy Discussion Group. http://www.ich.org/cache/compo/276-254-1.html.

17. EMEA. *CHMP Monthly Report, November 2005*. General-EMEA/CHMP/364660/2005. London: EMEA; 2005. http://www.emea.eu.int/pdfs/human/press/pr/36466005en.pdf.

18. Immonen A, Vapalahti M, Tyynelä K, et al. *AdvHSV*-tk gene therapy with intravenous ganciclovir improves survival in human malignant glioma: a randomised, controlled study. *Mol Ther*. 2004;10:967–972. http://www.arktherapeutics.com/main/index.php?content = products_cerepro.

19. Marshall E. Gene therapy death prompts review of adenovirus vector. *Science*. 1999; 286:2244–2245.

20. Cichon G, Boeckh-Herwig S, Schmidt HH, et al. Complement activation by recombinant adenoviruses. *Gene Ther*. 2001;8:1794–1800.

21. Check E. Gene therapy put on hold as third child develops cancer. *Nature*. 2005; 433:561

22. Thrasher A. Gene therapy: great expectations? Unrealistic expectations may over-shadow genuine advances and focus attention more on failures. *Med J Aust*. 2005; 182:440–441.

23. Fischer A, Cavazzana-Calvo M. Integration of retroviruses: a fine balance between efficiency and danger. *PLoS Med*. 2005;2:e10.

24. Hacein-Bey-Abina S, Von Kalle C, Schmidt M, et al. LMO2-associated clonal T cell proliferation in two patients after gene therapy for SCID-X1. *Science*. 2003;302: 415–419.

29 Venture Capital and Biotechnology Startups

DOUGLAS D. LIND

GBP Capital, Greenwich, Connecticut

The knowledge gap between the scientific entrepreneur and the venture capitalist is frequently wide. Scientific entrepreneurs are often focused on getting projects funded in order to maintain a technical and intellectual property edge, while venture capitalists are typically heavily focused on market strategy, return on investment, and liquidity strategies. The goal of this chapter is to provide scientific entrepreneurs with a brief introduction to financial concepts and issues that are typically encountered early in relationships with venture capitalists. Two primary topics are covered: principles of equity financing and execution of an equity financing.

PRINCIPLES OF EQUITY FINANCING

Of the two primary means of financing a startup venture, debt and equity, equity is the primary source of operating capital for venture-stage biotechnology companies.* The preparation for equity funding discussions is focused on drafting a business plan, validating the business plan, and valuing a business plan. These topics are described briefly in this section.

Drafting a Business Plan

A business plan is the what, who, and why of a business. What does the company propose to do? Who will do it? Why? These topics must be addressed in the plan directly and concisely. A typical business plan outline is presented below.

---

*To the extent that debt financing and research grants are available, they should be accessed. Debt and grant financing can take the form of state business development; small business innovation research and small business technology transfer (SBIR and SBTT, U.S. Small Business Administration) grants and loans are available that can provide a valuable supplement to equity financing.

Concepts in Genetic Medicine, Edited by Boro Dropulic and Barrie Carter
Copyright © 2008 John Wiley & Sons, Inc.

 i. Executive summary

 ii. Technology and intellectual property

 iii. Market(s)

 iv. Competition

 v. Business strategy

 vi. Management team

 vii. Collaborations

 viii. Financial projections

 ix. Liquidity strategy

The executive summary is perhaps the most important section and the most difficult to write. It is the only section that 90% of the audience will read. It must in less than two pages, make a compelling statement addressing the what, who, and Why questions, based on the more extensive detail provided in the sections that follow.

The technology and intellectual property section describes the asset that serves as the basis for proposing a business. It should be technical, fully referenced, and contain explanatory language, given the often nontechnical background of the audience. All patents, issued and filed, should be listed and explained.

The market(s) section describes a commercial need that can be filled using the technology. It should include answers and references to the following questions: Is it a new or existing market? How large is the market? How rapidly is it growing? How is the market currently being served? The question of how the market will evolve and be addressed in the future should be addressed in the section on competition, which will identify any known or potential competitors. For example, the fact that the HIV market in the United States is currently nearly $4 billion annually, growing at a rate of 12% and that it is currently served primarily by HIV reverse transcriptase inhibitors and HIV protease inhibitors belongs in the market(s) section. The analysis that future competition may include HIV integrase inhibitors, HIV vaccines, and HIV gene therapies belongs in the competition section.

The competition section is an important place to demonstrate firsthand knowledge of the competition. How is the competitive landscape likely to be shaped at the time the proposed product/technologies will be introduced? What intellectual property must be accessed by the company? Is it readily available? On what terms? What potential intellectual property conflicts may arise? What is the proposed strategy to manage or block other competitors? It is most important to identify the potential risks even if all of the strategic answers are not evident. Competition is a risk that any investor in health care technology must accept, but it must be as informed as possible. To a venture capitalist it is a sign of forthrightness and thoroughness for the competition section to be comprehensive and complete, leaving no future surprises to come during the due diligence phase (described later).

The business strategy section answers the how question. It incorporates the technology, intellectual property, market, and competition sections to explain fully how the proposed technology can be successfully introduced into the current or future market. It may also discuss potential stages of growth. For example, initial product candidates may be licensed at early stages to larger pharmaceutical partners in return for working capital to finance the full development of other product candidates in the pipeline. In other cases a company's technology may be offered as a service; a gene therapy company with its sights set on developing new gene therapies serving large global markets may initially serve the smaller, more immediate research market by supplying custom vectors. Well before a therapeutic product is developed and approved, consideration should be given to marketing strategy. Some markets, such as the cardiovascular or rheumatoid arthritis markets nearly always require partnership with large marketing organizations, whereas others, such as HIV and oncology, can often be addressed adequately with the resources of a smaller biotechnology company. Finally, a time line of strategic milestones should be presented, including product and technology development, future collaboration, scientific publication, and other commercial milestones.

The management team section provides an introduction to the members of the current and proposed management to the extent that they have been identified. Typically, information from each person's résumé is drafted into a biography that highlights the person's credentials and relevant prior experience. If the reader is enthusiastic about the potential business, the next question becomes: Can this team execute the plan?

The collaborations section provides details on any existing or expected near-term collaborations, including CRADAs (cooperative research and development agreements) and academic or industry collaborations.

The financial projections section addresses three important questions regarding return on investment: (1) what will the plan cost?, (2) what is the reward?, and (3) what is the time frame? On the question of cost, it should identify all required upfront capital expenditures, such as laboratory and office equipment and legal and licensing fees. It should then provide detailed revenue and expense projections for the first two years of operations and reasonable estimates for several years thereafter, taking into account projected growth in head count and research and development expenses. On the second question, it should quantify market sizes, product penetration rates, and timing consistent with the market section.

Finally, a liquidity strategy section should briefly outline the possible liquidity event or exit scenarios for the venture capitalist. Although venture capital investors invest in the long-term prospects for a business, in the case of biotechnology companies they do so with the understanding that they will probably have been liquidated at least partially by the time the prospect is realized. As a practical matter, their return on investment depends on a liquidity event at an attractive valuation, which in turn depends on convincing a new investor that they, too, will receive an attractive return on investment (ROI) based on the valuation at the time and expected appreciation based on the execution of future milestones. The liquidity strategy section identifies these investors and at what valuation one can reasonably expect an exit for the venture capital fund. Within the biotechnology industry, most venture funds achieve liquidity through either an initial public offering or through merger and acquisition activity. It is important for both the entrepreneur and the venture investor to have an understanding of and agreement regarding the preferred liquidity strategy.*

Validating the Business Plan

Investors purchase equity on the premise that it will become more valuable over time. Unlike most businesses, which justify their value based on revenues and revenue growth rates, venture-stage biotechnology companies typically must be valued on the prospect of future revenues. For the equity of the venture to increase in value this prospect must be increasingly validated. Validation requirements are dynamic. They are based on current industry views and trends, which evolve rapidly and account for much of the volatility in valuation seen in both the private and public equity markets. For example, it has been said in jest that in the early stages of development of the biotechnology industry, two lab coats and a centrifuge were the only requisite to attracting venture capital financing. Although the hurdle may never have been quite so low, clearly much more validation is required today than it was 20 years ago. There was a time when Wall Street analysts valued publicly traded early-stage companies based on the ratio of Ph.D.s on staff to company cash reserves or market capitalization. As the industry evolved throughout the mid-1990s, analysts continued using similarly questionable measures, such as quantity and stages of pipeline candidates, or numbers of patent applications or genes discovered, in attempt to quantify and justify the value attributed to them in the public markets. During this period the risk of becoming profitable was often acknowledged among industry analysts because the business is then valued as an operating entity, often to the detriment of its prior market valuation. As discussed in the next section, contemporary valuation methods have evolved to the use of discounted revenues, earnings, or cash flows, which may be more financially sound but remain highly subjective in their assumptions.

Thus, there is a continuous link between validation and valuation for all stages of a biotechnology company's development until revenues are in hand. For a company seeking its initial seed capital ("series A," prior to its first formal venture capital financing), validation may include the experience and pedigree of the management team, peer-reviewed scientific publications, patents issued,

---

*Many venture funds favor a near-term definitive liquidity event at a reasonable valuation if it meets their ROI criteria. This may pressure an entrepreneur, for the sake of the venture fund's ROI, to engage in an initial public offering well before he or she believes the company is prepared to do so. Alternatively, it could pressure the company into accepting an early acquisition offer ahead of an important milestone that could significantly increase the valuation in a future initial public offering (IPO).

SBIR or SBTT grants, CRADAs, academic research collaborations and initial service or supply agreements with academia or larger industry participants.

Validation requirements for the first formal round of venture financing (known as "Series B") often include the presence of a management and operating infrastructure, continued submission and issuance of relevant intellectual property, execution of existing and new collaborations, and designation of the ability to meet previously set goals and milestones.

Subsequent venture capital financings through to the IPO and life as a public company require increasingly robust validation, even though revenues may remain several years away. This validation includes product research and development milestones, such as lead identification and optimization, completion of preclinical research, submission and acceptance of regulatory milestones such as a U.S. Food and Drug Administration (FDA) investigational new drug (IND). Cover articles in *Science* and *Nature* are common at this stage, as is the ability to hire well-known industry managers. Further validation may include product-specific development and marketing industry collaborations, especially at and beyond the IPO stage. Finally, the perceived quality of the company's investor base itself becomes a source of validation. Companies that are able to attract investments from venture capital firms with perceived strong track records frequently find others ready to follow.

Valuing the Business Plan

The process of valuing a venture-stage biotechnology company is inherently subjective, due to uncertainties in execution, timing, and success of its associated business plan. Valuation is highly influenced by current conditions and sentiment toward similar companies in the public market. At a given point in time, valuation can be grossly defined as the price for which a buyer is willing to pruchase a given equity stake and the price at which a seller is willing to sell the equity stake. Proponents of the "inefficient market theory" commonly cite examples from public equity markets in which transient valuations bear little resemblance to those suggested by traditional valuation methodologies. During the peak of the "dot com" market in 2000, it was not uncommon to see private equity valuations exceeding those assigned to successful IPOs a mere two years prior. As public equity valuations fell during the following year, many venture-stage companies completed financing at a discount to their prior valuations despite the fact that many had achieved milestones that should have increased their valuation.

This can be understood, if not justified, by returning to the concept of *return on investment* which is simply the current value of an investment divided by the purchase price per unit of time as represented by the equation $ROI = R/(I \times t)$, where R represents the end value of investment (return), I the initial value of investment, and t the term of investment in years. In the example above, private equity valuations were highly correlated with public equity valuations because of the expected value and timing of the initial public offering liquidity event. When the public equity markets are exuberant, private equity investors often reflect the expectations of an early and attractively valued liquidity event in the price they are willing to pay for a company that they believe can provide the exit. Similarly, when the public markets are tepid, the prospect of a near-term IPO seems remote and is reflected in the fund's valuation calculation.

With respect to a particular financing of venture-stage biotechnology companies at any given point in time, valuation is as much a strategy of negotiation as it is a fundamental exercise. Each side, the buyer and the seller, uses theoretical valuation metrics to justify a lower or higher valuation, respectively. For lack of more precise methods, the two most common valuation approaches used are industry-comparable analysis and discounted revenues/earnings. The two approaches can be used in tandem and provide validation to the extent that one agrees the other. *Industry-comparable analysis* is achieved by the identification of companies with similar assets and business models that are at a similar or advanced stage of development as the subject company. The process involves identifying the similarities between the comparable companies and using the similarities to justify similar valuations. In the case of a more mature comparable company, the methodology is applied with the implication that the subject company will be at a similar stage of development and therefore valuation will be within a specified period of time. This projected valuation is then discounted on an annual basis to reflect execution and other risks to achieve the *present valuation* as depicted by the equation $PV = FV/(1 + d)^p$, where PV is the present value, FV the future value, d the annual discount rate, and p the number of periods (years). For example, a startup gene therapy company may identify a comparable company with a similar business model, similar technology, and a similar revenue projection that was recently assigned a valuation of $90 million in a recent venture capital financing. The startup founders will perhaps highlight their company's superior technology, intellectual property estate, or business strategy, which would suggest that the startup will be valued at a similar or higher level upon reaching the development stage of the comparable within four years. Because there is a degree of risk inherent in the execution of the startup's strategy (including risks related to the issuance of intellectual property, unforeseen changes in competitive landscape, expected future financial dilution, and operational risk), a discount factor of 60% is assigned that equates to the return on investment that the investor requires in return for assuming the risk. In this case, $PV = \$90$ million$/(1 + 0.6)^4$, or $13.7 million.

The discounted revenues/earnings method calculates present value based on discounted revenues or earnings. A market multiple is applied to expected future revenues or earnings, consistent with the multiple implied by current public market valuations. The multiples on revenues for high-growth publicly traded companies can exceed 10× revenues and multiples on earnings (price/earnings ratios) can exceed 60× revenues. The value of projected revenues or earnings in a given year is multiplied by the appropriate multiple to derive the projected value at that future point in time. The earlier equation is modified as follows:

$PV = RM/(1 + d)^p$, where PV is the present value, R the future revenue projection in a given year, M the market multiple, d the annual discount rate, and p the number of periods (years).

Using this method to value a venture-stage company, the future value is discounted back to the present in the same manner as described above. For example, a company may have a therapeutic product candidate with launch projected in two years and projected annual revenues of $80 million in its third year postlaunch. Thus, in five years the company could be expected to have a public market valuation of $640 million using an eightfold revenue multiple. If an investor requires 60% annual return to assume the risk associated with the investment (reflected as a discount factor of 0.6), the present value of the company suggested by this methodology is $61 million.

PROCESS OF EQUITY FINANCING

The process of equity financing generally follows four stages:

1. Introduction
2. Due diligence
3. Negotiation
4. Closing

The introductory phase begins by identifying potential investors. Most regions of the United States have developed angel networks and venture capital funds. Many investors maintain a bias toward investing locally, due either to charter or simply to geographic convenience. Many can be identified by conducting a simple Internet search. Others can be identified by reviewing recent financings of other regional biotechnology companies, many of which are listed in industry publications, local newspapers, and corporate Web sites. Industry conferences, including those sponsored by state development and industry associations and the national Biotechnology Industry Association (BIO) provide yet another source of funding prospects.

Venture funds commonly request submission of a business plan as the first step. Given the often large volume of plans submitted, it is important that the summary be both complete and concise, as discussed above. Any personal introduction to the fund at this point can be helpful in prioritizing the plan for review. Unfortunately, many plans are reviewed only superficially and are discarded because they do not meet a fund's technical investment criteria. Little if any feedback is provided to the entrepreneur, who must guard against giving that lack personal connotation.

Plans that pass the internal review usually lead to an introductory meeting with the management, where the plan can be presented in greater detail, usually under a confidentiality agreement. Slide presentations are advisable and should be kept to no more than 20 slides, summarizing the content and order of the business plan. Feedback during the introductory meeting is rare and should not be expected. Often, several weeks lapse before a fund forms a decision on the next step.

The second stage, due diligence, involves verification and evaluation of all operational aspects of the business, including contracts, collaborations, and employment and consulting agreements. Investors will probably further evaluate the science and technology, intellectual property, and market and competitive dynamics, often with a team of expert consultants. They will probably request interviews with management, employees, and external vendors such as attorneys and accountants and may conduct background checks on key employees. It is extremely important for management to be honest and forthright during this process. No company or strategy is without risk or flaws. Upfront acknowledgment of known risks, along with a plan to manage the risk, can serve as an important early sign of integrity.

The third stage, negotiation, is the process of negotiating the size and price of the equity stake. If it has not been done during the due diligence phase, an investor is identified who will lead the negotiation on behalf of a syndicate of other funds. Management will solicit input from prior investors, attorneys, accountants, and consultants during the process. Both sides will attempt to justify their respective positions on valuation based on various methodologies, as discussed above. The structure and timing of the investment must also be considered. For example, capital may be committed by a fund in specified amounts upon the achievement of specified milestone events. Valuation will also be influenced by the degree of interest by other funds, which may compete with each other on valuation for the opportunity to participate in the transaction. In this case, in choosing its investor base, the management team has an opportunity to consider other factors including industry expertise, expected contribution on the board of directors, ability to participate in future financings, and personal chemistry.

The final stage is the closing, where all related legal documents are finalized and capital is transferred to the company. Documents related to the establishment of a new company include the stock purchase agreement (including a disclosure schedule, a list of milestone event and a preliminary budget), voting agreement, investors' rights agreement, right of first refusal and co-sale agreement, certificate of incorporation, and employment and consulting agreements. Founders stock is issued and a corporate bank account is formed if not done previously.

CONCLUSIONS

Many venture funds favor a near-term definitive liquidity event at a reasonable valuation if it meets their ROI criteria. This may pressure an entrepreneur, for the sake of the venture fund's ROI to engage in an initial public offering well before he or she believes the company is prepared. Alternatively, it could pressure a company into accepting an early acquisition offer ahead of an important milestone that could significantly increase the company's valuation in a future IPO.

REFERENCES

1. Cardis J. et al. *Venture Capital: The Definitive Guide for Entrepreneurs, Investors, and Practitioners*. New York: Wiley; 2001.
2. Metrick A. *Venture Capital and the Finance of Innovation*. Hoboken, NJ: Wiley; 2006.
3. Wilmerding A. *Deal Terms: The Finer Points of Venture Capital Deal Structures, Valuations, Terms Sheets, Stock Options and Getting VC Deals Done*. Boston, MA: Aspatore; 2003.
4. Zider B. How venture capital works. *Harvard Business Review*. November–December 1998.

30 The Role of Investment Banking in the Growth of Biotechnology Companies

DOUGLAS J. SWIRSKY

GenVec, Inc., Gaithersburg, Maryland

Research and development of all novel technologies require capital. When support from academic institutions and government agencies are insufficient, biotechnology entrepreneurs seek access to capital from public and private investors. One approach to accessing such capital is through the services of an investment bank.

There are many shapes and sizes of investment banks, from small boutiques that work only with private companies, to international giants with full capabilities to assist private and public companies on a variety of transaction structures. Health care, and biotechnology in particular, attract much interest from investment banks. This interest stems from the frequent need to access capital and the high level of strategic activity in the industry. As a result, most biotechnology companies will be contacted by investment banks prior to there being a need for one. Other companies that require an introduction to an investment bank often gain such introductions through lawyers, accountants, or other advisors.

INVESTMENT BANKING'S ROLE IN RAISING CAPITAL

Investment banks should not be mistaken for providers or sources of capital, but rather, should be seen as middlemen. Most investment banks will not invest their own capital in their clients but instead, serve as a conduit to other sources of capital. This is so even when a bank has a venture capital or merchant banking division. These third-party sources of capital are typically venture capitalists, high-net-worth individuals, and institutional investors.

An investment bank can assist a biotechnology company in several ways. For example, a bank can work with the company to develop a business plan in the form of a private placement memorandum. Although the company may

Concepts in Genetic Medicine, Edited by Boro Dropulic and Barrie Carter
Copyright © 2008 John Wiley & Sons, Inc.

be capable of developing its own financing documents, working with an advisor will allow the company's management to focus on its technology. In addition, an experienced investment bank will know how best to position the company's value proposition to maximize the interest of investors.

Perhaps the most important way that an investment bank can add value to the financing process is through introductions to appropriate investors. First-time entrepreneurs will have a particular need for these introductions, as they typically have had only limited prior contact with the venture capital community. These introductions can be critical to a biotechnology company's financing success. In 2006, venture capitalists invested $7.2 billion into the life sciences sector, providing funding for 731 companies.*

At an early stage, most companies will not be raising enough money to justify engaging an investment bank. Because it is often just as difficult to raise $5 million as it is to raise $25 million, most investment banks will not become actively engaged on capital raises of less than $10 million.† Even if a biotechnology company does not have a current need to engage a bank, it is never too soon to begin meeting with investment bankers, as they can provide a source of market intelligence and often impart valuable free advice.

Unlike some other types of advisors, investment banks do not charge by the hour and will invest substantial time and effort in potential clients. A biotechnology company will often have developed two or three substantive relationships with investment banks prior to actually engaging one or more of them. A forward-thinking investment bank will often invest two or more years into a client relationship before there is an opportunity to be actively engaged in a transaction.

A typical fee structure for an investment bank on private financing is 7% or more of the amount raised.‡ Additionally, the investment bank may seek additional compensation in the form of warrants. These fees are not trivial. In a $10 million financing utilizing the services of an investment bank, at least $700,000 will not be available to fund a company's science. Paying such a fee can only be justified if a better outcome can be achieved with the assistance of an investment bank than could be achieved without one. The success of a financing process can be measured in several ways:

- *Completion of a financing.* Some companies may not have the ability to complete a financing process without professional help.
- *Pre-money valuation.* An investment bank should be able to conduct a financing process that attracts multiple term sheets from investors. A competitive process may provide a higher valuation than could otherwise be obtained.

*2006 MoneyTree Survey by PricewaterhouseCoopers, Thomson Venture Economics, and the National Venture Capital Association. Includes biotechnology and medical device companies.
†Larger banks typically will not be engaged in financing proposals under $20 million.
‡Based on the author's historical experience working for and with several investment banks.

- *Structure of financing.* Term sheets for private placements are complex and may contain pitfalls of which a company must be aware. Investment banks can help determine which provisions reflect market terms and which terms can and should be negotiated.
- *Quality of investors.* By providing additional validation of a company's business model, investment banks can often provide access to investors that might be less accessible to biotechnology entrepreneurs. Improving the quality of investors will enhance the prospects for both the transaction contemplated and future financings.
- *Amount of capital raised.* A company may be able to attract more capital with the help of an agent. Although this must be weighed carefully alongside valuation, additional proceeds will allow a company to advance its technology to a more advanced point before seeking additional investor funds.

ADVISORY SERVICES OF INVESTMENT BANKS

In between financings, investment banks provide strategic advice to companies and may suggest potential partners for mergers or other strategic relationships. Although investment banks may propose potential acquisitions for private company clients, a more typical scenario is the sale of a private company to a public acquirer. Although biotechnology entrepreneurs rarely prefer this option, the financing environment may require that a sale strategy be considered.

Private companies must choose continually between funding their science through the capital markets and gaining access to capital and resources through strategic transaction with better-capitalized companies. The optimal time to sell or license a company's technology is heavily influenced by the appetite of investors at a given point in time. Investment banks can, therefore, be a good source for evaluating both the financing markets and the availability of strategic alternatives.

SELECTING AN INVESTMENT BANK

Investment banking is a competitive industry, and companies often attract multiple investment banks with whom they can choose to work. Selected advisors and agents should bring skills and experience that complement the needs of the company. It is unlikely that any investment bank will outshine its competitors in every way, and companies are advised to optimize their selection by weighing the importance of various factors, including:

- *Experience with similar companies.* The bank selected should have prior experience in successful execution for similar companies of the type of financing or transaction contemplated. Investment banks with exposure to companies utilizing genetic medicine, for example, will be able to leverage their knowledge to achieve a better outcome for these companies or at least to achieve a given outcome more efficiently.

- *Attention from senior personnel.* It should not be assumed that the team of bankers that a particular firm presents to a company will be the same people who would actually work on the transaction being discussed. Like all professional service industries, investment banks must leverage their experienced bankers with less seasoned personnel. Rather than focusing on the most experienced banker presented by each firm, companies are encouraged to evaluate the qualifications of the entire team presented. In particular, the background and experience of the vice president or senior associate who will work most closely with the company should be evaluated.
- *Proficiency in relevant practice area.* Some investment banks are known for their ability to raise capital; others are mergers and acquisition specialists. It is important to work with a bank where the transaction contemplated is a strength.
- *Ability to assist the company on future transactions.* Ideally, the bank that a company chooses should be able to work with a company as its capital formation evolves. On the other hand, working with a firm that specializes in certain types of transactions will provide greater flexibility in selecting the most qualified agent or advisor for a future transaction.
- *Fees and engagement terms.* In general, fees tend to be similar between banks. The structure of the fees can, however, be quite different. A large upfront fee may be an indication of an investment bank's lack of confidence in completing a transaction. On the other hand, a minimal retainer may be indicative of minimal resources being dedicated to the effort. In addition to fees, engagement letters may contain provisions that require a firm to utilize the bank's services for future transactions for some period of time, often at least one year.
- *References.* Companies contemplating working with an investment bank are encouraged to check client references for the investment bank and selected banking team members. Inquiries should include a discussion of the investment bank's performance as well as of the level of attention provided after the transaction has been closed.

CONCLUSIONS

As financial middlemen, an investment bank's view on the attractiveness of a particular technology is dictated by the views of investors. The interest in genetic medicine has varied over time, and the availability of capital and valuations for companies utilizing these technologies has been equally volatile. Developing long-term relationships with selected investment banks will provide a source of ongoing advice and will make it easier for companies to tap into capital markets when they need to do so.

31 Managing Reimbursement for Gene Therapy Products

MARTIN GOLD

Technology Access Partners, LLC, Suffern, New York

Several years ago it was assumed that the function of reimbursement and all the activities involved were entirely the responsibility of health care providers and that companies need not concern themselves with this issue. Recently, companies and investors arrived at the understanding that many of the underlying functions of reimbursement are indeed the responsibility of the company and in many cases must be addressed long before product launch.

As is the case for all truly novel therapeutics, the commercial opportunity for gene therapy is difficult to determine. Gene therapy as a science is still early in its life cycle, and although many products are in clinical development, there are few examples of fully commercialized products. As a result, one must apply the basic principles of reimbursement to the science to identify the hurdles that companies will need to overcome in order to achieve long-term success. The term *reimbursement*, often considered a single financial concern, is actually a function of three distinct aspects of the health care system: coverage, coding, and payment. For health care providers to obtain reimbursement for gene therapy products, all three aspects of the system must be properly aligned.

Coverage refers to a third-party payer's willingness to include a product or service in its approved benefits structure, thereby making it available to its members or enrollees. The coverage process employed by payers usually necessitates an analysis of the therapeutics' clinical efficacy and cost-effectiveness. The clinical evaluation is generally referred to as *health technology assessment* (HTA). HTA is the systematic and comprehensive evaluation of available scientific evidence to identify the benefits and risks of a particular medical technology or treatment in relation to its potential clinical use for a defined group of patients.[1] HTA generally involves the review and analysis of published peer-reviewed journal articles, case studies, and other relevant clinical data. The results of HTA tend to indicate the degree to which reliable clinical data exist to support use of the technology and the degree to which it improves health

Concepts in Genetic Medicine, Edited by Boro Dropulic and Barrie Carter
Copyright © 2008 John Wiley & Sons, Inc.

outcomes. The determination of improved health outcomes is especially important to payers when the technology is either costly or has broad applicability to its subscribers. In either case, the payer feels compelled to clinically justify the adoption of a technology that may have a significant financial impact to its business.

The Blue Cross and Blue Shield Association's Technology Evaluation Center (TEC), an organization that provides HTA services to its member Blue Cross plans, has developed five criteria by which it assesses a technology. The criteria are intended to address issues such as off-label use by clinicians, inconclusive clinical evidence, the clinical value generated by the financial investment, and overall applicability of outcome evidence to the general population. The TEC evaluation criteria are as follows[2]:

1. The technology must have final approval from the appropriate governmental regulatory bodies.

    a. This criterion applies to drugs, biological products, devices and any other product or procedure that must have final approval to market from the U.S. Food and Drug Administration or any other federal governmental body with authority to regulate the technology.

    b. Any approval that is granted as an interim step in the U.S. Food and Drug Administration's or any other federal governmental body's regulatory process is not sufficient.

    c. The indications for which the technology is approved need not be the same as those which Blue Cross and Blue Shield Association's Technology Evaluation Center is evaluating.

2. The scientific evidence must permit conclusions concerning the effect of the technology on health outcomes.

    a. The evidence should consist of well-designed and well-conducted investigations published in peer-reviewed journals. The quality of the body of studies and the consistency of the results are considered in evaluating the evidence.

    b. The evidence should demonstrate that the technology can measure or alter the physiological changes related to a disease, injury, illness, or condition. In addition, there should be evidence or a convincing argument based on established medical facts that such measurement or alteration affects health outcomes.

    c. Opinions and evaluations by national medical associations, consensus panels, or other technology evaluation bodies are evaluated according to the scientific quality of the supporting evidence and rationale.

3. The technology must improve the net health outcome.

a. The technology's beneficial effects on health outcomes should outweigh any harmful effects on health outcomes.

4. The technology must be as beneficial as any established alternatives.

a. The technology should improve the net health outcome as much as, or more than, established alternatives.

5. The improvement must be attainable outside the investigational settings.

a. When used under the usual conditions of medical practice, the technology should be reasonably expected to satisfy TEC criteria 3 and 4.

The requirement that conclusive scientific evidence be available speaks to the large number of clinical studies conducted that are poorly structured and report questionable results. To conduct HTA properly, researchers evaluate the reliability and importance of clinical data based upon the study design and methodology used to generate the data. The Centers for Medicare and Medicaid Services (CMS), the agency responsible for administering the Medicare program, places greater emphasis on randomized controlled studies than on single-case reports when performing coverage analyses. CMS bases its valuation of a study design on its ability to minimize systematic bias in the data results.[3] The following outlines CMS's hierarchy of study designs from most to least reliable:

1. Randomized controlled trials
2. Nonrandomized controlled trials
3. Prospective cohort studies
4. Retrospective case–control studies
5. Cross-sectional studies
6. Surveillance studies (e.g., using registries or surveys)
7. Consecutive case series
8. Single case reports

In actuality, the HTA is a component of a broader analysis, the results of which are communicated to medical providers and patients through a formal medical policy that states the intention of the payers to either approve or deny coverage for the particular therapy being studied. In a medical coverage policy published by the Regence Group (a Blue Cross Blue Shield plan insuring 3 million people across four Pacific Northwest states), the policy concluded that Regence would not provide coverage for gene therapies since it has not yet been "established that gene therapy for any indication results in improved health outcomes, nor is it established that the health outcomes from gene therapy are as good as or better than the health outcomes from existing therapies."[4]

It is important to recognize that in the early stages of a technology's development the availability of peer-reviewed clinical data will be limited. This is the case with gene therapy. But given the data needs of payers, it is important to incorporate these data requirements into the structure of gene therapy clinical trials and publication plans to accommodate their decision-making processes.

For accurate assessment by payers of the clinical value of a therapeutic, reliable data must be provided in a manner that allows for scrutiny of both the study methodologies and results. The standard method for disseminating clinical data is through publication of the study results in well-recognized peer-reviewed clinical journals. Therefore, it is also important to publish the results of trials conducted outside the United States in U.S. medical journals.

In an HTA published by the National Coordinating Centre for Health Technology Assessment (NCCHTA), an agency that supports the medical policy decisions for the United Kingdom's National Health Service, it identified three factors that would strongly affect the commercial success of gene therapies: (1) the cost of manufacturing the products, (2) the market size of the treatment population, and (3) the resolution of patient issues related to gene sequences, viral vectors, cell lines, and other gene transfer systems.[5] All three factors relate to the cost-effectiveness, clinical effectiveness, and safety of the products. The determination as to whether a particular gene therapy product meets these requirements would result from an analysis by NCCHTA of reliable data published in well-recognized peer-reviewed clinical journals.

In addition to coverage, companies must address the challenges associated with coding and payment. *Coding* refers to the alphanumerical structure used by health care providers to communicate to payers and other interested parties specifics about a patient's condition as well as the services rendered and products provided to the patient. *Payment* refers to the payment from a payer to a health care provider to compensate the provider for the reasonable costs of providing care to a patient, including the use of separately purchased therapeutics. Without accurate coding, the tracking and payment for gene therapy products would be difficult.

The issue of payment must be addressed from both the payer's and the provider's perspectives. From the provider's perspective, payment from third-party payers must provide reasonable compensation for the cost of providing care to patients, including therapeutics and other products. Payment can vary substantially among individual payers. Therefore, it falls to the company to ensure that its products are reimbursed appropriately in the marketplace.

From the payers' perspective, the price paid for a gene therapy product will be weighed against the perceived clinical and economic value provided by the therapeutic. The perceived value is often influenced by the target treatment market and the indication chosen. A costly gene therapy product would be accepted by payers more easily if the target indication could not be managed effectively with a less costly alternative. Hence, it meets the Blue Cross Blue Shield TEC criteria that "the technology must be as beneficial as any established alternatives."

In addition to the direct cost of the product, the *degree* of clinical benefit is important. Payers would more easily provide coverage for an expensive product that represents a lifesaving treatment than for a product that merely provides improvement in a patient's quality of life. Needless to say, a gene therapy product that could not make a claim for a significant improvement in health outcomes and was at the same time costly to produce would not be well received by payers and would encounter a difficult market adoption process.

Although gene therapy products will face a variety of reimbursement barriers as products are introduced into the health care marketplace, many of the more common reimbursement problems can be minimized through appropriate reimbursement planning. Due to the lengthy development time lines for gene therapy products, it is important to integrate reimbursement planning into the business and regulatory planning process as early as possible.

REFERENCES

1. Hayes, Inc. www.hayesinc.com.
2. Blue Cross and Blue Shield Association's Technology Evaluation Center. *Technology Evaluation Center Criteria*. http://www.bcbs.com/tec/teccriteria.html. Accessed June 21, 2006.
3. Gold M. Clinical data can make or break your product. *Med Prod Outsourc*. April 2005;24–25.
4. The Regence Group. *Gene Therapy Medical Policy*. http://www.regence.com/trgmedpol/medicine/med13.html. Accessed June 25, 2006.
5. When and how to assess fast-changing technologies: a comparative study of medical applications of four generic technologies. *Health Technol Assess*. 1997;1(14). NHS R&D HTA Programme. http://www.hta.nhsweb.nhs.uk/fullmono/mon114.pdf. Accessed June 1, 2006.

INDEX

A549 cells, engineered, 247

AADC expression, 157

AAV5 capsid vectors, 149. *See also* Adeno-associated virus (AAV) vectors

AAV9 capsid, 131

AAV capsids, 64
variants of, 125

AAV DNA genomes, 62
structures of, 63

AAV serotype 2 (AAV2)-based vectors, 64, 65, 140. *See also* Ad2/5 serotypes
for cystic fibrosis, 148

AAV serotypes, 131
exposure to, 126

AAV vector-mediated delivery, feasibility and efficacy of, 140. *See also* Ad/AAV hybrid-based production method; Adeno-associated virus (AAV) vectors

Aβ (amyloid β) levels, reducing, 155

"Accessory" viral genes, 239

Acute cardiovascular event toxicities, 51

Ad2/5 serotypes, 52

Ad35 (group B) fiber vectors, 49

Ad/AAV hybrid-based production method, 248–249

Adaptive immune responses, 170–172
role in eliminating transgene expression, 170–171

Adaptor-based targeting, 224

Adeno-associated virus (AAV) vectors, 61–67, 238. *See also* AAV entries; Ad/AAV hybrid-based production method; rAAV vectors; Recombinant adeno-associated virus (rAAV)
characteristics/properties of, 62, 245–246
elements influencing vector properties, 64
generation of, 62
genome design of, 61–63, 64
immune responses and, 147
for intraarticular RA gene therapy, 140

manufacture of, 245–252

payload capacity of, 63

persistence, safety, and clinical applications of, 65–66

therapeutic proteins and, 149

Adenosine deaminase deficiency SCID (ADA-SCID), 2–3. *See also* X-linked severe combined immunodeficiency disease (X-SCID)

Adenoviral (Ad) vectors, 39–59, 226, 236–238. *See also* AAV entries; Ad entries; Adeno-associated virus (AAV) vectors; Adenoviruses
company programs using, 44–45
current use of, 52–53
early clinical applications of, 52
evolution of, 47–50
first-generation, 169
future of, 53
immune response to, 147, 169, 170
manufacturing methods for, 47, 236–237
oncolytic, 269–273
properties attracting widespread use of, 43–47
systemic delivery of, 51–52
toxicity of, 50–51, 336
as a vector system, 223–224

Adenoviral genome transcription/replication, 42–43

Adenoviral-mediated synovial gene transfer, 139–140

Adenoviral targeting, 48
improving, 224–225

Adenoviruses. *See also* Adenoviral (Ad) vectors
biology of, 41–42
characteristics of, 39–41
immune system and, 41
labeling of, 226
life cycle of, 41–43
viral attachment and entry of, 42
virions of, 39, 40

Adenovirus replication, assessing, 226

Concepts in Genetic Medicine, Edited by Boro Dropulic and Barrie Carter
Copyright © 2008 John Wiley & Sons, Inc.

Gene replacement, 26
"Generic" packaging cell line, 248
Gene silencing, 22, 24–25, 27, 258
  transcriptional, 210–211
Gene therapy, 223
  advances in, 4–5
  brain as a target for, 153–165
  clinical, 25–27
  clinical promise of, 2
  combination, 72
  consequences for the central nervous system,
    172–173
  evolution of, 1–6
  goal of, 69
  regulatory documents relating to, 270
  results of, 2
  worldwide effort related to, 4
Gene therapy approaches
  for brain tumors, 157–158
  for cardiovascular disease, 129–135
  for HIV-1 treatment, 212–213
  for Parkinson's disease, 156
Gene therapy clinical trials, 280
Gene therapy product development, critical
    issues in, 336–337
Gene therapy products, xiii
  classification of, 331–332
  defined, 329
  diversity of, 330–332
  EU licensing of, 332–333
  EU regulation of, 329–339
  health outcomes of, 358–359
  human and xenogeneic, 329–330
  managing reimbursement for, 355–359
  toxicology challenges for, 324–327
  toxicology for, 319–327
Genetically modified T cells, for human gene
    therapy, 193–205
Genetic modification
  of capsids, 224
  of T cells, 195–196
Genetic retargeting strategies, combination
    approaches to, 225
Genetic viral vector products, manufacture of,
    229–244
Gene transfer approaches, 53–54. See also
    Therapeutic gene transfer
  technologies for, 123
Gene transfer efficiency, 72
  maximizing, 14
Gene transfer vector, direct intraarticular
    administration of, 139
Genome integrity, persistence of expression
    without disrupting, 127–128

Genome transcription/replication, adenoviral,
    42–43
Genomic DNA, isolation of, 294
Genomic RNA, packaging, 293
Genotoxicity, of lentiviral vectors, 29
Gibbon ape leukemia virus (GALV), 284
Glial cell-derived neurotrophic factor (GDNF),
    95, 156
Glioblastoma multiforme, 156–158
α-Glucosidase (Gaa), 129, 130–131
β-Glucuronidase (GUSB) activity, 132
Glycosaminoglycans (GAGs), catabolism of, 132
GM-CSF (granulocyte macrophage
    colony-stimulating factor), 188
GM-CSF/IL-2 receptors, chimeric, 195
GMP-compliant plasmid DNA, 300. See also
    Good manufacturing practice (GMP)
GMP implementation, 235–236
Gold, Martin, x, 355
Good laboratory practice (GLP), 333
Good manufacturing practice (GMP), 28, 61,
    230, 308, 333. See also GMP entries
Gradient purification, 260
Graft versus host disease (GVHD), 196
Granulomatous immune response, 183
Gregorevic, Paul, x, 123
Growth factor expression, 156–157
Guidance documents, 316–317
  GTWP, 335
GVAX vaccine, 27

Health technology assessment (HTA), 355–356,
    358
  conducting, 357
Heat shock protein 27 (hsp27), 95–96
Heat-shock proteins, 182
HEK293 cell line. See Human embryonic
    kidney-derived 293 (HEK283; 293HEK)
    cell line
HeLa cells, engineered, 247
HeLa-*tat* cells, 262
Helper-dependent adenoviruses, 53
helper plasmid, 246
Hematologic malignancies, 188
Hematopoietic progenitor cells, 214
Hematopoietic stem cell (HSC)-based gene
    therapy, 212
Hematopoietic stem cells
  relative safety of, 193–195
  retrovirus transduction of, 239
Her-2/*neu*+ allogeneic breast cancer cell line,
    187
Herceptin, 232
Hereditary emphysema, 148